CT Colonography

Guest Editors

SUBHAS BANERJEE, MD
JACQUES VAN DAM, MD, PhD

GASTROINTESTINAL ENDOSCOPY CLINICS OF NORTH AMERICA

www.giendo.theclinics.com

Consulting Editor
CHARLES J. LIGHTDALE, MD

April 2010 • Volume 20 • Number 2

SAUNDERS an imprint of ELSEVIER, Inc.

W.B. SAUNDERS COMPANY
A Division of Elsevier Inc.

1600 John F. Kennedy Blvd. ● Suite 1800 ● Philadelphia, Pennsylvania 19103-2899

http://www.giendo.theclinics.com

GASTROINTESTINAL ENDOSCOPY CLINICS OF NORTH AMERICA Volume 20, Number 2
April 2010 ISSN 1052-5157, ISBN-13: 978-1-4377-1913-0

Editor: Kerry Holland

Gastrointestinal Endoscopy Clinics of North America (ISSN 1052-5157) is published quarterly by Elsevier Inc., 360 Park Avenue South, New York, NY 10010-1710. Months of issue are January, April, July, and October. Business and Editorial Offices: 1600 John F. Kennedy Blvd., Suite 1800, Philadelphia, PA, 19103-2899. Periodicals postage paid at New York, NY and additional mailing offices. Subscription prices are $290.00 per year for US individuals, $394.00 per year for US institutions, $149.00 per year for US students and residents, $320.00 per year for Canadian individuals, $481.00 per year for Canadian institutions, $405.00 per year for international individuals, $481.00 per year for international institutions, and $207.00 per year for Canadian and foreign students/residents. To receive student/resident rate, orders must be accompanied by name of affiliated institution, date of term, and the *signature* of program/residency coordinator on institution letterhead. Orders will be billed at individual rate until proof of status is received. Foreign air speed delivery is included in all *Clinics* subscription prices. All prices are subject to change without notice. **POSTMASTER:** Send address change to *Gastrointestinal Endoscopy Clinics of North America*, Elsevier Health Sciences Division, Subscription Customer Service, 3251 Riverport Lane, Maryland Heights, MO 63043. **Customer Service: 1-800-654-2452 (US). From outside the United States, call 1-314-447-8871. Fax: 1-314-447-8029. E-mail: JournalsCustomerService-usa@elsevier.com (for print support) or JournalsOnlineSupport-usa@elsevier.com (for online support).**

Reprints. For copies of 100 or more, of articles in this publication, please contact the Commercial Reprints Department, Elsevier Inc., 360 Park Avenue South, New York, NY 10010-1710. Tel. (212) 633-3812; Fax: (212) 482-1935; E-mail: reprints@elsevier.com.

Gastrointestinal Endoscopy Clinics of North America is covered in *Excerpta Medica, MEDLINE/PubMed (Index Medicus), and MEDLINE/MEDLARS.*

Printed and bound by CPI Group (UK) Ltd, Croydon, CR0 4YY

Transferred to Digital Print 2011

Contributors

CONSULTING EDITOR

CHARLES J. LIGHTDALE, MD
Professor, Department of Medicine, Columbia University Medical Center, New York, New York

GUEST EDITORS

SUBHAS BANERJEE, MD
Co-Director of Endoscopy; Associate Professor of Medicine, Division of Gastroenterology and Hepatology, Stanford University School of Medicine, Stanford, California

JACQUES VAN DAM, MD, PhD
Professor of Medicine, Division of Gastroenterology and Hepatology, Stanford University School of Medicine, Stanford, California

AUTHORS

RIZWAN ASLAM, MD
Chief of Computed Tomography, San Francisco Veterans Affairs Medical Center; Associate Professor of Radiology and Biomedical Imaging, University of California, San Francisco, California

CHRISTOPHER F. BEAULIEU, MD, PhD
Professor of Radiology, Department of Radiology, Stanford University School of Medicine, Stanford, California

STEVE CARPENTER, MD
Associate Professor of Medicine, Chair and Program Director, Department of Internal Medicine, Mercer University School of Medicine, Memorial University Medical Center, Savannah, Georgia

CAPT (SEL) BROOKS D. CASH, MD, FACP, FACG, AGAF, MC, USN
Associate Professor of Medicine, Uniformed Services University of the Health Sciences; Integrated Chief of Medicine, Gastroenterology Service, National Naval Medical Center, Bethesda, Maryland; Integrated Chief of Medicine, Walter Reed Army Medical Center, Washington, DC

AMY BERRINGTON DE GONZALEZ, DPhil
Investigator, Division of Cancer Epidemiology and Genetics, Radiation Epidemiology Branch, National Cancer Institute, Bethesda, Maryland

R. BROOKE JEFFREY, MD
Professor of Radiology, Department of Radiology, Stanford University School of Medicine; Section Chief, Abdominal Imaging, Department of Radiology, Stanford University Medical Center, Stanford, California

DAVID H. KIM, MD
Associate Professor of Radiology, Department of Radiology, University of Wisconsin School of Medicine and Public Health, Madison, Wisconsin

KWANG PYO KIM, PhD
Assistant Professor, Department of Nuclear Engineering, Kyung Hee University, Giheung-gu, Yongin-si, Gyeonggi-do, Republic of Korea

DIPTI K. LENHART, MD
Division of Abdominal Imaging and Intervention, Department of Radiology, Massachusetts General Hospital, Boston, Massachusetts

DAVID LIEBERMAN, MD
Professor of Medicine and Chief, Division of Gastroenterology and Hepatology, Oregon Health and Science University, Portland, Oregon

KLAUS MERGENER, MD, PhD
Digestive Health Specialists, Tacoma, Washington

PERRY J. PICKHARDT, MD
Professor of Radiology, Department of Radiology, University of Wisconsin School of Medicine and Public Health, Madison, Wisconsin; Department of Radiology, Uniformed Services University of the Health Sciences, Bethesda, Maryland

PETER D. POULLOS, MD
Clinical Instructor of Radiology, Department of Radiology, Stanford University School of Medicine, Stanford, California

VASSILIOS RAPTOPOULOS, MD
Professor of Radiology, Department of Radiology, Beth Israel Deaconess Medical Center, Boston, Massachusetts

JONATHAN A. ROSENBERG, MD
Clinical Research Fellow, Section of Gastroenterology, Hepatology and Nutrition, Department of Medicine, University of Chicago Medical Center, Chicago, Illinois

DAVID T. RUBIN, MD
Associate Professor of Medicine, Section of Gastroenterology, Hepatology and Nutrition, Department of Medicine, University of Chicago Medical Center, Chicago, Illinois

SRIKANT SADDA, MD
Department of Radiology and Biomedical Imaging, Mount Sinai Medical Center, Miami Beach, Florida

LEWIS K. SHIN, MD
Assistant Professor of Radiology, Department of Radiology, Stanford University School of Medicine; Department of Radiology, The Lucas Center for MR Spectroscopy and Imaging, Stanford University, Stanford, California

RONALD M. SUMMERS, MD, PhD
Imaging Biomarkers and Computer-Aided Diagnosis Laboratory, Radiology and Imaging Sciences, National Institutes of Health Clinical Center, Bethesda, Maryland

JEROME D. WAYE, MD
Clinical Professor of Medicine, Department of Medicine, Mount Sinai Medical Center, New York, New York

JUDY YEE, MD
Chief of Radiology, San Francisco Veterans Affairs Medical Center; Professor and Vice Chair of Radiology and Biomedical Imaging, University of California, San Francisco, California

BENJAMIN YEH, MD
Assistant Chief of Radiology, San Francisco Veterans Affairs Medical Center; Associate Professor of Radiology and Biomedical Imaging, University of California, San Francisco, California

MICHAEL E. ZALIS, MD
Director CT Colonography/QPID Informatics, Division of Abdominal Imaging and Intervention, Department of Radiology, Massachusetts General Hospital; Associate Professor, Harvard Medical School, Boston, Massachusetts

GIULIA A. ZAMBONI, MD
Istituto di Radiologia, Policlinico GB Rossi, Verona, Italy

Contents

> The technical objective of computed tomographic colonography (CTC) is
> to acquire high-quality computed tomography images of the cleansed,
> well-distended colon for polyp detection. In this article the authors provide
> an overview of the technical components of CTC, from preparation of the
> patient to acquisition of the imaging data and basic methods of interpreta-
> tion. In each section, the best evidence for current practices and recom-
> mendations is reviewed. Each of the technical components must be
> optimized to achieve high sensitivity in polyp detection.

> The amount of data accumulated in trials of CT colonography (CTC) has
> greatly increased in the past decade. The information from these studies
> is shaping clinical practice and public health policy regarding screening
> for colorectal cancer (CRC). This article examines the performance of
> CTC in clinical trials for individuals at average risk and increased risk for
> CRC. It also addresses the efficacy of CTC after incomplete colonoscopy,
> when colon preparations are reduced or eliminated, and in academic ver-
> sus nonacademic environments. The data suggest that CTC is effective
> especially for the detection of larger lesions and when more advanced im-
> aging technology is used.

> The primary goal of colorectal cancer screening and prevention is the de-
> tection and removal of advanced neoplasia. Computerized tomography
> (CT) colonography is now well established as an effective screening test.
> Areas of greater uncertainty include the performance characteristics of
> CT colonography for detecting small (6–9 mm), diminutive (≤5 mm), and
> flat (nonpolypoid) lesions. However, the actual clinical relevance of small,

diminutive, and flat polyps has also been the source of debate. This article addresses these controversial and often misunderstood issues.

Dipti K. Lenhart and Michael E. Zalis

Colorectal polyps less than 6 mm in size pose a negligible risk to the development of colorectal carcinoma. The sensitivity and specificity for detection of diminutive lesions on all available examinations including CT colonography (CTC) and optical colonoscopy (OC) is relatively low. In the context of regular screening, the low clinical significance and slow to negligible growth of diminutive polyps, as well as the low detection performance of CTC and OC for these lesions, would contribute to wasted health care resource and excess morbidity if each diminutive polyp were referred for potential resection. Respect for patient safety, attention to proper use of resources, and appropriate focus on larger, clinically significant polyps lead the authors to the conclusion that colonic polyps of less than 6 mm should not be separately reported.

David Lieberman

New diagnostic technologies can visualize colon polyps, but not remove them. There is clear consensus that polyps 10 mm or larger need to be removed. There is still controversy surrounding the appropriate reporting and management of small 1 to 5 mm and 6 to 9 mm polyps. The author recommends that patients whose largest polyp is 6 mm or larger should be offered colonoscopy. If the largest polyp is less than 6 mm in size, and imaged with high reliability, the author recommends reporting the finding, and individualizing the decision to pursue colonoscopy versus repeat imaging.

Ronald M. Summers

Computer-aided polyp detection aims to improve the accuracy of the colonography interpretation. The computer searches the colonic wall to look for polyplike protrusions and presents a list of suspicious areas to a physician for further analysis. Computer-aided polyp detection has developed rapidly in the past decade in the laboratory setting and has sensitivities comparable with those of experts. Computer-aided polyp detection tends to help inexperienced readers more than experienced ones and may also lead to small reductions in specificity. In its currently proposed use as an adjunct to standard image interpretation, computer-aided polyp detection serves as a spellchecker rather than an efficiency enhancer.

David H. Kim and Perry J. Pickhardt

This article defines the necessary skill set and knowledge base required for accurate computed tomography colonography (CTC) interpretation. The components of the interpretative process as well as the various strategies currently employed are discussed. The role of extracolonic evaluation as an integral part of this examination is also covered. Within this context, the question of whether a radiologist or gastroenterologist is better suited to interpret this examination is explored.

Screening for colorectal neoplasms has become the standard of care in advanced medical settings worldwide. Identifying asymptomatic colorectal neoplastic lesions has been shown to reduce colorectal cancer incidence and the overall cost of medical care. Clinicians have several alternatives at their disposal as they consider screening for their respective patient population. Two important methods to consider are optical colonoscopy and computed tomographic colonography (CTC). The purpose of this article is to make the case that gastroenterologists should read CTC. Central to the argument that gastroenterologists read CTC is the benefit of experience with video-assisted colonic imaging and the physician-patient relationship.

Computed tomographic colonography (CTC) has emerged as an alternative screening tool for colorectal cancer due to the potential to provide good efficacy combined with greater acceptability than optical colonoscopy or fecal occult blood testing. However, some organizations have raised concerns about the potential harms, including perforation rates and radiation-related cancer risks, and have not recommended that it currently be used as a screening tool in the general population in the US. In this article the authors review the current evidence for these potential harms from CTC and compare them to the potential harms from the alternatives including colonoscopy and double-contrast barium enema.

Colon screening examinations have been shown to discover neoplastic lesions at an early stage. Even the most careful studies by colonoscopy and by computed tomographic colonography (CTC) can overlook tumors with a diameter greater than 5 mm. Advances in technology have continually improved the ability to find polyps, which will lead to a real decrease in colorectal cancer incidence.

Computed tomographic colonography (CTC) is a validated tool for the evaluation of the colon for polyps and cancer. The technique employed for CTC includes a low-dose CT scan of the abdomen and pelvis that is typically performed without the administration of intravenous contrast. Using this technique it is possible to discover findings outside of the colon. By far, most extracolonic findings are determined to be clinically inconsequential on CTC and most patients are not recommended for further testing. However, some findings may result in additional diagnostic evaluation or intervention, which can lead to patient anxiety and increased morbidity and health care costs. Alternatively, some findings can lead to the earlier diagnosis of a clinically significant lesion, which could result in decreased patient morbidity and mortality as well as overall savings in downstream health care costs. The controversies of detecting and evaluating these incidental extracolonic findings on CTC are discussed.

The bowel is a common site for pathologic processes, including malignancies and inflammatory disease. Colorectal cancer accounts for 10% of all new cancers and 9% of cancer deaths. A significant decrease in the incidence of colorectal cancer and cancer death rates has been attributed to screening measures, earlier detection, and improved therapies. Virtual colonoscopy (VC), also known as computed tomography colonography, is an effective method for detecting polyps. However, in light of increasing concerns about ionizing radiation exposure from medical imaging and potential increased risk of future radiation-induced malignancies, magnetic resonance imaging (MRI) is seen as an increasingly attractive alternative. Improvements in MRI technology now permit three-dimensional volumetric imaging of the entire colon in a single breath hold at high spatial resolution, making VC with MRI possible.

Conventional radiologic and endoscopic evaluations of the small bowel are often limited by the length, caliber, and motility of the small bowel loops. The development of new multidetector-row CT scanners, with faster scan times and isotropic spatial resolution, allows high-resolution multiphasic and multiplanar assessment of the bowel, bowel wall, and lumen. CT Enterography (CTE) is a variant of routine abdominal scanning, geared toward more sustained bowel filling with oral contrast material, and the use of multiplanar images, that can enhance gastrointestinal (GI) tract imaging. This article examines the techniques and clinical applications of CTE in comparison with CT enteroclysis, focusing on Crohn disease, obscure GI bleeding, GI tumors, acute abdominal pain, and bowel obstruction.

Computed tomography colonography (CTC) has the potential to become a major component of colorectal cancer (CRC) screening programs and to have a significant effect on CRC prevention. This article describes the potential role of CTC within the framework of colorectal cancer screening. Current screening recommendations and traditional screening tests are reviewed, followed by a summary of recent study results on the use of CTC as a screening tool. Several factors that are affecting the acceptance and adoption of CTC are outlined. Although CTC is valuable and holds considerable promise as a way to increase the use of CRC screening, these issues need to be addressed before CTC becomes more widely disseminated as a screening modality.

Brooks D. Cash

This article describes the steps involved in establishing a screening computed tomographic colonography (CTC) practice and integrating that practice within a gastroenterology practice. The standard operating procedures followed at the National Naval Medical Center's Colon Health Initiative are presented and are followed by a discussion of practical aspects of establishing a CTC practice, such as equipment specifications, CTC performance, and interpretation training requirements for radiologists and nonradiologists. Regulatory considerations involved in establishing a screening CTC program are examined along with the salient features of a CTC business plan. Finally, reimbursement issues, quality control, and the potential impact of screening CTC on colonoscopy practice are discussed.

THE CLINICS ARE NOW AVAILABLE ONLINE!

Access your subscription at:
www.theclinics.com

Foreword

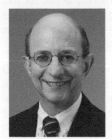

Charles J. Lightdale, MD
Consulting Editor

Anyone who might be surprised to find an issue of the *Gastrointestinal Endoscopy Clinics of North America* devoted entirely to a nonendoscopic method, computed tomographic colonography (CTC), should be reassured that I had a similar reaction when our Guest Editor, Jacques Van Dam, proposed the idea to me. However, as I listened to Dr Van Dam's presentation on the telephone, it quickly became clear that this was precisely the right thing to do. Dr Van Dam, the current President of the American Society for Gastrointestinal Endoscopy, has always had a wonderful grasp of the strategic big picture issues affecting our field, and how to assimilate "virtual colonoscopy" into colorectal cancer screening has become an important consideration.

Some gastroenterologists have already integrated CTC into their practices. Most remain skeptical, however, particularly in light of data that show a lower detection rate for smaller polyps, the continued need for rigorous bowel cleansing, and the significant radiation dose involved. There is also the need to follow up positive findings on CTC with real or optical colonoscopy for confirmation and polypectomy. Another issue for gastroenterologists was how responsible they would be for abnormalities detected on CT outside the colon. The decision taken last year by the US Centers for Medicare and Medicaid Services (CMS) to deny coverage for CTC was certainly a major setback for proponents. The CMS cited the relatively low sensitivity of CTC compared with optical colonoscopy, the increased costs involved with follow-up colonoscopy for positive findings, and the lack of data to support the claim that the less-invasive CTC would be more acceptable to patients and therefore would increase screening rates.

Nonetheless, there is no doubt that CTC will continue to evolve and improve. The possibility of a "virtual prep" remains tantalizing. Imagine being able to achieve a pristine clean colon by pushing the delete button on the CTC machine. There are many questions for the future. Will CTC or possibly magnetic resonance colonography attract the 50% of Americans who are eligible for colon cancer screening but are not being screened? Will quality CTC improve screening of the right colon, a well-documented problem in community-based screening with optical colonoscopy? How will

Gastrointest Endoscopy Clin N Am 20 (2010) xiii–xiv
doi:10.1016/j.giec.2010.02.014

CTC fit in with new screening options, such as more accurate and reliable fecal immunochemical tests or the new blood tests just emerging from the laboratory?

I am very grateful to Dr Van Dam and co-Guest Editor, Dr Subhas Banerjee, for this superb, comprehensive publication. CTC is an important, evolving modality that needs to be thoroughly understood by all those involved with colorectal cancer screening, as we move forward with whatever it takes to save lives from this preventable disease.

Charles J. Lightdale, MD
Department of Medicine
Columbia University Medical Center
161 Fort Washington Avenue, Room 812
New York, NY 10032, USA

E-mail address:
CJL18@columbia.edu

Preface

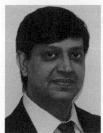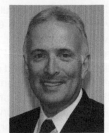

Subhas Banerjee, MD   Jacques Van Dam, MD, PhD
Guest Editors

There is widespread consensus among gastroenterologists in the United States that conventional colonoscopy is the best screening modality for colorectal cancer (CRC). However, a large segment of the population at risk for the disease remains unscreened. Although there are many purported reasons for such underutilization fear of invasive testing is among the most commonly offered. Also contributing to the screening shortfall is the fact that there are too few endoscopists in the United States to meet current and projected needs for CRC screening by conventional colonoscopy.

One of the most compelling and significant advances in CRC screening of the past decade has been the rapid evolution of computed tomography colonography (CTC). The use of CTC as a primary CRC screening exam, however, has generated controversy relating to its clinical and cost effectiveness, its potential performance as it devolves from academic centers into the community, the cost and risks associated with reporting of extracolonic lesions, the amount of training necessary to read CTC, the qualifications of gastroenterologists to read CTC, the magnitude of the associated radiation risk, and so forth.

Initially, CTC was viewed as a strong competitor to colonoscopy. Like colonoscopy, CTC enables imaging of the entire colon, yet it does so without the same degree of invasiveness. Despite fears of competition, some gastroenterologists embraced the use of CTC believing that screening by any modality is better than no screening at all. Many gastroenterologists even felt they could incorporate reading CTCs into their clinical practices.

Acceptance of CTC as a primary CRC screening modality gained momentum late in the last decade. The American Gastroenterological Association convened a CTC Task Force in 2004, published standards for gastroenterologists for performing and interpreting CTC in October 2007, and began hosting courses on CTC for gastroenterologists. In March 2008, CTC was included in the joint colorectal screening guideline issued by the US Multi-Society Task Force, American Cancer Society, and American College of Radiology. This was followed in September 2008 by the publication of National CTC Trial (ACRIN 6664), funded by the National Institutes of Health, that indicated colonoscopy and CTC performed similarly in the detection of large polyps.

Gastrointest Endoscopy Clin N Am 20 (2010) xv–xvi
doi:10.1016/j.giec.2010.02.015
1052-5157/10/$ – see front matter © 2010 Elsevier Inc. All rights reserved.

However, the quest to become part of the standard of care halted abruptly in 2009 when the Centers for Medicare and Medicaid Services (CMS) decided not to approve reimbursement coverage for CTC. The decision was based predominantly on data that showed inadequate performance in the Medicare-age population; however, radiologists, with the support of their specialty societies, can be expected to continue to refine the technology until it is ready for widespread use.

What are the current arguments that accompany this test? In this issue of *Gastrointestinal Endoscopy Clinics of North America*, we assembled a renowned collection of radiologists and gastroenterologists, celebrated for their contributions to the field, to comprehensively review and report on the current "state-of-the-art" as well as the controversies related to CTC and magnetic-resonance colonography.

We would like to thank all of our authors for their superlative contributions. We would also like to thank Dr Charles Lightdale for the opportunity to guest edit this volume and Kerry Holland for her support in bringing this volume to completion.

Subhas Banerjee, MD
Stanford University School of Medicine
A175, MC 5309
300 Pasteur Drive, Stanford
CA 94305, USA

Jacques Van Dam, MD, PhD
Division of Gastroenterology and Hepatology
Stanford University School of Medicine
A175, MC 5309
300 Pasteur Drive, Stanford
CA 94305, USA

E-mail address:
sbanerje@stanford.edu (S. Banerjee)

Current Techniques in the Performance, Interpretation, and Reporting of CT Colonography

Peter D. Poullos, MD[a],*, Christopher F. Beaulieu, MD, PhD[b]

KEYWORDS

• CT colonography • Virtual colonoscopy • Colorectal carcinoma
• Colorectal polyp • Cancer screening • Stool tagging

As early as 1983, Computed tomography (CT) was recognized as a potential colon cancer screening technique.[1] By 1994, technological advances allowed realization of what is now called CT colonography (CTC) or virtual colonoscopy.[2] The technical objective of CTC is to acquire high-quality CT images of the cleansed, well-distended colon for polyp detection.[3,4] Since the mid 1990s, many studies have confirmed the ability of CTC to accurately detect polyps and colorectal cancer.[5–7] and there exist well over 1000 peer-reviewed articles on various aspects of CTC. The ultimate clinical implementation of CTC, however, continues to be controversial, most recently manifest in the fierce debate over Medicare coverage.

In this article the authors provide an overview of the technical components of CTC, from preparation of the patient to acquisition of the imaging data and basic methods of interpretation. In each section, the best evidence for current practices and recommendations is reviewed. Each of the technical components must be optimized to achieve high sensitivity in polyp detection.[8] That being said, the tremendous research and technical advances that have occurred over the last decade should now enable any modern CT imaging center to perform high-quality examinations.

[a] Department of Radiology, Stanford University School of Medicine, 300 Pasteur Drive, Room H-1307, Stanford, CA 94305-5105, USA
[b] Department of Radiology, Stanford University School of Medicine, 300 Pasteur Drive, S078, Stanford, CA 94305-5105, USA
* Corresponding author.
E-mail address: ppoullos@stanford.edu

Gastrointest Endoscopy Clin N Am 20 (2010) 169–192
doi:10.1016/j.giec.2010.02.007
1052-5157/10/$ – see front matter © 2010 Elsevier Inc. All rights reserved.

BOWEL PREPARATION
Background

Adequate bowel preparation may be even more critical for CTC than for colonoscopy. Whereas in colonoscopy, rinsing and suction may be used to remove residual stool and/or liquid, there is no such opportunity to alter the colonic contents once the CTC images have been acquired. Imaging the patient in both supine and prone positions is helpful,[9] but does not substitute for an adequate preparation. Adherent stool is the most common cause of false-positive findings on CTC.[10] Retained liquid and stool can also obscure lesions, especially small ones, resulting in false-negative diagnoses. Interpretation times also increase when a large number of false lesions must be interrogated and documented.[11]

Diet

Dietary restriction is a prerequisite to a good pharmacologic bowel preparation, and should begin at least 1 day before CTC. Low-residue solids may be consumed that morning, followed by a purely liquid diet the remainder of the day. It is important to avoid high residue foods and dairy products.

Pharmacologic Laxatives: Wet and Dry

There is a multitude of pharmacologic colon cleansing preparations, reflecting the difficulty in perfecting one that balances strength with safety, taking into account patient acceptance and tolerance.[12] Among those available, the major distinction lies between so-called dry preps and wet preps.

Dry prep

The central ingredient of a dry prep usually consists of a low-volume, hyperosmotic preparation with either sodium phosphate (NaP) or magnesium citrate.[13] The dry preps cause an osmotic catharsis as intraluminal saline draws plasma water into the bowel lumen. Macari and colleagues[14] reported that on average, a phospho-soda preparation provided significantly less residual fluid than a polyethylene glycol preparation, which is advantageous in CTC.

Sodium phosphate Oral NaP products include the prescription products Visicol and OsmoPrep, and over-the-counter laxatives (eg, Fleet Phospho-soda).[15] The liquid form is packaged in a 45-mL bottle, which is mixed with 4 ounces of water and taken late in the afternoon with 8 additional ounces of water on the day before CTC.[16] The taste is considerably salty. Onset to catharsis is approximately 1 hour. Four bisacodyl tablets are also taken orally in the evening after the NaP is finished, and a bisacodyl rectal suppository is inserted the morning of the examination. Some have advocated double dose (90 mL) of NaP, but a single dose is just as effective.[17] NaP also comes in pill form. The tablet-based formulation bypasses the problem of flavor and also enables oral intake with any clear liquid.

The routine use of NaP is controversial due to its history of causing serious electrolyte abnormalities.[18] Patients may become dehydrated and develop hyperphosphatemia, hypocalcemia, hypernatremia, and hypokalemia.[19,20] Metabolic acidosis, tetany, and death have been reported.[21,22] In addition, rare reports of acute phosphate nephropathy have been published. Acute phosphate nephropathy is associated with calcium-phosphate crystal deposition in the renal tubules that may result in permanent renal dysfunction, sometimes requiring dialysis.[15] The risk appears to be related to factors such as advanced age, hypovolemia, baseline renal insufficiency, increased bowel transit time, colonic mucosal injury from colitis, or the use of nephrotoxic medications such as diuretics, angiotensin-converting enzyme inhibitors, angiotensin receptor blockers, and possibly nonsteroidal anti-inflammatory drugs (NSAIDs).[15,16,18] As such, the Food and Drug Administration (FDA) has required the manufacturer of Visicol and OsmoPrep to add a Boxed Warning to their labeling.[15,16]

A 2008 review by Belsey and colleagues[18] analyzed all available published sources of adverse events reported for both NaP and polyethylene glycol (PEG). These investigators highlighted a 1998 meta-analysis of 8 trials investigating the adequacy of NaP versus PEG preparation for optical colonoscopy.[23] The quality of cleansing was similar, but NaP was superior in terms of patient tolerance and cost. Another meta-analysis, looking at 16 studies, also demonstrated superiority of NaP.[24] However, the largest meta-analysis, based on 24 studies, showed no significant difference between NaP and PEG.[25] None of the 3 meta-analyses demonstrated any significant difference in adverse events. In fact, in the largest analysis neither group suffered any clinically significant serious adverse events.[25] Some CTC programs have screening questionnaires to triage at-risk patients away from NaP. However, such systems are imperfect, as one study showed that 2% of cases with contraindication to NaP could not have been prospectively excluded based on their clinical history alone.[26] Many CTC programs have thus decided to terminate its use. If used, however, the manufacturers have advised that the dose be restricted or split and that the patient drink sufficient liquids.[18]

Magnesium citrate Magnesium citrate can be dispensed in powder or liquid form. The powder form is mixed with 16 ounces of liquid. The liquid form comes ready to drink in a 10-ounce bottle. Like NaP, magnesium citrate is taken in the late afternoon 1 day before the examination. Time to onset of catharsis is around 1 hour. Oral hydration should be maintained to prevent dehydration.[16]

As with NaP, bisacodyl tablets are taken the night before, and a bisacodyl suppository on the morning of the examination. The sodium content of magnesium citrate is much less than NaP and therefore may be preferred in patients at risk for electrolyte abnormalities.[12,16] In a 2005 study by Delegge and Kaplan,[12] 506 patients undergoing optical colonoscopy were randomized to receive either a magnesium citrate (LoSo Prep, containing magnesium citrate, bisacodyl tablets and a bisacodyl suppository) or NaP-based prep (double dose NaP). The group that received magnesium citrate demonstrated superior colon cleansing, and frequency of reported side effects was similar for both groups (59% vs 58% for NaP and Neutra prep/LoSo prep, respectively).

Wet prep
A wet prep refers to a high-volume, iso-osmotic preparation based on PEG. PEG is a washout lavage preparation that is nonabsorbable and is osmotically balanced. PEG does not cause fluid shifts from the intracellular to the extracellular space. A disadvantage of this preparation is considerable residual fluid in the colon, which is easily suctioned at optical colonoscopy but obscures portions of the bowel wall in CTC (**Fig. 1**).[14]

PEG Standard preparation with PEG is usually accomplished by drinking 4 L of the solution the afternoon before the examination. Although popular for colonoscopy preparation, PEG has progressively fallen out of favor for use in CTC, for both technical and patient-related reasons. A PEG preparation not infrequently leaves liquid in the colon, potentially obscuring lesions. PEG also has the poorest adherence of the preparations, due to its consistency and taste as well as the imposing volume. At one experienced center, PEG accounts for less than 1% of CTC preparations.[27] However,

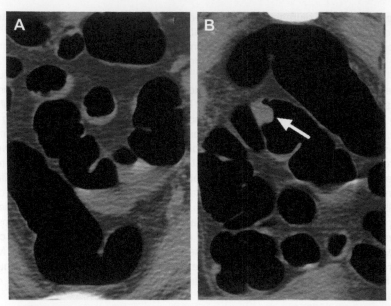

Fig. 1. (A) 2D supine axial view of the abdomen demonstrates fluid layering dependently within a loop of colon. No lesion is visible. (B) The corresponding prone view demonstrates that the fluid has redistributed, revealing a large polyp.

PEG does have the advantage of not causing fluid shifts and is safe for those in fragile health.[28] Trials examining the relative efficacies of NaP versus PEG have yielded varying results. A 2009 Japanese study compared the performance and safety of the NaP tablet (with and without laxatives) and PEG bowel preparations prior to colonoscopy, and found the quality of colon cleansing equivalent. Although serum levels of inorganic phosphorus were abnormally increased in the NaP groups, these increases were only transitory.[29] A study performed on a population with a high-residue diet showed better colonic cleansing and shorter CTC interpretation times with a PEG-based preparation compared with the NaP-based preparation.[30]

Side effects associated with PEG are not as alarming, but data suggests that it too is potentially associated with electrolyte disturbances, albeit to a lesser extent than with NaP. Reported adverse events attributable to oral PEG generally reflect sodium imbalance, gastrointestinal injury caused by vomiting, allergic reactions, and aspiration.[18] Regardless of the type of bowel preparation, the majority of patients experience discomfort and inconvenience.[31,32] Ongoing research to perform low-prep or no-prep CTC with fecal tagging has the potential to eliminate the most onerous part of the examination.

Fecal Tagging

Background

Many CTC programs now routinely employ fecal tagging.[33,34] Fecal tagging refers to the oral ingestion of high-density oral contrast agents so that residual colonic contents, liquid and solid, are homogeneously high in attenuation and can therefore be differentiated easily from soft tissue density polyps (**Fig. 2**). Tagging may therefore help improve the performance of CTC for polyp detection. Many different contrast agents and combinations of agents have been used for fecal tagging.[9,10,32,35–39] In

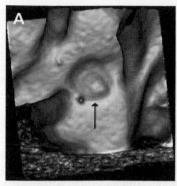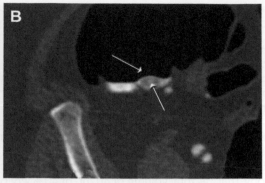

Fig. 2. (*A*) 3D endoluminal cube view of a segment of the right colon demonstrates a mucosal lesion (*arrow*) suspicious for polyp. Differentiation of true polyps from adherent stool on 3D endoluminal images is difficult. (*B*) 2D supine axial image demonstrates the same lesion (*large arrow*), highlighted by surrounding tagged liquid. There is central high attenuation (*small arrow*) within the filling defect, consistent with tagged stool.

general, there are 2 main classes in common use: barium-based and iodine-based (both ionic and nonionic).

Barium

Many different densities of barium-based tagging agents have been proposed,[32] and tagging protocols using barium alone have been reported to be effective.[40–42] Barium-based formulations (eg, Tagitol V 40% w/v) are similar to those regularly used in standard abdominal CT scanning, have an excellent safety record, and are familiar to radiologists. There is some evidence that barium selectively adheres to polyps with villous histology, which may prove beneficial in polyp diagnosis.[43] On the other hand, high-density barium, particularly if the density is heterogeneous, produces problems for electronic cleansing regimens, discussed later.[44] In addition, barium can cause constipation or even impaction.[45]

Iodinated

Iodine-based agents are similarly safe and familiar. Studies have demonstrated that iodinated contrast ingested alone may also be used to tag residual material in the colon.[35,37,46] Iodinated agents are hypertonic, can cause fluid shifts into the bowel lumen, and thus have an additional cathartic effect.[46] In a 2009 retrospective study of nonlaxative or minimum-laxative regimens, Nagata and colleagues[34] found the homogeneity of tagged fecal matter was better with iodine-based regimens then with barium.

Ionic iodinated

Iodinated contrast agents come in 2 varieties, ionic and nonionic. Both are water soluble, which promotes more homogeneous tagging.[27] Diatrizoate meglumine and diatrizoate sodium (Gastrografin 37% organically bound iodine) is an ionic iodinated contrast agent that is commonly used as oral contrast in standard CT examinations, as well as for fluid/stool tagging in CTC[37]; it is less expensive than nonionic.[32] However, the taste is not palatable, especially when drinking large amounts.[47] Although oral ionic iodinated contrast agents are generally safe, they can induce gastrointestinal complaints and dehydration, and rare anaphylactic reactions have been reported.[48] Sodium diatrizoate is contraindicated in those with iodine allergies. Doses as low as 20 mL of been shown to be adequate for tagging purposes.[32]

Nonionic iodinated

Nonionic iodinated contrast (ie, iopromide, iohexol) has a low risk for causing dehydration and diarrhea. Unlike sodium diatrizoate, it is almost tasteless and has good patient acceptance.[49] However, this contrast agent is more expensive than both barium and ionic iodinated contrast.[34]

Of course, the use of barium and iodine-based tagging agents are not mutually exclusive. The strategy behind combined tagging is to achieve opacification of residual solids with barium, and of fluid with iodine. These agents have been successfully used in combination, as was done in the multicenter ACRIN National CT Colonography Trial.[7] A total volume of 40 mL of 40% w/v barium (Tagitol V) was administered orally the day before the CT scan in 3 divided doses. A total volume of 60 mL of sodium diatrizoate was administered in 3 doses of 20 mL starting the evening before the CT scan.

Although there is no consensus regimen, the European Society of Gastrointestinal and Abdominal Radiology suggests that the choice of tagging agent should be based on local experience, taking into account any history of allergy.[33]

Limited prep and noncathartic CTC

Preparation is one of the most unpleasant aspects of CTC,[50] and patients would have the examination more frequently if bowel preparation was not required.[51,52] Interest in developing tagging regimens is rooted in improving patient experience and compliance by decreasing or eliminating the need for a cathartic. Noncathartic or reduced cathartic CTC is more tolerable, especially for those with impaired mobility or those who have a poor response to laxatives.[32] Polyp detection in noncathartic or reduced cathartic preparations with fecal tagging is an area of intense ongoing research, with early studies reporting encouraging results.[39,53,54]

In a 2008 study of 40 patients who underwent the same fecal tagging regimen before CTC, the patients were randomized to 4 different cathartic regimens of varying intensity. There was no difference in image quality between the different cathartic groups. Bisacodyl, 30 mg and magnesium citrate, 16.4 g did not provide better image quality than bisacodyl alone, 20 mg. Patient acceptance rates were lower in the more aggressive cathartic groups.[55]

In a 2008 study by Jensch and colleagues,[39] CTC with fecal tagging without stool subtraction and a bisacodyl-only prep was compared with colonoscopy. Despite homogeneous fecal tagging, there was a large number of false-positive findings (specificity 79%) when 6 mm was used as a size threshold. In a 2009 study by Nagata and colleagues,[32] minimum laxative fecal tagging CTC demonstrated equally high sensitivity to full laxative examination. However, the full laxative fecal tagged CTC yielded a higher specificity. The investigators concluded that it might be desirable to offer patients the option of the full prep for highest accuracy and the ability to perform a same-day colonoscopy, or a minimum laxative CTC for those willing to accept an increased risk of false positives and attendant unnecessary colonoscopy, which not only is inconvenient, but increases risk and costs.

Electronic Subtraction of Tagged Material

"Electronic cleansing" or "electronic subtraction" of fluid and fecal contents is an area of active research, with the goal of manipulating the images such that the high-density tagging material is removed, but without interfering with polyp detection.[44] This manipulation is important for visualization as well as for computer-aided polyp detection, whether the prep is a full prep with fecal tagging or a less rigorous limited or noncathartic one. Several commercial platforms now employ algorithms for electronic cleansing.[56] At present, electronic subtraction is technically challenging, principally because of heterogeneous fecal tagging, variable colonic transit times, and normal stool desiccation as it progresses toward the rectum. Also, interfaces of stool, air, and tissue are prone to partial volume artifacts.[51] "Oversubtraction," where normal tissue or polyps are subtracted along with stool, must be avoided. Although stool subtraction has been shown to improve sensitivity of CTC, studies have also shown that the specificity can decrease, especially for the detection of moderate-sized polyps.[51]

One of the main issues with noncathartic preps is difficulty in performing a primary 3-dimensional (3D) interpretation without the ability to perform electronic cleansing. Residual stool and artifacts render the 3D virtual colonoscopic view unreadable, as the colonic mucosa is essentially "buried." A large number of filling defects would have to be addressed one by one.[51] Even with stool subtraction, optimal fecal tagging would be needed to make 3D interpretation possible.[6] Without stool subtraction, a primary 2-dimensional (2D) method must be employed with 3D problem solving. A primary 2D approach permits the reader to quickly examine the internal density of filling defects and decide if they are truly soft tissue polyps or if they contain air or tagging agent consistent with stool.[51]

As part of a 2006 study by Zalis and colleagues,[46] a group of CTC patients who ingested magnesium citrate preparation and iodinated fecal tagging agent without dietary restriction were compared with a group of patients who took PEG prep with standard dietary restrictions. Electronic subtraction was applied. Readability was equal between the 2 groups, and discomfort was less in the magnesium citrate group. In a 2008 study of a group of patients drawn from the Walter Reed Army Medical Center public database, Serlie and colleagues[57] found that electronic cleansing shortened interpretation time, lowered assessment effort, and had a positive effect on observer confidence.

Same-Day CTC and Colonoscopy Service: Impact on Selection of Bowel Prep

In an ideal setting, positive CTC examinations could be followed up with same-day colonoscopy, thereby avoiding a second bowel cleansing for the patient. This procedure requires close coordination with the gastroenterology department at each particular institution. Patients should be scheduled for CTC in the early morning while their colon remains freshly prepared. For appropriate triage, the studies need to be interpreted within 1 to 2 hours following data acquisition, while the patient remains NPO (nil by mouth) and awaits further instructions. Positive findings can then be communicated directly to the patient and to the gastroenterologist. Some flexibility in the colonoscopy schedule is needed so that CTC patients can be accommodated when needed. The amount of flexibility is determined by the work flow of the CTC program as well as the referral rate. The referral rate is in turn determined by the size threshold for referral. This threshold must be chosen in consultation with the local gastroenterologists. For example, if a size threshold of 5 mm is chosen for referral to colonoscopy, more patients will be referred than if the threshold were 1 cm.

The issue of patient preparation must also be addressed by consensus. The preparation for CTC must be acceptable to the gastroenterologist as adequate for colonoscopy. In some instances, as in a 2002 study by Lefere and colleagues,[41] additional preparation is performed between CTC and colonoscopy. In that study, a preparation regimen of magnesium citrate and fecal tagging agents was compared with PEG solution without fecal tagging. Because the preparation for CTC was less aggressive, patients underwent additional colonic cleansing with PEG before colonoscopy. The time between CTC and colonoscopy was 2 to 3 hours. Patients who get their CTC with the option of same-day colonoscopy must adhere to guidelines intended for colonoscopy patients, who are prepared for potential polypectomy; this includes stopping aspirin and NSAIDs. The images of the CTC should be available to the gastroenterologist, in a format which is intuitive and informative. Polyp size, location, and distance from the rectum should be easily attainable (**Fig. 3**). 3D endoluminal and "virtual barium enema" (**Fig. 4**) are excellent views to include. These images can be reconstructed on a 3D workstation and either sent back to PACS (picture archiving and communications system) or be made available on the 3D server.

BOWEL INSUFFLATION AND SPASMOLYTICS
Patient Arrival

The patient arrives in the CT suite approximately 2 to 3 hours after completion of the bowel preparation, at a time when evacuation of as much residual liquid as possible has been achieved. The technologist inquires about compliance with the preparation as well as appearance of the stool. If the patient has not finished the preparation or is

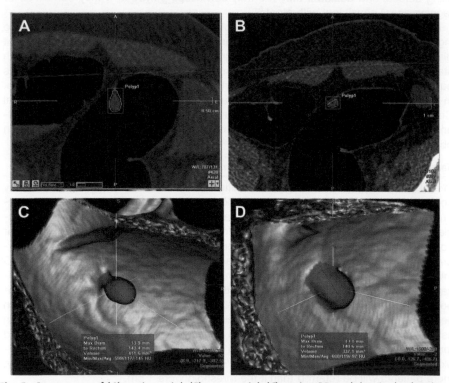

Fig. 3. Screen save of (A) supine axial, (B) prone axial, (C) supine 3D endoluminal cube view, and (D) prone 3D endoluminal cube view demonstrates a pedunculated polyp in the sigmoid colon. When the reader identifies and marks the polyp, the software automatically measures the diameter, volume, distance to rectum, and internal density. Note the apparent difference in morphology between the supine and prone images, a result of the polyp's mobility.

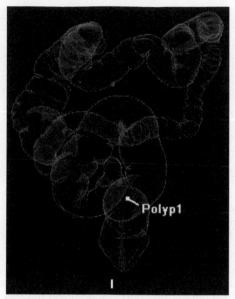

Fig. 4. "Virtual barium enema" 3D reconstruction of the colon demonstrates that the locations of polyps can be labeled as an aid to the gastroenterologist who will be performing the subsequent colonoscopy. "Polyp 1" is seen in the distal sigmoid colon.

continuing to have semisolid stools, rather than rescheduling the examination, more cathartic agents may be administered in the department. Before the examination, the patient is encouraged to use the restroom one last time.

Insufflation

Adequate colonic distention is of fundamental importance for CTC. Collapsed bowel segments may reduce sensitivity and specificity, obscuring disease or mimicking pathology.[9,10] Diagnostic confidence can be reduced[58] and interpretation times increased.[9,10,59] Distention can be achieved by staff or patient administration of either room air or carbon dioxide (CO_2), via a manual pump or electronic insufflator. The simplest and least expensive technique is room air insufflation using a hand-held plastic bulb.[59] This method can even be performed by patients themselves.[6] Of the possible combinations, electronic insufflation of CO_2 is favored for the reasons given below.

Burling and colleagues[59] demonstrated that automated CO_2 insufflation significantly improved colonic distention compared with manual CO_2 insufflation for CTC, particularly the left colon in the supine position and the transverse colon when both supine and prone scans were combined. Slow administration of CO_2 at continuous low pressures likely decreases colonic spasm, especially in segments with diverticular disease **(Fig. 5)**.[27] CO_2 is, because of its superior lipid solubility and higher partial pressure gradient, more rapidly absorbed by the colon than room air.[60] Thus, compared with room air, postprocedural gaseous discomfort is reduced.[61] Complications are also likely reduced, as close to all of the reported perforations from CTC have involved staff-controlled manual insufflation of room air. The perforation risk with electronic CO_2 insufflation is negligible in the screening population.[62]

A physician, radiology technician, or nurse inserts a thin, flexible rectal catheter that is connected to the electronic CO_2 insufflator (PROTOCO2L; Bracco Diagnostics,

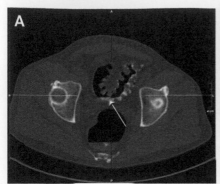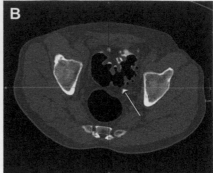

Fig. 5. (*A*) Axial supine view of the sigmoid colon demonstrates multiple sigmoid diverticula and muscular hypertrophy with poor sigmoid distention. (*B*) The prone image demonstrates that the sigmoid colon is better distended, making the reader more confident that this segment of colon can be adequately evaluated. A change in positioning is often helpful in this regard.

Princeton, NJ, USA). Larger catheters, such as those used at barium enema, are not typically used unless the patient has difficulty retaining the gas. The balloon may or may not be inflated. The target pressure, usually around 25 mmHg, is programmed and the CO_2 is insufflated, titrating to pressure and patient comfort. Because of differences in colonic anatomy, patient tolerance, ileocecal reflux, and anal incontinence, the total volume of CO_2 delivery can vary a great deal, and thus has little significance.[59] Anywhere from 3 to 10 L may be needed for adequate distention.[16,27] Cooperation with gas retention is essential.

Insufflation techniques vary between centers,[16,27] but often start with the patient in the right-side down decubitus position to facilitate rectosigmoid and descending colon distention. Insufflation is continued in the supine position until the patient reports fullness in the right side of the abdomen, usually indicating cecal distention. It is crucial to acquire the CT images during active replacement of CO_2 at equilibrium pressures.[27] A scout radiograph is then used to assess colonic distention (**Fig. 6**). If adequate, supine CT images are obtained. The scout, however, is sometimes unreliable for evaluation of distention. At some institutions technologists or research assistants are trained to assess the adequacy of distention by reviewing the CT images on the scanner console. This assessment allows for problem solving in real time, and reduces the need for callbacks.

After supine acquisition, the patient is then turned prone and the scout is then repeated. More CO_2 may or may not need to be insufflated. Elevation of the torso and hips with pillows, especially in overweight patients, can improve distention of the transverse colon.[11,16] Axial prone images are then obtained. The supine and prone scans are obtained at end expiration, elevating the diaphragm, and allowing more room for the splenic flexure and transverse colon.[27] The rationale of dual positioning is to redistribute residual fluid and as well as to help redistribute air (**Fig. 7**).[10,63] Polyp detection sensitivity has been proven to improve when both supine and prone acquisitions are performed (**Fig. 8**).[9,10,63]

Glucagon

Some investigators have studied spasmolytic agents such as glucagon with the goal of reducing bowel peristalsis and resulting motion artifact. Part of the justification for

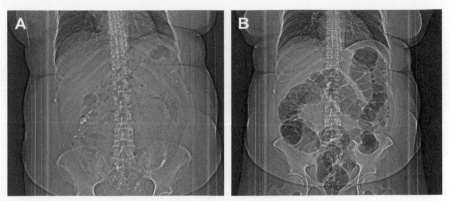

Fig. 6. (*A*) Supine scout topogram demonstrates no significant colonic distention. The rectal tubing had been disconnected from the CO_2 insufflator. Approximately 5 L of CO_2 was wasted. (*B*) After connecting the tubing and restarting the electronic CO_2 insufflator, excellent colonic distention is seen.

using glucagon in CTC arises from its role as an antiperistaltic agent in barium enema studies.[64] The data regarding glucagon's efficacy in colonic radiology is conflicting. Lappas and colleagues,[65] in a placebo-controlled study of glucagon effects in patients having double-contrast barium enemas, demonstrated that glucagon improved patient discomfort. However, an effect was not noted until after 8 minutes post administration. On a practical level, because of the speed of the CTC, patients will have already completed the examination before glucagon achieves its maximum effect.[66] Moreover, waiting for maximum effect increases duration of the CTC examination[61] and decreases efficiency. Other studies of glucagon have shown no beneficial effect. Yee and colleagues[67] performed a blinded, nonrandomized study of 60 patients undergoing CTC. The 33 patients who were administered glucagon did not show any difference and segmental or overall colonic distention. Morrin and colleagues[66]

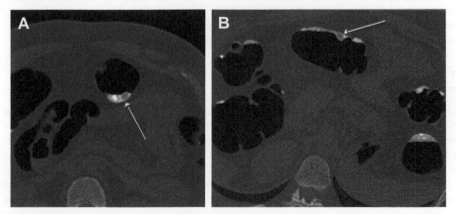

Fig. 7. (*A*) Axial supine view of the abdomen demonstrates a filling defect in the transverse colon (*arrow*). The defect is located dependently on the posterior wall and is surrounded by high-density tagged liquid; this could represent a polyp or stool. (*B*) Axial prone view of the abdomen demonstrates that the filling defect is mobile, and is seen now on the anterior wall (*arrow*); this is consistent with stool.

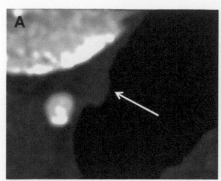 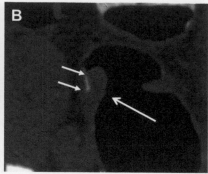

Fig. 8. (*A*) Axial supine view of the sigmoid colon demonstrates a mucosal lesion (*arrow*) suspicious for polyp. (*B*) Axial prone view demonstrates that the lesion (*large arrow*) changes morphology. Tagged liquid can be seen between the lesion and the colonic wall (*small arrows*), and a pedunculated polyp can be confidently diagnosed.

studied 74 patients who were administered glucagon before CTC and found that distention scores for the glucagon and nonglucagon patients were similar. In addition, Glucagon is costly (wholesale cost is US$48–66 per 1-mg vial) and requires an intra-venous or intramuscular injection.[66] Also, glucagon carries a risk of side effects.[61]

Glucagon's lack of proven effectiveness in CTC is not surprising from a physiologic standpoint, given that the colon is recognized as the least responsive part of the bowel to the antiperistaltic effects.[68] Thus, routine administration of glucagon is not recom-mended. However, glucagon may be given in the setting of significant abdominal discomfort or if there is persistent spasm or poor distention not improved by dual positioning.[16]

Though not available in the United States, the spasmolytic hyoscine-*N*-butylbro-mide (Buscopan) is available in Europe, and has been suggested to be more effective than glucagon as an antiperistaltic agent.[69] However, despite improved colonic distension in certain segments, Buscopan did not necessarily translate into improved polyp detection, thus is not routinely used in CTC.

Based on the literature and personal experience, there does not appear to be justi-fication for routine use of spasmolytics in CTC. At the same time, a small percentage of patients may have cramping and pain that significantly limit tolerance of bowel insuf-flation, and in these cases ad hoc administration of glucagon may be worthwhile.

CT DATA ACQUISITION
Introduction

A key technical advance in imaging which enabled CTC was the introduction of spiral or helical CT in the early 1990s. For the first time, this allowed continuous movement of the patient through the CT gantry during scanning, producing a spatially registered set of transverse slices during a single breath-hold. Since then, CT scanning has sped up by another factor of about 500, such that the CT acquisition portion of the examination is not limited whatsoever in the overall process. There remain, however, important considerations related to slice thickness, reconstruction interval, and radiation dose.

Section Thickness

Initial work with single-detector CTC typically used 3- to 5-mm thick sections with a high degree of image overlap for data acquisition[70–72] With the advent of multidetector-row CT scanners, data can be acquired with much thinner slices, with faster scan times. The acquisition of thin sections decreases partial volume averaging and improves image quality of the multiplanar reformats (MPR) and the 3D endoluminal images.[16,73] CT images of the entire abdomen and pelvis can be now obtained with a single breath-hold, which decreases respiratory motion artifacts. The use of multi-detector CT also results in better colonic distention when compared with single detector.[74]

Lui and colleagues[72] investigated how the performance characteristics of CTC would change in 25 patients by reconstructing their data sets with 2 different slice thicknesses. Sections of 1.25 mm were reconstructed every 1 mm, and 5-mm sections were reconstructed every 2 mm. Although no significant difference was found in polyp detection sensitivity comparing thin and thick sections, the specificity was superior for the thin ones.[16,72] A 2007 study by Johnson and colleagues[75] demonstrated that for both conventional 2D image displays and 3D virtual dissection image displays, there was no significant difference in polyp detection between 2.5- and 1.25-mm slice thicknesses. The investigators concluded that selecting the thickest possible slice collimation that preserves filling defect attenuation, while not degrading spatial resolution, is most favorable.

When using a 64-row multidetector CT scanner, the collimation typically ranges between 0.5 and 0.625 mm. The American College of Radiology Practice Guidelines for the Performance of CTC suggest a collimation of 3 mm or less with a reconstruction interval of 1.5 mm or less. Other CT scan parameters include: an effective mAs = 50; kV = 120; rotation time = 0.5 seconds; and reconstruction interval = 1 to 1.25 mm. Acquisition times in each position will be less than 10 seconds.[16] In addition, automatic tube current modulation has been shown to significantly reduce CTC dose.[76]

Another advantage of multidetector CT is that images can be reconstructed at thicknesses larger than the collimator width, for example, at 2.5-or 5-mm thickness, if desired by the radiologist. This option is very helpful for efficient interpretation of extracolonic structures.[16]

Radiation Dose

Increasing collimation or decreasing tube current (mAs) or voltage (kVp) will decrease radiation dose. Yet, although thinner sections improve polyp depiction, each time the slice thickness is reduced by half the radiation dose must be doubled to maintain constant image noise.[77] Some scanners may automatically increase radiation doses to maintain image noise as slice thickness is decreased. Thus careful setting of the dose parameters, influenced by the current (mAs) and voltage (kVp) of the CT beam, is needed to minimize radiation dose. Because image noise increases as dose is decreased, image noise can, at a certain point, degrade image quality and may decrease diagnostic performance, especially for smaller polyps.[78] It may be more difficult to differentiate stool from polyps because the attenuation of polyps becomes more heterogeneous as noise increases. Alternatively, radiologists must be willing to accept images with higher noise levels.

Radiologists should make every effort to maintain radiation exposure As Low As Reasonably Achievable (ALARA), especially so for elective screening examinations, where the benefit/risk ratio must be high.[79] As CTC becomes increasingly accepted and recommended for colon cancer screening, the radiology community must consider any potential radiation risk to the population that these potential millions of scans will have.[79] Summed over all organs at risk, the estimated absolute lifetime risk of cancer induction from 2 CTC scans (with the scanner parameters at 65 mAs, 120 kVp, 10 mm collimation, and pitch 1.35) in a 50-year-old is 0.14%, or roughly 1 in 700. Clearly the estimated risk of cancer death would be less, but this order of magnitude of potential cancer induction from a screening examination must be taken very seriously.[79]

Fortunately, because of the large difference in the attenuation between the bowel wall and the intraluminal air, as well as the lack of need to visualize solid organs well, there is great potential for dose reduction. The dose/noise trade-off can be very much weighted toward low-dose higher-noise images, while still maintaining sensitivity and specificity, at least for polyps larger than 10 mm in diameter.[79–82]

Concern over radiation exposure was one of the reasons given why Medicare declined reimbursement of screening CTC in 2009. A 2005 study by Brenner and Georgsson[83] estimated the radiation dose for CTC with prone and supine images at around 13 mSv. However, this study used data from older-generation 8- and 16-row scanners. In comparison, the ACRIN trial used newer multidetector scanners with low-dose technique and was able to limit radiation dose to approximately 5 mSv per examination.[7] This value is close to the 4.5 mSv annual background exposure at high altitude.[11] In addition, a 2008 study by Liedenbaum and colleagues[84] surveyed CTC providers about their equipment and dose parameters. These investigators found that 62% of their questionnaire respondents were using 64-row scanners and 50% used dose modulation. The average dose of their respondents was 5.7 mSv. The recently released 2009 ACR Practice Guidelines recommend that scan parameters should be modified such that desired image quality is achieved at or below the suggested CTDIvol values (6.25 mGy per scan position or 12.5 mGy total for supine and prone data sets). The dose may have to be increased in a morbidly obese patients in order to maintain image quality (gories/quality_safety/guidelines/dx/gastro/ct_colonography.aspx).

Ultralow-dose scans have been shown to be able to deliver an effective radiation dose of 1.8 mSv for males and 2.4 mSv for females while preserving excellent sensitivity (100% for polyps >10 mm and 100% for cancers).[85] In a 2004 feasibility study, Van Gelder and colleagues[78] studied 15 patients with doses ranging from 0.05 to 12 mSv. Overall sensitivity for polyps 5 mm or larger decreased at lower doses, but was 74% or higher down to 1.6 mAs (0.2 mSv).

Further discussion of the safety of CTC (see the article by Berrington and colleagues elsewhere in this issue for further exploration of this topic).

INTERPRETATION
Background

Assuming a cephalocaudal extent 35 cm for the colon, images at 1-mm intervals, and full supine and prone datasets, the initial scan data from a CTC study contains at least 700 images for interpretation. Compounding this, there are now a large number of techniques for 2D reformation and 3D reconstruction of the scan data, leading to even more images for review. Given this daunting task, there has been considerable investigation into how to most accurately and efficiently interpret CTC studies, which is the focus of this section. Note that computer-aided detection of polyps has also been an active area of research, (see the article by Summers elsewhere in this issue for further exploration of this topic).

One other issue that must be kept in mind is that advanced adenomas are relatively uncommon in a screening population, approximately 4% in incidence,[7] so the expectation is that the majority of CTC studies will be "negative" regarding detecting such a polyp. This "needle in a haystack" issue is one that substantially motivates methods for the most efficient and accurate means of study interpretation.

Polyp Identification

Polyps are homogeneous soft tissue attenuation, ovoid or round in shape. Sessile lesions should not change position with respect to the colonic wall in different positions.[16] Polyps may be located anywhere along the mucosal surface, including on haustral folds or the ileocecal valve. Residual stool, on the other hand, is often heterogeneous in attenuation, irregular in shape, and tends to change position between supine and prone scans. On 2D images, thickened folds may be mistaken for polyps. However, interpretive pitfalls are abundant, a point that underscores the importance of systematic reader training and experience. Through training, readers need to recognize that stool may be homogeneous in density, and that pedunculated polyps may trap air and appear heterogeneous in attenuation, or may appear to be mobile on prone and supine data sets, amongst other pitfalls.[16]

2D and 3D Interpretation

Alongside the technological advancements in CT imaging, computer graphics technology has rapidly evolved over the past 15 years, such that there now exist on the order of 10 commercial workstations with FDA-approved software targeted at CTC interpretation, among other applications. Some systems are thin-client web based, some stand-alone work stations, and others are integrated into PACS, and while many features are common, there is considerable variety in capabilities and ease of use. All are capable of MPR and 3D endoluminal reconstructions. Additional features may include panoramic views or "virtual dissection," translucency rendering, and wide-angle views, among others. All of these tools are aimed at improving sensitivity and specificity, as well as increasing reader confidence and interpretation efficiency, although one "optimal" means of CTC interpretation is not applicable to all readers, and thus some debate persists.

One issue that all can agree on is that comprehensive assessment of CTC data requires a dedicated software platform and that both 2D and 3D views are necessary. Having said this, the primary method of interpretation of CTC can begin with either 2D or 3D. The choice of method depends somewhat on personal preference, although multiple investigations have been made regarding the sensitivity and specificity of the different methods. Despite controversy regarding the optimal display,[8] endoluminal reformats have been demonstrated to improve the sensitivity for polyp detection at CTC,[6,86] and the 2 displays are undoubtedly complementary.

The 2D data set is the standard gray-scale display, optimized for CTC viewing and polyp detection by employing high-contrast window settings (width =1400, level = −350).[16] MPR such as coronal and sagittal views fall under the umbrella of 2D. The 3D data set refers to other reformats such as virtual endoluminal views. A "primary 2D reader" reviews the data in the axial plane with interrogation and problem solving of suspected findings using 3D reconstructions. In this mode, it is critical to perform a systematic analysis of the colon from rectum to cecum, or vice versa. A "primary 3D reader" interrogates the colon using the 3D endoluminal view and uses the gray-scale CT data to further investigate suspected findings.

There are advantages and disadvantages to each method. Primary 3D interpretation is often easier for inexperienced readers, and the views are intuitive to gastroenterologists. Small polyps in particular are more easily separated from haustral folds. In addition, proponents contend that performance is superior compared with primary 2D interpretation. Furthermore, interobserver variability is lower with the 3D technique.[6,87] However, 3D reads can require longer interpretation times compared with 2D reads.[7]

Advantages of primary 2D interpretation include shorter interpretation times,[7] caused by the lack of necessity to perform a total of 4 fly-throughs, 2 in each direction in both the supine and prone data sets. With interpretation times ranging from about 10 minutes[71,73,88] to more than 30 minutes,[89,90] speed is essential. The density of filling defects is readily discernible on the 2D data sets. The bowel wall integrity and fold contour are also more readily assessed (**Fig. 9**).[75,89,91]

A newer technique called the "virtual dissection" or "filet" view has been developed, which allows the entire colonic mucosal surface to be visualized at once (**Fig. 10**). These types of views grew out of laboratory work demonstrating the efficacy of various wide-angle and panoramic views designed to improve the visualized surface area in virtual endoscopy.[92] A center line is generated, then the colon is virtually straightened along the center line and "sliced" open as if it were a pathologic specimen.[93] The advantage of this technique is that entire segments of colonic mucosa can be visualized on a single image without obscuration by folds.[75] Disadvantages include anatomic distortion, as well as the need for 2D problem solving. Johnson and colleagues[93] demonstrated that distortion is predictable, and the need for 2D problem solving applies not only to the filet view but to all 3D techniques.[94] 3D filet is comparable to 2D in detection rates for both experienced[75,95,96] and inexperienced[97] readers. Moreover, Johnson and colleagues[75] showed that interpretation times for virtual dissection were 28% faster than with the conventional 2D method (10.4 vs 14.5 minutes, respectively). In addition, double review using both conventional and virtual dissection can compensate for poorer performing reviewers, decreasing interobserver variability and improving sensitivity, even surpassing the sensitivity of colonoscopy for adenomatous lesions greater than or equal to 1 cm.[75]

Computer software for CTC is available that offers a translucency rendering or color map overlay based on the attenuation of the lesion detected on 3D images. The translucency view is typically used to help differentiate tagged stool from the soft tissue density of a true polyp.[98]

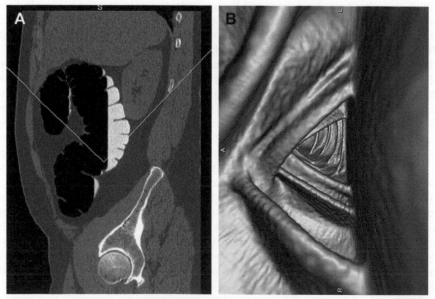

Fig. 9. (*A*) 2D supine sagittal MPR view of the ascending colon demonstrates layering high-density tagged liquid. The soft tissue density colonic wall remains visible. (*B*) 3D endoluminal view of the same segment of colon demonstrates that the layering high density liquid is opaque, obscuring the dependent part of the colonic wall.

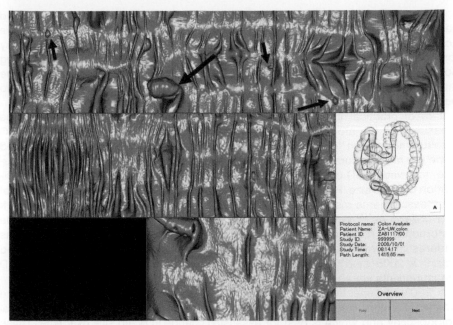

Fig. 10. "Virtual dissection" or "filet" view of the colon demonstrates a possible large polyp (*large arrow*) as well as 3 possible diminutive polyps (*smaller arrows*). The entire colon can be visualized at once, giving the reader an overview of potential pathology. Each of these potential lesions can be interrogated separately using 2D multiplanar reformats. (*Courtesy of* Ziosoft Inc; with permission.)

Despite the exciting technology and innovative displays, interpretation time remains a limiting issue in widespread use of CTC. As stated above, this is one of the motivations for computer-aided detection, (see article by Summers elsewhere in this issue for further exploration of this topic). In addition, some have advocated that trained radiologic technologists may play a role in initial interpretation of CTC studies, leading to more efficient double checking by a radiologist.[88]

REPORTING
Polyp Measurements, Volume Versus Diameter to Detect Incremental Changes

Background
The size of an adenomatous polyp correlates directly with its malignant potential.[99] For this reason, accurate polyp measurement is essential for proper patient management.[100] In addition, proper measurements are important for matching at colonoscopy, as well as for CTC research and polyp follow-up over time. MPR and 3D volumetric images allow the interpreter several ways of measuring a polyp, including 2D axial source images, 2D MPR images, or endoluminal 3D images, each of which has been demonstrated to give differing measurements, as does the window-level setting used to view the images.[101,102] Polyp measurement and matching are not always straightforward, and standardization across research studies is lacking.[102] Although polyp size-matching algorithms have been designed to allow for a systematic method of comparison of CTC with colonoscopy,[103] inexact polyp matching is still likely a factor in error and uncertainty in the appraisal of the performance of CTC.[102,104]

Both CTC and colonoscopy have intrinsic limitations in measurement accuracy and capability.[103,105–107] It is likely, however, that polyp measurements on CTC are more accurate and reliable than colonoscopy. Colonoscopists usually use open biopsy forceps, which have been shown to be inaccurate by, for example, underestimating polyp size.[103] In a 2007 direct comparison of CTC and optical colonoscopy in the measurement of 86 simulated polyps in pig colonic specimens, CTC was shown to be superior in both accuracy and interobserver agreement.[103]

It is of practical interest to understand by which method a polyp should be measured. In the aforementioned 2007 study by Park and colleagues,[103] 2D CTC measurements in an "optimized MPR view," the longest 2D measurement, were found to be the most accurate. 3D volumetric measurements were the second most accurate, followed by 2D orthogonal MPR. 3D measurements resulted in a slight overestimation of polyp size. However, the investigators concluded that the speed and ease of 3D measurements made up for the inaccuracy, and were preferred in practice. Park and colleagues[103] acknowledge the limitations of 3D measurement, which include distortion with nontraditional 3D techniques such as "virtual dissection," as well as underestimation of size when the polyp is partially obscured by fluid or collapsed colon. A 2005 study by Pickhardt and colleagues[108] also demonstrated that 3D measurements were superior to 2D in vitro and in vivo.

A 2006 retrospective study by Yeshwant and colleagues[109] aimed to determine which CT colonographic polyp measurement method most approximated optical colonoscopy and which is best for assessing change in polyp size over time. These investigators found that, compared with optical colonoscopy, manual measurement of the length from 3D endoluminal images has the least variability. The investigators postulate that this may be because this measurement most closely replicates a linear probe size measurement at optical colonoscopy. Linear size measurement, however, is difficult and inconsistent when evaluating change in size over time because, at least in theory, polyps grow at different rates along multiple axes. Volume measurements are better able to account for changes in polyp shape that are not accompanied by changes in size. Consequently, linear diameter calculated from automated volume measurements may be the best way to assess polyp size changes over time.[109] In a 2006 study of interobserver error for linear and volumetric measurements by Pickhardt and colleagues,[110] it was also concluded that volume is a more reliable indicator of size change. Moreover, because changes in linear size are accompanied by an even greater change in the corresponding volume, volume measurements need not be as precise as linear measurements to demonstrate the same change in polyp size.[109]

Systematic reporting

A system for structured reporting of CTC studies has been proposed by a panel of experts, with the aim of replicating the benefits of the BI-RADS system used in mammography. The C-Rads system[111] captures information about preparation quality, polyp presence and size, and extracolonic findings, and places the overall study into 1 of 5 categories including recommendations for follow-up. Such a system will be very useful for large-scale research both for epidemiologic and cost-effectiveness purposes.

SUMMARY

CTC has several inherent technical components—preparation, insufflation, CT data acquisition, interpretation, and reporting—all of which must be optimized to ensure high-quality patient care. This field is an excellent example of collaborative research between radiologists and gastroenterologists moving forward to advance technology and reduce the morbidity and mortality of a common disease. As the authors have discussed, these extensive efforts have established a very solid foundation on which to base a clinical program in CTC.

REFERENCES

1. Coin CG, Wollett FC, Coin JT, et al. Computerized radiology of the colon: a potential screening technique. Comput Radiol 1983;7:215.
2. Vining DJ, Shifrin RY, Grishaw EK, et al. Virtual colonoscopy. Radiology 1994; 193(P):446.
3. Hara AK, Johnson CD, Reed JE, et al. Detection of colorectal polyps by computed tomographic colography: feasibility of a novel technique. Gastroenterology 1996;110:284.
4. Dachman AH, Lieberman J, Osnis RB, et al. Small simulated polyps in pig colon: sensitivity of CT virtual colography. Radiology 1997;203:427.
5. Kim DH, Pickhardt PJ, Taylor AJ, et al. CT Colonography versus colonoscopy for the detection of advanced neoplasia. N Engl J Med 2007;357:1403.
6. Pickhardt PJ, Choi JR, Hwang I, et al. Computed tomographic virtual colonoscopy to screen for colorectal neoplasia in asymptomatic adults. N Engl J Med 2003;349:2191.
7. Johnson CD, Chen M-H, Toledano AY, et al. Accuracy of CT colonography for detection of large adenomas and cancers. N Engl J Med 2008;359:1207.
8. Fletcher JG, Booya F, Johnson CD, et al. CT colonography: unraveling the twists and turns. Curr Opin Gastroenterol 2005;21:90.
9. Yee J, Kumar NN, Hung RK, et al. Comparison of supine and prone scanning separately and in combination at CT colonography. Radiology 2003;226:653.
10. Fletcher JG, Johnson CD, Welch TJ, et al. Optimization of CT colonography technique: prospective trial in 180 patients. Radiology 2000;216:704.
11. Yee J. Virtual colonoscopy workshop lecture. In: San Francisco (CA); 2009.
12. Delegge M, Kaplan R. Efficacy of bowel preparation with the use of a prepackaged, low fibre diet with a low sodium, magnesium citrate cathartic vs. a clear liquid diet with a standard sodium phosphate cathartic. Aliment Pharmacol Ther 2005;21:1491.
13. Nelson DB, Barkun AN, Block KP, et al. Technology status evaluation report. Colonoscopy preparations. May 2001. Gastrointest Endosc 2001;54:829.
14. Macari M, Lavelle M, Pedrosa I, et al. Effect of different bowel preparations on residual fluid at CT colonography. Radiology 2001;218:274.
15. FDA. Oral sodium phosphate (OSP) products for bowel cleansing (marketed as Visicol and OsmoPrep, and oral sodium phosphate products available without a prescription); 2008. Available at: http://www.fda.gov/Safety/MedWatch/SafetyInformation/SafetyAlertsforHumanMedicalProducts/ucm094900.htm. Accessed February 11, 2010.
16. Yee J. CT colonography: techniques and applications. Radiol Clin North Am 2009;47:133.
17. Kim DH, Pickhardt PJ, Hinshaw JL, et al. Prospective blinded trial comparing 45-mL and 90-mL doses of oral sodium phosphate for bowel preparation before computed tomographic colonography. J Comput Assist Tomogr 2007;31:53.
18. Belsey J, Epstein O, Heresbach D. Systematic review: adverse event reports for oral sodium phosphate and polyethylene glycol. Aliment Pharmacol Ther 2008. [Epub ahead of print].

19. Ehrenpreis ED, Nogueras JJ, Botoman VA, et al. Serum electrolyte abnormalities secondary to Fleet's Phospho-Soda colonoscopy prep. A review of three cases. Surg Endosc 1996;10:1022.

20. Vukasin P, Weston LA, Beart RW. Oral Fleet Phospho-Soda laxative-induced hyperphosphatemia and hypocalcemic tetany in an adult: report of a case. Dis Colon Rectum 1997;40:497.

21. Markowitz GS, Stokes MB, Radhakrishnan J, et al. Acute phosphate nephropathy following oral sodium phosphate bowel purgative: an underrecognized cause of chronic renal failure. J Am Soc Nephrol 2005;16:3389.

22. Khurana A, McLean L, Atkinson S, et al. The effect of oral sodium phosphate drug products on renal function in adults undergoing bowel endoscopy. Arch Intern Med 2008;168:593.

23. Hsu C-W, Imperiale TF. Meta-analysis and cost comparison of polyethylene glycol lavage versus sodium phosphate for colonoscopy preparation. Gastrointest Endosc 1998;48:276.

24. Tan JJ, Tjandra JJ. Which is the optimal bowel preparation for colonoscopy— a meta-analysis. Colorectal Dis 2006;8:247.

25. Belsey J, Epstein O, Heresbach D. Systematic review: oral bowel preparation for colonoscopy. Aliment Pharmacol Ther 2007;25:373.

26. Mathus-Vliegen EM, Kemble UM. A prospective randomized blinded comparison of sodium phosphate and polyethylene glycol-electrolyte solution for safe bowel cleansing. Aliment Pharmacol Ther 2006;23:543.

27. Pickhardt PJ. Screening CT colonography: how I do it. AJR Am J Roentgenol 2007;189:290.

28. Ell C, Fischbach W, Keller R, et al. A randomized, blinded, prospective trial to compare the safety and efficacy of three bowel-cleansing solutions for colonoscopy (HSG-01*). Endoscopy 2003;35:300.

29. Aihara H, Saito S, Arakawa H, et al. Comparison of two sodium phosphate tablet-based regimens and a polyethylene glycol regimen for colon cleansing prior to colonoscopy: a randomized prospective pilot study. Int J Colorectal Dis 2009; 24:1023–30.

30. Kim SH, Choi BI, Han JK, et al. CT colonography in a Korean population with a high residue diet: comparison between wet and dry preparations. Clin Radiol 2006;61:483.

31. Gluecker TM, Johnson CD, Harmsen WS, et al. Colorectal cancer screening with CT colonography, colonoscopy, and double-contrast barium enema examination: prospective assessment of patient perceptions and preferences. Radiology 2003;227:378.

32. Nagata K, Okawa T, Honma A, et al. Full-laxative versus minimum-laxative fecal-tagging CT colonography using 64-detector row CT: prospective blinded comparison of diagnostic performance, tagging quality, and patient acceptance. Acad Radiol 2009;16:780.

33. Taylor S, Laghi A, Lefere P, et al. European society of gastrointestinal and abdominal radiology (ESGAR): Consensus statement on CT colonography. Eur Radiol 2007;17:575.

34. Nagata K, Singh AK, Sangwaiya MJ, et al. Comparative evaluation of the fecal-tagging quality in CT colonography: barium vs. iodinated oral contrast agent. Acad Radiol 2009;16:1393–9.

35. Bielen D, Thomeer M, Vanbeckevoort D, et al. Dry preparation for virtual CT colonography with fecal tagging using water-soluble contrast medium: initial results. Eur Radiol 2003;13:453.

36. Lefere P, Gryspeerdt S, Baekelandt M, et al. Laxative-free CT colonography. AJR Am J Roentgenol 2004;183:945.
37. Iannaccone R, Laghi A, Catalano C, et al. Computed tomographic colonography without cathartic preparation for the detection of colorectal polyps. Gastroenterology 2004;127:1300.
38. Nagata K, Endo S, Ichikawa T, et al. Polyethylene glycol solution (PEG) plus contrast medium vs PEG alone preparation for CT colonography and conventional colonoscopy in preoperative colorectal cancer staging. Int J Colorectal Dis 2007;22:69–76.
39. Jensch S, de Vries AH, Peringa J, et al. CT colonography with limited bowel preparation: performance characteristics in an increased-risk population. Radiology 2008;247:122.
40. Taylor SA, Slater A, Burling DN, et al. CT colonography: optimisation, diagnostic performance and patient acceptability of reduced-laxative regimens using barium-based faecal tagging. Eur Radiol 2008;18:32.
41. Lefere PA, Gryspeerdt SS, Dewyspelaere J, et al. Dietary fecal tagging as a cleansing method before CT colonography: initial results polyp detection and patient acceptance. Radiology 2002;224:393.
42. Gryspeerdt S, Lefere P, Herman M, et al. CT colonography with fecal tagging after incomplete colonoscopy. Eur Radiol 2005;15:1192.
43. O'Connor SD, Summers RM. Revisiting oral barium sulfate contrast agents. Acad Radiol 2007;14:72.
44. Zalis ME, Hahn PF. Digital subtraction bowel cleansing in CT colonography. AJR Am J Roentgenol 2001;176:646.
45. Horton KM, Fishman EK, Gayler B. The use of iohexol as oral contrast for computed tomography of the abdomen and pelvis. J Comput Assist Tomogr 2008;32:207.
46. Zalis ME, Perumpillichira JJ, Magee C, et al. Tagging-based, electronically cleansed CT colonography: evaluation of patient comfort and image readability. Radiology 2006;239:149.
47. Davis GR, Santa Ana CA, Morawski SG, et al. Inhibition of water and electrolyte absorption by polyethylene glycol (PEG). Gastroenterology 1980;79:35.
48. Seymour CW, Pryor JP, Gupta R, et al. Anaphylactoid reaction to oral contrast for computed tomography. J Trauma 2004;57:1105.
49. Stordahl A, Laerum F, Gjølberg T, et al. Water-soluble contrast media in radiography of small bowel obstruction—comparison of ionic and non-ionic contrast media. Acta Radiol 1988;29:53.
50. Ristvedt SL, McFarland EG, Weinstock LB, et al. Patient preferences for CT colonography, conventional colonoscopy, and bowel preparation. Am J Gastroenterol 2003;98:578.
51. Johnson CD, Manduca A, Fletcher JG, et al. Noncathartic CT colonography with stool tagging: performance with and without electronic stool subtraction. AJR Am J Roentgenol 2008;190:361.
52. Beebe TJ, Johnson CD, Stoner SM, et al. Assessing attitudes toward laxative preparation in colorectal cancer screening and effects on future testing: potential receptivity to computed tomographic colonography. Mayo Clin Proc 2007;82:666.
53. Callstrom MR, Johnson CD, Fletcher JG, et al. CT colonography without cathartic preparation: feasibility study. Radiology 2001;219:693.
54. Lefere P, Gryspeerdt S, Marrannes J, et al. CT colonography after fecal tagging with a reduced cathartic cleansing and a reduced volume of barium. AJR Am J Roentgenol 2005;184:1836.

55. Jensch S, de Vries AH, Pot D, et al. Image quality and patient acceptance of four regimens with different amounts of mild laxatives for CT colonography. Am J Roentgenol 2008;191:158.
56. Pochaczevsky R. Digital subtraction bowel cleansing in CT colonography. AJR Am J Roentgenol 2002;178:241.
57. Serlie IW, de Vries AH, van Vliet LJ, et al. Lesion conspicuity and efficiency of CT colonography with electronic cleansing based on a three-material transition model. AJR Am J Roentgenol 2008;191:1493.
58. Pickhardt PJ, Choi JR, Nugent PA, et al. The effect of diagnostic confidence on the probability of optical colonoscopic confirmation of potential polyps detected on CT colonography: prospective assessment in 1,339 asymptomatic adults. AJR Am J Roentgenol 2004;183:1661.
59. Burling D, Taylor SA, Halligan S, et al. Automated insufflation of carbon dioxide for MDCT colonography: distension and patient experience compared with manual insufflation. AJR Am J Roentgenol 2006;186:96.
60. Vining DJ. Virtual colonoscopy. Semin Ultrasound CT MR 1999;20:56.
61. Shinners TJ, Pickhardt PJ, Taylor AJ, et al. Patient-controlled room air insufflation versus automated carbon dioxide delivery for CT colonography. AJR Am J Roentgenol 2006;186:1491.
62. Pickhardt PJ. Incidence of colonic perforation at CT colonography: review of existing data and implications for screening of asymptomatic adults. Radiology 2006;239:313.
63. Chen SC, Lu DS, Hecht JR, et al. CT colonography: value of scanning in both the supine and prone positions. AJR Am J Roentgenol 1999;172:595.
64. Skucas J. The use of antispasmodic drugs during barium enemas. AJR Am J Roentgenol 1994;162:1323.
65. Lappas JC, Maglinte DD, Chernish SM, et al. Discomfort during double-contrast barium enema examination: a placebo-controlled double-blind evaluation of the effect of glucagon and diazepam. Radiology 1995;197:95.
66. Morrin MM, Farrell RJ, Keogan MT, et al. CT colonography: colonic distention improved by dual positioning but not intravenous glucagon. Eur Radiol 2002;12:525.
67. Yee J, Hung RK, Akerkar GA, et al. The usefulness of glucagon hydrochloride for colonic distention in CT colonography [comments]. AJR Am J Roentgenol 1999; 173:169.
68. Chernish SM, Maglinte DD. Glucagon: common untoward reactions—review and recommendations. Radiology 1990;177:145.
69. Bruzzi JF, Moss AC, Brennan DD, et al. Efficacy of IV Buscopan as a muscle relaxant in CT colonography. Eur Radiol 2003;13(10):2264–70.
70. Hara AK, Johnson CD, Reed JE. CT colography (CTC) for clinical use: a new method to reduce evaluation time. Radiology 1997;205(P):718.
71. Fenlon HM, Nunes DP, Schroy PC 3rd, et al. A comparison of virtual and conventional colonoscopy for the detection of colorectal polyps [comments]. N Engl J Med 1999;341:1496.
72. Lui YW, Macari M, Israel G, et al. CT colonography data interpretation: effect of different section thicknesses—preliminary observations. Radiology 2003;229: 791.
73. Macari M, Bini EJ, Xue X, et al. Colorectal neoplasms: prospective comparison of thin-section low-dose multi-detector row CT colonography and conventional colonoscopy for detection. Radiology 2002;224:383.
74. Hara AK, Johnson CD, MacCarty RL, et al. CT colonography: single- versus multi-detector row imaging. Radiology 2001;219:461.

75. Johnson CD, Fletcher JG, MacCarty RL, et al. Effect of slice thickness and primary 2D versus 3D virtual dissection on colorectal lesion detection at CT colonography in 452 asymptomatic adults. Am J Roentgenol 2007;189:672.
76. Graser A, Wintersperger BJ, Suess C, et al. Dose reduction and image quality in MDCT colonography using tube current modulation. AJR Am J Roentgenol 2006;187:695.
77. McCollough CH. Optimization of multidetector array CT acquisition parameters for CT colonography. Abdom Imaging 2002;27:253.
78. van Gelder RE, Venema HW, Florie J, et al. CT colonography: feasibility of substantial dose reduction—comparison of medium to very low doses in identical patients. Radiology 2004;232:611.
79. Hall EJ, Brenner DJ. Cancer risks from diagnostic radiology. Br J Radiol 2008; 81:362.
80. van Gelder RE, Venema HW, Serlie IW, et al. CT colonography at different radiation dose levels: feasibility of dose reduction. Radiology 2002;224:25.
81. Luz O, Buchgeister M, Klabunde M, et al. Evaluation of dose exposure in 64-slice CT colonography. Eur Radiol 2007;17:2616.
82. Hara AK, Johnson CD, Reed JE, et al. Reducing data size and radiation dose for CT colonography. AJR Am J Roentgenol 1997;168:1181.
83. Brenner DJ, Georgsson MA. Mass screening with CT colonography: should the radiation exposure be of concern? Gastroenterology 2005;129:328.
84. Liedenbaum MH, Venema HW, Stoker J. Radiation dose in CT colonography—trends in time and differences between daily practice and screening protocols. Eur Radiol 2008;18:2222.
85. Iannaccone R, Laghi A, Catalano C, et al. Feasibility of ultra-low-dose multislice CT colonography for the detection of colorectal lesions: preliminary experience. Eur Radiol 2003;13:1297.
86. Beaulieu CF, Jeffrey RB Jr, Karadi C, et al. Display modes for CT colonography. Part II. Blinded comparison of axial CT and virtual endoscopic and panoramic endoscopic volume-rendered studies. Radiology 1999;212:203.
87. Cotton PB, Durkalski VL, Pineau BC, et al. Computed tomographic colonography (virtual colonoscopy): a multicenter comparison with standard colonoscopy for detection of colorectal neoplasia. JAMA 2004;291:1713.
88. Burling D, Halligan S, Altman DG, et al. CT colonography interpretation times: effect of reader experience, fatigue, and scan findings in a multi-centre setting. Eur Radiol 2006;16(8):1745–9.
89. Macari M, Milano A, Lavelle M, et al. Comparison of time-efficient CT colonography with two- and three-dimensional colonic evaluation for detecting colorectal polyps. AJR Am J Roentgenol 2000;174:1543.
90. Royster AP, Fenlon HM, Clarke PD, et al. CT colonoscopy of colorectal neoplasms: two-dimensional and three-dimensional virtual-reality techniques with colonoscopic correlation. AJR Am J Roentgenol 1997;169:1237.
91. Dachman AH, Kuniyoshi JK, Boyle CM, et al. CT colonography with three-dimensional problem solving for detection of colonic polyps. AJR Am J Roentgenol 1998;171:989.
92. Paik DS, Beaulieu CF, Jeffrey RB Jr, et al. Visualization modes for CT colonography using cylindrical and planar map projections. J Comput Assist Tomogr 2000;24:179.
93. Johnson KT, Johnson CD, Fletcher JG, et al. CT colonography using 360-degree virtual dissection: a feasibility study. AJR Am J Roentgenol 2006; 186:90.

94. Rottgen R, Fischbach F, Plotkin M, et al. CT colonography using different reconstruction modi. Clin Imaging 2005;29:195.
95. Kim SH, Lee JM, Eun HW, et al. Two- versus three-dimensional colon evaluation with recently developed virtual dissection software for CT colonography. Radiology 2007;244:852.
96. Hoppe H, Quattropani C, Spreng A, et al. Virtual colon dissection with CT colonography compared with axial interpretation and conventional colonoscopy: preliminary results. AJR Am J Roentgenol 2004;182:1151.
97. Fisichella VA, Jaderling F, Horvath S, et al. Primary three-dimensional analysis with perspective-filet view versus primary two-dimensional analysis: evaluation of lesion detection by inexperienced readers at computed tomographic colonography in symptomatic patients. Acta Radiol 2009;50:244.
98. Pickhardt PJ. Translucency rendering in 3D endoluminal CT colonography: a useful tool for increasing polyp specificity and decreasing interpretation time. AJR Am J Roentgenol 2004;183:429.
99. Ferrucci JT. Colon cancer screening with virtual colonoscopy: promise, polyps, politics. AJR Am J Roentgenol 2001;177:975.
100. Dachman AH, Zalis ME. Quality and consistency in CT colonography and research reporting. Radiology 2004;230:319.
101. Burling D, Halligan S, Taylor S, et al. Polyp measurement using CT colonography: agreement with colonoscopy and effect of viewing conditions on interobserver and intraobserver agreement. AJR Am J Roentgenol 2006;186:1597.
102. Halligan S, Altman DG, Taylor SA, et al. CT colonography in the detection of colorectal polyps and cancer: systematic review, meta-analysis, and proposed minimum data set for study level reporting. Radiology 2005;237:893.
103. Park SH, Choi EK, Lee SS, et al. Polyp measurement reliability, accuracy, and discrepancy: optical colonoscopy versus CT colonography with pig colonic specimens. Radiology 2007;244:157.
104. Halligan S, Park SH, Ha HK. Causes of false-negative findings at CT colonography. Radiology 2006;238:1075.
105. Morales TG, Sampliner RE, Garewal HS, et al. The difference in colon polyp size before and after removal. Gastrointest Endosc 1996;43:25.
106. Debatin JF, Schoenenberger AW, Luboldt W, et al. In vivo exoscopic and endoscopic MR imaging of the colon. AJR Am J Roentgenol 1997;169:1085.
107. Fennerty MB, Davidson J, Emerson SS, et al. Are endoscopic measurements of colonic polyps reliable? Am J Gastroenterol 1993;88:496.
108. Pickhardt PJ, Lee AD, McFarland EG, et al. Linear polyp measurement at CT colonography: in vitro and in vivo comparison of two-dimensional and three-dimensional displays. Radiology 2005;236:872.
109. Yeshwant SC, Summers RM, Yao J, et al. Polyps: linear and volumetric measurement at CT colonography. Radiology 2006;241:802.
110. Pickhardt PJ, Lehman VT, Winter TC, et al. Polyp volume versus linear size measurements at CT colonography: implications for noninvasive surveillance of unresected colorectal lesions. AJR Am J Roentgenol 2006;186:1605.
111. Zalis ME, Barish MA, Choi JR, et al. CT colonography reporting and data system: a consensus proposal. Radiology 2005;236:3.

Performance of CT Colonography in Clinical Trials

Jonathan A. Rosenberg, MD, David T. Rubin, MD*

KEYWORDS

- CT colonography • Colorectal cancer screening
- Clinical trials • High-risk colon cancer surveillance
- Incomplete colonoscopy

The performance of computed tomography colonography (CTC) in clinical trials has improved in the past decade and is now providing the basis for the recommendations for its use by various professional and payer organizations. However, these groups have come to different conclusions following review of the available data. For instance, the American Cancer Society, US Multisociety Task Force on Colorectal Cancer, and American College of Radiology in 2008 recommended CTC as an appropriate screening modality for average-risk individuals.[1] In contrast, the Centers for Medicare and Medicaid (CMS) stated in a recent decision memo that the available evidence was insufficient to recommend CTC as screening modality for average-risk individuals, and instead concluded that it remain noncovered.[2] The US Preventative Task Force recently determined that the evidence for screening with CTC was inadequate (grade I) to assess the benefits and harms of the test.[3] These disparate recommendations, generally derived from the same available data, have resulted in mixed messages to patients, health care providers, and third-party payer organizations.

This article summarizes the performance of CTC in major trials for a variety of clinical indications. It focuses on major clinical trials of CTC for average-risk colon cancer screening, including issues of precision, sensitivity, and specificity. The CTC clinical trials for patients at increased risk for colorectal cancer are also discussed. Other topics include the data for CTC use after incomplete colonoscopy, reduced preparation or unprepped CTC, and academic versus nonacademic environments for interpretation of CTC studies.

Section of Gastroenterology, Hepatology and Nutrition, Department of Medicine, University of Chicago Medical Center, 5841 South Maryland Avenue, MC 4076, Chicago, IL 60637-1463, USA
* Corresponding author.
E-mail address: drubin@medicine.bsd.uchicago.edu

Gastrointest Endoscopy Clin N Am 20 (2010) 193–207
doi:10.1016/j.giec.2010.02.009
1052-5157/10/$ – see front matter © 2010 Elsevier Inc. All rights reserved.

GENERAL CONSIDERATIONS REGARDING PERFORMANCE IN CLINICAL TRIALS

There are several general considerations regarding assessment of performance of an evolving technology like CTC across different clinical trials. These must be taken into consideration to fully appreciate potential differences in results. First, the approach to performance of CTC has evolved with improved technology and understanding of how to use it appropriately. Second, there is variation in the years of experience of the investigators or observers in the trials, as well as in the way trials are designed to minimize interobserver variability. Third, the patient population included in the trial must be considered when reviewing the trial results. Some studies have focused on average-risk individuals, whereas others enhanced the trial population by selecting those with previous polyps and therefore a greater likelihood of having positive findings (but biasing the radiologists). It is therefore not surprising that the interpretation of available clinical trial results varies by specialty, society, or third-party payer.

PERFORMANCE OF CTC IN PATIENTS AT AVERAGE RISK FOR COLON CANCER

The first major study published in 2003 by Pickhardt and colleagues[4] on this topic involved same-day CTC and optical colonoscopy, and used proprietary three-dimensional (3D) CTC reading techniques and endoluminal fly-though views. Three different medical centers contributed 1233 asymptomatic average-risk adult patients to the study. The mean age in the study was 57.8 years, and men represented 59% of the study population. Exclusion criteria for the study included a positive fecal occult blood test, anemia, rectal bleeding, history of polyps or cancer, or an optical colonoscopy within the previous 10 years. In a process termed segmental unblinding, colonoscopists were first blinded to the CTC results when encountering a new segment of bowel, but then the CTC findings were revealed after assessing each subsequent colonic segment. For large polyps (10 mm or >) the investigators reported a per-patient sensitivity of 93.8% and specificity of 96%. These percentages decreased when smaller polyps were considered. For 6-mm polyps the per-patient sensitivity was 88.7% and per-patient specificity was 79.6%. The 2 patients with malignant polyps in this average-risk cohort were detected by CTC. An 11-mm malignant polyp was missed on optical colonoscopy before the results of the colonic segment were unblinded.

Macari and colleagues[5] published a case series in 2004 of 68 asymptomatic average-risk men who underwent CTC followed by same-day optical colonoscopy. In this study, polyps were grouped in size categories of 1 to 5 mm, 6 to 9 mm, and greater than 10 mm. A total of 98 polyps were described at the time of colonoscopy. CTC detected 21 of the 98 polyps. CTC did identify all 3 of the polyps that measured 10 mm or greater by conventional colonoscopy. The detection sensitivity decreased as polyp size diminished from 9/17 (52.9%) for 6- to 9-mm polyps and 9/78 (11.5%) for diminutive polyps (1–5 mm). The investigators concluded that CTC was a sensitive and specific test for polyps greater than 10 mm. This study may have been limited by using a CT with only 4-detector rows, two-dimensional (2D) rather than 3D views, and because the performance and interpretation of CTC and optical colonoscopy was carried out by a limited number of individuals.

A major study by Kim and colleagues[6] in 2007 compared parallel screening cohorts to compare CTC and optical colonoscopy in a general screening population. They compared 3163 individuals in a traditional screening colonoscopy protocol with 3120 participants in a separate CTC program. Patients in this study were excluded for a history of polyps, a history of a bowel disorder, and hereditary nonpolyposis colorectal cancer syndrome. The primary outcomes of the study were the detection of advanced neoplasia (defined as advanced adenomas and carcinomas) and total number of polyps removed. In this study more advanced CT scanners were used (8- and 16-detector rows). There were slightly more men than women in both cohorts and there was no significant difference in age between the 2 groups. Ninety-eight percent of patients in both groups were asymptomatic individuals, and 92% of subjects had no family history of colorectal cancer. The investigators found that there were identical rates of advanced neoplasm (4%) and advanced adenoma (3%) detection in the CTC and optical colonoscopy groups. The investigators reported that 7.9% of patients were offered referral to optical colonoscopy because they had polyps greater than 6 mm. As expected, many more polyps were removed in the optical colonoscopy group (2434) than in the CTC patients subsequently referred for therapeutic polypectomy (561).

Cornett and colleagues[7] in 2008 reported a cohort of 159 asymptomatic adults with polyps greater than 5 mm seen on CTC who underwent a planned therapeutic optical colonoscopy. In this study the endoscopists were aware of the findings of the prior CTC. Eight- and 16-detector row CT machines were used and, again, there were slightly more men than women in the study population (51%). The average age of participants was 59.3 years. Two hundred and thirty polyps were reported on CTC and a total of 359 polyps were identified at subsequent optical colonoscopy. CTC missed 6.2% of polyps greater than 9 mm and 18.2% of polyps 6 to 9 mm. Seventy-two percent of the polyps detected on therapeutic colonoscopy, but not on CTC, were less than 6 mm. The investigators reported a false-positive rate of 5% for CTC (normal colonoscopy despite CTC finding).

In 2008, Johnson and colleagues,[8] in conjunction with the American College of Radiology Imaging Network (ACRIN), reported their findings of a multicenter trial of CTC versus optical colonoscopy in 2600 average-risk adults, with a primary end point of the detection of large (>10 mm) colorectal adenomas and cancers. Patients enrolled in this trial were all aged 50 years or older, reported no major bowel symptoms or diseases, and were otherwise considered normal candidates for screening colono-scopy. All studies were performed on 16-detector row machines. The average age of the participants was 58 years and, unlike other major CTC clinical trials, most of the study subjects were women (52%). In the per-patient analysis, the investigators reported a sensitivity of 90% for polyps greater than 10 mm and a specificity of 86%. The sensitivity and specificity of CTC for smaller lesions was less, as noted in all previous studies. The positive predictive value of CTC, or the proportion of patients with positive test results who were correctly diagnosed by traditional colonoscopy, for polyps greater than 10 mm was 23%. The negative predictive value for lesions of this size was 99%.

In one of the more recent trials performed in Germany, Graser and colleagues[9] reported the findings in 311 asymptomatic average-risk adults who underwent 5 sepa-rate but parallel screening modalities for colorectal cancer. These included CTC, colo-noscopy, sigmoidoscopy, and fecal occult blood/immunochemical testing. All patients had their colonoscopy performed after CTC in a segmental, unblinded fashion. The CT scanners used in the study had 64-detector row capability, which was higher than any of the previous major trials. The enrolled patients were more than 50 years of age and did not report any gastrointestinal (GI) warning signs (blood in stool, change in bowel habits, abdominal pain), and were excluded from the study if they had a history of inflammatory bowel disease or family history of colon cancer. Of the 307 who completed CTC and optical colonoscopy, a total of 221 adenomas were reported. Approximately two-thirds of the overall adenomas detected were 5 mm or greater. Similar to previous clinical trials, the per-polyp and per-patient sensitivity and specificity increased in concert with the increasing size of the lesions. For adenomas greater than 9 mm the per-polyp sensitivity was 93.9% and per-patient sensitivity was 92%. Of the 46 advanced lesions detected, almost 30% were less than or equal to 9 mm.

These clinical trials are summarized in **Table 1**. There are many important similarities between these trials. The studies relied on traditional colonoscopy as their reference standard. All studies used bowel preparation and stool tagging to aid in the diagnosis of polyps on CTC. All but the 2 earliest studies used higher-resolution CT scanners. All studied provided a real-world group of patients who could be considered as average-risk colon cancer screening candidates. Most of the studies used several highly trained gastroenterologists and radiologists to carry out the performance and interpretation of CTC and optical colonoscopies. CTC was considered to be a simple test to carry out on widely available machines without the use of sedation.

Several investigators have attempted to draw conclusions from well-designed systematic reviews of CTC and average-risk colon cancer screening. Winawer[10] published a systematic review of colorectal cancer screening in 2007. In his analysis of CTC studies he found a high detection rate for large polyps (>10 mm), with an average sensitivity of 93% and specificity of 97%. When polyps greater than 6 mm were included in the analysis, the sensitivity decreased to 86% and the specificity to 86%. When all polyps were considered in the studies under review, the sensitivity decreased to as low as 45%, and specificity to 26%. Whitlock and colleagues[11] published a systematic review of colorectal cancer screening in 2008. A total of 4312 average-risk patients across 4 studies were described. In general, these investigators found a lack statistical heterogeneity in the pooled analysis for large polyps, suggesting that the high sensitivities (>90%) are accurate. However, the investigators stated that they did not pool estimates for smaller polyps because of the statistical heterogeneity of the studies.

CTC by various techniques is effective at the identification of large (>10 mm) lesions, and the sensitivity to smaller lesions decreases with the size of the polyps. The clinical significance of missing smaller lesions, and the effect on patient adherence with colorectal screening or overall mortality benefits, remain unknown. In addition, issues of radiation risk, extracolonic findings, and size and type of findings all contribute to the overall health outcomes of CTC, and must be factored into the overall interpretation of the benefit seen in these trials.

PERFORMANCE OF CTC FOR INDIVIDUALS AT INCREASED RISK FOR COLORECTAL CANCER

One of the first multicenter trials to examine a cohort of subjects with increased risk for colorectal cancer was reported by Cotton and colleagues[12] in 2004. This study involved 615 patients at 9 sites who were referred for a clinically indicated elective colonoscopy. This study did not enroll a screening population, so all were considered at increased risk for neoplastic lesions. Two- and 4-section CT scanners were used in this study, representing an earlier generation of machines. The average age of participants was 61 years, and men comprised 45% of the study population. A total of 824 lesions were found in 308 participants. For lesions of at least 10 mm, the sensitivity and specificity of CTC were 55% and 96% respectively. For similarly sized lesions, optical colonoscopy showed a sensitivity and specificity of 100%. For medium-sized lesions greater than 6 mm, CTC and conventional colonoscopy had sensitivities of 39% and 99%, whereas the respective specificities were 90.5% and 100%. Of the 8 cancers found by optical colonoscopy, CTC only identified 6.

Also in 2004, Van Gelder and colleagues[13] reported a cohort of 249 subjects at increased risk for colorectal cancer who underwent CTC before colonoscopy. The

Table 1
CTC performance in average-risk individuals

Author	Year	Number of Subjects	% Men	Type of Practice	CTC Technique	Sensitivity (>10 mm) (%)	Sensitivity (>6-9 mm) (%)	Sensitivity (<5 mm) (%)	PPV (%)	NPV (%)
Pickhardt et al[4]	2003	1233	59	Multicenter, academic	4,8-row MDCT	94	89	NR	30	NR
Macari et al[5]	2004	68	100	Single center, academic	4-row MDCT	100	53	12	NR	NR
Kim et al[6]	2007	6283	44	Single center, academic	8,16-row MDCT	NR	NR	NR	NR	NR
Cornett et al[7]	2008	159	51	Single center, academic	8,16-row MDCT	NR	NR	NR	NR	NR
Johnson et al[8]	2008	2600	48	Multicenter, mixed	>16-row MDCT	90	78	NR	45	95
Graser et al[9]	2009	311	55	Single center, academic	64-row MDCT	92 (>9 mm)	921 (>5 mm)	NR	48	83.6

Per-patient sensitivity is noted for various sized lesions; overall PPV and NPV are noted.
Abbreviations: MDCT, multidetector computed tomography; NPV, negative predictive value; NR, not reported; PPV, positive predictive value.

investigators defined increased risk as having a personal or family history of colorectal polyps or cancer. The participants underwent same-day CTC and colonoscopy. Two experienced radiologists used 3D views with 2D problem solving for interpretation of images. The radiologist and endoscopist were blinded to each other's findings, and a third party reviewed both examinations using colonoscopy as the comparative reference standard. Forty-one percent of the participants were women, and the average age was 56 years. Eight percent of patients had GI symptoms (abdominal pain, hematochezia, or alteration in bowel habits.) The per-patient sensitivity for lesions 10 mm or greater (n = 31) was 84%, for lesions 6 to 9 mm (n = 45) 78%, and for lesions of any size (n = 141) 62%. The reported per-patient specificity was 92% for lesions 10 mm or greater, 70% for lesions 6 to 9 mm, and 31% for lesions of any size. The positive predictive value of CTC was approximately 60%, whereas the negative predictive value was 98%.

Another multicenter trial that examined a cohort of patients with an increased risk for colorectal cancer was published by Rockey and colleagues[14] in 2005. Six hundred and fourteen patients with positive fecal occult blood testing, hematochezia, iron-deficiency anemia, or family history of colorectal cancer were enrolled in this trial. Every subject underwent an air-contrast barium enema followed 2 weeks later by a CTC and then same-day optical colonoscopy. The endoscopists were subject to segmental unblinding of the CTC results. Four- and 8-detector row CT scanners were used and radiologists used 2D images with 3D problem-solving capability. For the largest category of lesions (>10 mm, n = 63) the per-patient sensitivity for air-contrast barium enema was 48%, for CTC 59% ($P = 0.11$ for CTC vs air-contrast barium enema), and 98% for optical colonoscopy ($P<.0001$ for colonoscopy vs CTC). For medium-sized lesions (6–9 mm, n = 116), air-contrast barium enema showed a sensitivity of 35%, CTC had 51% sensitivity ($P<.05$ for CTC vs air-contrast barium enema), and 99% sensitivity for colonoscopy ($P<.0001$ for colonoscopy vs CTC). The specificity for larger lesions (>10 mm) was 99.6% for optical colonoscopy, 96% for CTC, and 90% for air-contrast barium enema. This trial was halted early at the planned interim analysis because of the statistical superiority of optical colonoscopy.

Another study of patients at high risk for colon cancer was reported in 2005 by Chung and colleagues.[15] Fifty-one patients who were deemed to be at high risk for colon cancer by the presence of altered bowel habits, anemia of unknown cause, abdominal pain, positive fecal occult blood testing, and hematochezia were prospectively enrolled. Sixty-three percent of the participants were men, and the mean age was 63 years. Of 21 colorectal cancers that were ultimately confirmed at the time of surgical intervention, the sensitivity and specificity for CTC and optical colonoscopy were 100%. Forty-one true polyps were found at surgery or during colonoscopy, and the investigators reported a statistical superiority of CTC over optical colonoscopy in terms of overall sensitivity ($P = .001$). However, of the 9 lesions that were missed at initial colonoscopy, 7/9 were due to obstructing lesions preventing discovery, and 2 were false negatives, but traditional colonoscopy maintained a positive predictive value of 100%. CTC detected 37 of 41 polyps for a higher sensitivity of 90%; however, the positive predictive value was 74%. The sensitivity and positive predictive values were reported for diminutive polyps (≤5 mm, n = 19, 84% and 67% respectively), small polyps (6–9 mm, n = 16, 94% and 75% respectively) and large polyps (>10 mm, n = 6, 100% and 100%).

An article from Finland in 2007 specifically discussed a cohort of patients with hereditary nonpolyposis colorectal cancer syndrome with a confirmed DNA mismatch repair gene mutation.[16] The average age of subjects was 41 years and none had previous evidence of colon cancer (1 had a history of rectal cancer treated with abdominoperineal resection and permanent colostomy.) Subjects underwent CTC just before colonoscopy. Fecal tagging was not performed, multiplanar 2D reformation in 3 directions of images was used, and a 4-row multidetector scanner was used. The radiologist and endoscopist were blinded to each other's findings. Of the 78 subjects enrolled in the study, 37 lesions were found in 28 subjects. The per-patient sensitivity and specificity of all lesions averaged 27% and 79%. When only lesions of 10 mm or more were considered, the average sensitivity and specificity were 80% and 96% respectively. No cancers (n = 2) were missed by CTC. The investigators concluded that CTC should remain a second-line diagnostic test for surveillance in patients with hereditary nonpolyposis colorectal cancer syndrome. The findings and conclusions of these investigators may have been limited by early-generation technology and single-center reporting.

A recent study by White and colleagues[17] examined a prospective cohort of 150 individuals at high risk for the development of colorectal cancer. Individuals were considered at high risk (per British Department of Health guidelines) if they met the following criteria: age more than 40 years; bright red/dark blood per rectum bleed, or unexplained anemia and altered bowel habit/family history of colorectal cancer.[18] Forty-nine percent of the participants were men and the average age was 61 years. CTC was performed first, followed by same-day optical colonoscopy. Radiologists used 2D views with 3D problem solving. The endoscopists were blinded to the CTC findings and the radiologists were unaware of the colonoscopy finding at the time of their review of findings. For the 18 cancers found, CTC showed a sensitivity of 100% and specificity of 99.2%. A total of 42 polyps were identified in 33 patients. For large polyps (>10 mm, n = 11), CTC had a sensitivity of 91% and specificity of 99.2%. A potential advantage of CTC recognized by the investigators was that CTC detected 4 polyps proximal to stenosing carcinomas that could not be traversed by the colonoscope. The κ score for interobserver agreement of findings was 0.78.

A trial conducted in the Netherlands by Liedenbaum and colleagues[19] published in 2009 reported on a cohort of fecal occult blood test–positive patients who were scheduled for a colonoscopy and also underwent a CTC. Three hundred and two patients with a positive guaiac fecal occult blood test or immunochemical fecal occult blood test who referred for colonoscopy underwent CTC. The 2 procedures were not performed on the same day (CTC preceded colonoscopy by an average of 11 days) and the study used segmental unblinding for the endoscopist. The trial used 64-slice CT scanners and the radiologists used 2D image views with 3D problem solving for the detection of polyps. The cohort consisted of 62% male participants, and the average age was 61 years. Using a 6-mm CTC lesion cutoff limit, the per-patient sensitivity of CTC was 91% and the specificity was 69% with a positive predictive value of 87%. Using a 10-mm CTC lesion cutoff size, the per-patient sensitivity of CTC was 82% and the specificity was 86% with a positive predictive value of 84%. The investigators concluded that using CTC as a triage examination for patients with a positive fecal occult blood test would prevent the need for colonoscopy in 28 patients but would miss 2 lesions greater than or equal to 10 mm.

The largest multicenter trial of 1103 participants at increased risk for colorectal cancer was described by Regge and colleagues[20] in 2009. Participants with a family history of advanced neoplasia in first-degree relatives, personal history of colorectal adenomas, or positive results from fecal occult blood testing were eligible for inclusion in this study. Each participant had a same-day CTC and colonoscopy. The types of CT scanner ranged widely at the 21 European centers (minimum requirement was a 4-slice machine) and radiologists used 2D or 3D image interpretation depending on their own preferences. The colonoscopy was performed with segmental unblinding, allowing the unblinded colonoscopy to serve as the reference standard. Fifty-five percent of the participants were men, and the median age was 60 years. One hundred and seventy-seven patients with advanced neoplasia 6 mm or larger and the 667 subjects without these lesions were included in the analysis. The overall sensitivity (85.3%), specificity (87.8%), positive predictive value (61.9%), and negative predictive value (96.3%) were reported. The negative predictive value of the subgroup of patients enrolled into the study because of a positive fecal occult blood test (84.9%) was statistically significantly lower than that of those with a personal or family history of colorectal polyps or cancer (97.7% and 98.5% respectively, $P<.001$.)

These studies are summarized in **Table 2**. Pooled analyses of clinical trials have been published and have included populations of high-risk or symptomatic patients. Mulhall and colleagues[21] in 2005 performed a systematic review of 33 studies comprising 6393 patients who had undergone CTC. This study population also included a few subjects with no relevant medical problems, and there was heterogeneity in the type of CT scanners used, as well as the use of stool tagging and the use of 2D versus 3D image interpretation. The investigators found that the pooled per-patient sensitivity of CTC was 70% overall and specificity 86% overall. For polyps greater than 9 mm, the pooled per-patient sensitivity was 86% and specificity was 97%. A meta-analysis published in 2005 by Halligan and colleagues[22] examined 4181 patients across 24 studies. The sensitivity for polyp detection for lesions larger than 9 mm was 93% and the specificity was 97%. For smaller lesions of 6 to 9 mm, the sensitivity dropped to 86%, and the specificity to 86%. Rosman and colleagues[23] published a meta-analysis in 2007 of 30 studies that had been published between 1996 and 2005. They included studies in which subjects underwent CTC and optical colonoscopy and had large sample sizes. Again, high-risk symptomatic patients were in these studies, but so were patients with little or no risk for colon cancer. These investigators reported overall CTC per-patient sensitivity of 74% and per-patient specificity of 77%. For large polyps (>10 mm) the per-patient sensitivity was reported as 82%, for small polyps (6–9 mm) 63%, and for diminutive polyps (≤5 mm) 56%.

The performance of CTC in trials of subjects with an increased risk of colorectal cancer seems to show several common patterns. First, the statistical accuracy in these particular cohorts is dependent on the strength of the CT scanners used. The earlier-generation machines do not seem to generate the same degree of polyp detection as newer machines. Overall, the sensitivity of CTC for larger lesions in patients with an increased risk of colorectal cancer is at, or only slightly less than, the performance of CTC in a general screening population. Results of CTC for the subgroup of patients with positive fecal occult blood tests do not yet seem to warrant its use in preference to diagnostic (optical) colonoscopy.

PERFORMANCE OF CTC FOR INCOMPLETE COLONOSCOPY

One of the first studies to examine the role of CTC after an incomplete colonoscopy was published in 1999 by Morrin and colleagues.[24] They described a prospective cohort of 40 individuals who underwent same-day CTC after incomplete colonoscopy with adequate preparation. Twenty-six (65%) participants also underwent the additional test of a barium enema after CTC. The reasons for colonoscopy included rectal bleeding, family history of colon cancer, positive fecal occult blood testing, personal history of polyps, and alteration of bowel habits. CTC was able to delineate the cause of incomplete colonoscopy in 30 (74%) cases (tortuous redundant colon, severe diverticular disease, and obstructing sigmoid masses were the most common). CTC adequately revealed 96% of all colonic segments, whereas barium enema revealed

Table 2
CTC performance in increased-risk individuals

Author	Year	Number of Subjects	% Men	Type of Practice	CTC Technique	Sensitivity (>10 mm) (%)	Sensitivity (>6-9 mm) (%)	Sensitivity (<5 mm) (%)	PPV (%)	NPV (%)
Cotton et al[12]	2004	615	45	Multicenter, academic	2,4-row MDCT	55	39	14	46	88
Van Gelder et al[13]	2004	249	59	2 centers, academic	4-row MDCT	76	70	35	54	39
Rockey et al[14]	2005	614	70	Multicenter, academic	4,8-row MDCT	59	55	NR	NR	NR
Chung et al[15]	2005	51	63	Single center, academic	16-row MDCT	100	94	84	NR	NR
Renkonen-Sinisalo et al[16]	2007	78	54	Single center, academic	4-row MDCT	80	NR	NR	42	66
White et al[17]	2009	150	79	Single center, academic	16-row MDCT	91	86	46	NR	NR
Liedenbaum et al[19]	2009	302	62	Multicenter, academic	64-row MDCT	82	91	NR	87	77
Regge et al[20]	2009	1103	55	Multicenter, academic	>4-row MDCT (70% 16-row MDCT)	84	59	NR	62	93

Per-patient sensitivity is noted for various sized lesions; overall PPV and NPV are noted.
Abbreviations: MDCT, multidetector computed tomography; NR, not reported; NPV, negative predictive value; PPV, positive predictive value.

only 91% of colonic segments (*P*<.05). CTC successfully showed the previously non-traversed colon in 36 (90%) patients.

Kim and colleagues[25] in 2007 described the clinical usefulness of CTC after incomplete optical colonoscopy for occlusive colorectal cancer. The study prospectively enrolled 75 individuals with occlusive colorectal cancer, which resulted in an incomplete colonoscopy, to have a same-day CTC. After excluding 7 patients with peritoneal or extensive hepatic metastasis, 67 patients underwent 4-channel multidetector row CTC. Sixty-seven percent of participants were men and the mean age was 58 years. By performing the CTC, an additional 23 polyps were found on CTC. Six synchronous carcinomas were detected on CTC (3 proximal to obstruction and 3 distal to obstruction). Clinically significant errors of tumor localization by colonoscopy were noted in 12% of cases. The surgeons at this institution altered their surgical management based on the results of the CTC in 16% of the cases.

A retrospective chart review by Copel and colleagues[26] in 2007 included the largest number of patients for an evaluation of CTC after an incomplete colonoscopy. They reviewed the charts of 546 consecutive patients who underwent CTC after incomplete colonoscopy. The average age of participants was 64.1 years, and women comprised 73.4% of the cohort. They found that 90.1% were at increased risk for colorectal cancer, with the remainder as average risk. Patients were excluded if there was a suspicion of a familial polyposis syndrome or inflammatory bowel disease. Most (94.9%) of the CTCs were performed on the same day as the colonoscopy. Four- or 8-detector row scanners were used in this study. The most common reasons for incomplete colonoscopy were redundant or tortuous loops (39.9%), excessive bowel spasm (26.2%), severe diverticulosis (13.9%), and obstructive tumors (7.5%). They found that 13.2% of patients had 88 lesions of 6 mm or more that were not seen at colonoscopy. Sixty-three percent of these patients had follow-up colonoscopy at a median time of 31 months. Masses (lesions ≥20 mm), large polyps (10–19 mm), and small polyps (6–9 mm) were detected at these follow-up examinations 100%, 94%, and 45% of the time, respectively. The per-patient positive predictive values for these lesions were 90.9%, 91.7%, and 64.7%, respectively. The per-lesion positive predictive values were 70%, 33.3%, and 30.4%, respectively.

Yucel and colleagues[27] in 2008 sought to describe the performance of CTC in an older population (>60 years old) who were referred for CTC because of incomplete or contraindicated colonoscopy. Of the 42 patients considered in the final analysis, 30 participants had CTC for an incomplete colonoscopy. The reasons for incomplete colonoscopy included diverticular disease (n = 10), colonic redundancy (n = 10), adhesions (n = 3), residual colonic content (n = 3), sigmoid stricture (n = 1), ventral hernia (n = 1), and unknown cause (n = 2). In 90% of the patients adequate visualization of the entire bowel was obtained.

Sali and colleagues[28] in 2008 reported a cohort of patients who had positive fecal occult blood test and underwent diagnostic colonoscopy and, if incomplete, CTC. Of the 903 colonoscopies performed, 65 were incomplete (7.2%). Of these 65 participants, 42 underwent CTC. Sixteen-multidetector row CT scanners were used and CTC was performed within 6 weeks of incomplete CTC (mean time 16 days). Twenty-six percent of participants were men and the average age was approximately 61 years. Twenty-one of the CTCs (505) showed polyps (N = 20) or masses (N = 2) and 15/21 of these patients underwent a repeat colonoscopy, whereas 2/21 proceeded directly to surgery. The positive predictive value of CTC for polyps and masses greater than 9 mm was reported to be 87.5%. The per-lesion positive predictive value for 6 to 9 mm masses was 77.8%.

The data clearly support the use of CTC after an incomplete colonoscopy. CTC seemed to have a high rate of detection of nonvisualized lesions on colonoscopy, as well as the ability to determine the cause of incomplete colonoscopy. Although a tortuous colon or severe diverticular disease seem to be common causes for incomplete colonoscopy necessitating a CTC, the most useful role of CTC may be in cases of obstructing carcinomas for which synchronous lesions, tumor localization, and surgical planning can potentially be greatly refined with the use of CTC.

PERFORMANCE OF CTC IN TRIALS WITH UNPREPPED OR REDUCED PREPARATION PROTOCOLS

To examine the effects of dietary fecal tagging in a reduced colonic cleansing scenario, Lefere and colleagues[29] in 2002 studied the resultant sensitivity and specificity of CTC in such a trial. The 100 subjects were patients referred for conventional colonoscopy, most of whom were to have average-risk screening. Patients underwent same-day CTC and colonoscopy (those patients with a reduced CTC preparation underwent additional polyethylene glycol cleansing until stools were watery and clear). Fifty subjects received a low-residue diet, magnesium citrate, bisacodyl tablets/suppository, and a barium suspension the day before procedure. The other 50 patients received 3 L of polyethylene glycol the day before the test. The investigators found that the reduced preparation group had more fecal residue but improved differentiation from polyps (specificity of reduced prep group 88%, conventional prep group 77%). There was no difference in sensitivities (reduced prep group 88%, conventional prep group 85%). In addition to reporting differences between CT interpretation time, colonic distention, and residual stool, the investigators noted that 3 polyps in 3 subjects in the unprepped group were noted at the time of endoscopy and were not noted at CTC. In the prepped group, CTC detected 2 of 3 polyps noted at colonoscopy.

Dachman and colleagues[30] in 2007 described a pilot study comparing unprepped CTC with a reduced prep CTC using same-day conventional colonoscopy as the reference standard. One group of 14 subjects consumed barium with a low-fiber diet, and the other group of 14 subjects consumed barium, low-fiber diet, and magnesium citrate. All patients drank 4 L of polyethylene glycol after CTC and before colonoscopy. Although the investigators described relevant findings such as ease of CT read, amount of stool, and residual fluid, they also commented on polyp identification. There were 3 polyps (all >5 mm) that were identified during colonoscopy and that were not visualized on an unprepped CTC. An additional 3 polyps (all >5 mm) were identified during colonoscopy in the prepped CTC group of which the CTC only detected 2 of the 3. The investigators suggested that unprepped CTC warrants further study because small and large polyps were missed.

Patients' preference for CTC rather than optical colonoscopy has been described in the literature.[31-33] The attempt to improve the experience of prepping for a CTC without sacrificing the overall quality of the examination would be a major advance in screening technology. The 2 studies reviewed suggest that reduced preparation is an intriguing methodology for the detection of polyps, but that unprepped regimens cannot be recommended at this time. Other studies of reduced-preparation CTC have mainly focused on image quality and patient satisfaction.[34,35] Larger multicenter studies focusing on the performance of CTC in the detection of neoplasms in a reduced-preparation environment are needed.

PERFORMANCE OF CTC IN ACADEMIC VERSUS NONACADEMIC ENVIRONMENTS

Little is known about the use and outcomes of CTC in the community setting. The National CT Colonography Survey in Israel published in 2008 found that 86% of all

CTC taking place in that country were performed in private clinics rather than in academic institutions.[36] Burling and colleagues[37] in 2006 presented a dataset of 15 CTC studies that had been used in a previous trial to a group of 13 radiologists from 7 nonacademic clinical practice centers to assess diagnostic accuracy compared with formally trained radiographic technicians (50 cases) and experienced radiologists in an academic environment.[38] The dataset included studies with cancer, small to large polyps, and normal examinations. All of the subjects used CTC in their clinical practice, and considered themselves to be nonacademic subspecialists in GI radiology, but none had formal training in CTC. The mean accuracy overall of nonacademicians versus experienced academicians was statistically significant (75% vs 88%, $P = .04$), but there was no difference between the study subjects and formally trained radiology technicians.

One of the reasons that CTC is an attractive diagnostic modality is that adherence to screening and follow-up colonoscopy is poor and presents an alternative option for health care practitioners and patients.[39–43] Presumably most eligible patients in need of such examinations receive their medical care in the community as opposed to in academic environments. Thus the performance of CTC in academic versus nonacademic environments may have important health care outcomes downstream. The reviewed data suggest that experienced readers at academic institutions are superior at reading CTC studies; however, this gap may close as nonacademicians improve their learning or have greater access to newer CTC technologies.

SUMMARY

Since the first description of CTC by Vining and colleagues[44] in 1994, the technology, methodology, and experience of CTC has improved greatly, and has translated into improved performance in several important clinical arenas for which CTC is emerging as an important diagnostic modality. Given poor population colorectal cancer screening rates,[39] the greatest need is for CTC to function effectively in a screening population. The existing trials in average-risk and increased-risk individuals consistently show accuracy for large (>10-mm) lesions, but diminishing sensitivity and specificity for the small and diminutive lesions. Thus, decisions about embracing CTC as a screening or diagnostic modality may be based on the relative effectiveness of this test compared with the risk of missed smaller lesions, or intentionally following smaller lesions rather than triggering polypectomy. The formula ([acceptable screening sensitivity + increased population acceptance] – [risks of missed lesions + risk of ionizing radiation exposure]) has not been fully calculated yet. However, CTC for incomplete colonoscopy seems reasonable given its usefulness and superiority to other imaging alternatives. Other areas, such as CTC for high-risk screening populations or in reduced/nonprepped protocols that may improve patient compliance, do not yet seem ready for prime time. The existing trials do not adequately address the learning process or the incorporation of CTC into community practices, so more work in this area will be welcome.

REFERENCES

1. McFarland E, Levin B, Lieberman D, et al. Revised colorectal screening guidelines: joint effort of the American Cancer Society, U.S. Multisociety Task Force on Colorectal Cancer, and American College of Radiology. Radiology 2008; 248:717–20.
2. Centers for Medicare and Medicaid Services. Decision memo for screening computed tomography colonography (CTC) for colorectal cancer (CAG-00396N).

Available at: https://www.cms.hhs.gov/mcd/viewdecisionmemo.asp?id=220. Accessed May 19, 2009.

3. U.S. Preventative Services Task Force. Screening for colorectal cancer: U.S. Preventative Services Task Force recommendation statement. Ann Intern Med 2008;149:627–37.

4. Pickhardt PJ, Choi RJ, Hwang I, et al. Computed tomographic virtual colonoscopy to screen for colorectal neoplasia in asymptomatic results. N Engl J Med 2003;349:2191–200.

5. Macari M, Bini EJ, Jacobs SL, et al. Colorectal polyps and cancers in asymptomatic average-risk patients: evaluation with CT colonography. Radiology 2004;230:629–36.

6. Kim DH, Pickhardt PJ, Taylor AJ, et al. CT colonography versus colonoscopy for the detection of advanced neoplasia. N Engl J Med 2007;357:1403–12.

7. Cornett D, Baracin C, Roeder B, et al. Findings on optical colonoscopy after positive CT colonography exam. Am J Gastroenterol 2008;103:2068–74.

8. Johnson CD, Chen MH, Toledano AY, et al. Accuracy of CT colonography for the detection of large adenomas and cancer. N Engl J Med 2008;359:1207–17.

9. Graser A, Steiber P, Nagel D, et al. Comparison of CT colonography, colonoscopy, sigmoidoscopy, and fecal occult blood tests for the detection of advanced adenoma in an average risk population. Gut 2009;58:241–8.

10. Winawer SJ. The multidisciplinary management of gastrointestinal cancer. Colorectal cancer screening. Best Pract Res Clin Gastroenterol 2007;21(6):1031–48.

11. Whitlock EP, Lin JS, Liles E, et al. Screening for colorectal cancer: a targeted, updated systematic review for the U.S. Preventive Task Force. Ann Intern Med 2008; 149:638–58.

12. Cotton PB, Durkalski VL, Pineau BC, et al. Computed tomographic colonography (virtual colonoscopy): a multicenter comparison with standard colonoscopy for detection of colorectal neoplasia. JAMA 2004;291:1713–9.

13. Van Gelder RE, Nio CY, Florie J, et al. Computed tomographic colonography compared with colonoscopy in patients at increased risk for colorectal cancer. Gastroenterology 2004;127:41–8.

14. Rockey DC, Paulson E, Niedzwiecki D, et al. Analysis of air contrast barium enema, computed tomographic colonography, and colonoscopy: prospective comparison. Lancet 2005;365:301–11.

15. Chung DJ, Huh KC, Choi WJ, et al. CT colonography using 16-MDCT in the evaluation of colorectal cancer. Am J Roentgenol 2005;184:98–103.

16. Renkonen-Sinisalo L, Kivisaari A, Kivisaari L, et al. Utility of computed tomographic colonography in surveillance for hereditary nonpolyposis colorectal cancer syndrome. Fam Cancer 2007;6:135–40.

17. White TJ, Avery GR, Kennan N, et al. Virtual colonoscopy vs. conventional colonoscopy in patients at high risk of colorectal cancer – a prospective trial of 150 patients. Colorectal Dis 2009;11:138–45.

18. Thompson MR. ACPGBI referral guidelines for colorectal cancer. Colorectal Dis 2002;4:287–97.

19. Liedenbaum MH, van Rijn AF, de Vries AH, et al. Using CT colonography as a triage technique after a positive faecal occult blood test in colorectal cancer screening. Gut 2009;58:1242–9.

20. Regge D, Laudi C, Galatola G. Diagnostic accuracy of computed tomographic colonography for the detection of advanced neoplasia in individuals at increased risk of colorectal cancer. JAMA 2009;301:2453–61.

21. Mulhall BP, Veerappan GR, Jackson JL. Meta-analysis: computed tomographic colonography. Ann Intern Med 2005;142:635–50.

22. Halligan S, Altman DG, Taylor SA, et al. CT colonography in the detection of colorectal polyps and cancer: systematic review, meta-analysis, and proposed minimum data set for study level reporting. Radiology 2005;237:893–904.
23. Rosman AS, Korsten MA. Meta-analysis comparing CT colonography, air contrast barium enema, and colonoscopy. Am J Med 2007;120:203–10.
24. Morrin MM, Kruskal JB, Farrell RJ, et al. Endoluminal CT colonography after an incomplete endoscopic colonoscopy. Am J Roentgenol 1999;172:913–8.
25. Kim JH, Kim WH, Kim TI, et al. Incomplete colonoscopy in patients with occlusive colorectal cancer: usefulness of CT colonography according to tumor location. Yonsei Med J 2007;48:934–41.
26. Copel L, Sosna J, Kruskal JB, et al. CT colonography in 546 patients with incomplete colonoscopy. Radiology 2007;244:471–8.
27. Yucel C, Lev-Toaff AS, Moussa N, et al. CT colonography for incomplete or contraindicated optical colonoscopy in older patients. Am J Roentgenol 2008;190:145–50.
28. Sali L, Falchini M, Bonanomi AG, et al. CT colonography after incomplete colonoscopy in subjects with positive faecal occult blood test. World J Gastroenterol 2008;14:4499–504.
29. Lefere PA, Gryspeerdt SS, Dewyspelaere J, et al. Dietary fecal tagging as a cleansing method before CT colonography: initial results - polyp detection and patient acceptance. Radiology 2002;224:393–403.
30. Dachman AH, Dawson DO, Lefere P, et al. Comparison of routine and unprepped CT colonography augmented by low fiber diet and stool tagging: a pilot study. Abdom Imaging 2007;32:96–104.
31. Rajapaksa RC, Macari M, Bini EJ. Racial/ethnic differences in patient experience with and preferences for computed tomography colonography and optical colonoscopy. Clin Gastroenterol Hepatol 2007;5(11):1306–12.
32. van Gelder RE, Birnie E, Florie J, et al. CT colonography and colonoscopy: assessment of patient preference in a 5-week follow-up study. Radiology 2004; 233(2):328–37.
33. Juchems MS, Ehmann J, Brambs HJ, et al. A retrospective evaluation of patient acceptance of computed tomography colonoscopy ("virtual colonoscopy") in comparison with conventional colonoscopy in an average risk screening population. Acta Radiol 2005;46(7):664–70.
34. Taylor SA, Slater A, Burling DN, et al. CT colonography: optimisation, diagnostic performance and patient acceptability of reduced-laxative regimens using barium-based faecal tagging. Eur Radiol 2008;18:32–42.
35. Jensch S, de Vries AH, Pot D, et al. Image quality and patient acceptance of four regimens with different amounts of mild laxatives for CT colonography. Am J Roentgenol 2008;191:158–67.
36. Blachar A, Levy G, Graif M, et al. Computed tomography colonography ("virtual colonoscopy") in Israel: results of the national CT colonography survey of the Israeli association of abdominal imaging and the Israeli radiological association. Isr Med Assoc J 2008;10:707–12.
37. Burling D, Halligan S, Atchley J, et al. CT colonography: interpretative performance in a non-academic environment. Clin Radiol 2007;62:424–9.
38. European Society of Gastrointestinal and Abdominal Radiologists (ESGAR) CT colonography study group investigators. Effect of directed training on reader performance for CT colonography: a multi-center study. Radiology 2007;242:152–61.
39. Baxter NN, Goldwasser MA, Paszat LF, et al. Association of colonoscopy and death from colorectal cancer: a population-based, case-controlled study. Ann Intern Med 2009;150:1–8.

40. Subramanian S, Amonkar MM, Hunt TL. Use of colonoscopy for colorectal cancer screening: evidence from the 2000 national health interview survey. Cancer Epidemiol Biomarkers Prev 2005;14:409–16.
41. Bujanda L, Sarasqueta C, Zubiaurre I, et al. EPICOLON group. Low adherence to colonoscopy in the screening of first-degree relatives of patients with colorectal cancer. Gut 2007;56(12):1714–8.
42. Nadel MR, Shapiro JA, Klabunde CN, et al. A national survey of primary care physicians' methods for screening for fecal occult blood. Ann Intern Med 2005; 142(2):86–94.
43. Rapuri S, Spencer J, Eckels D. Importance of postpolypectomy surveillance and postpolypectomy compliance to follow-up screening: review of literature. Int J Colorectal Dis 2008;23(5):453–9.
44. Vining DJ, Gelfand DW, Bechthold RE, et al. Technical feasibility of colon imaging with helical CT and virtual reality [abstract]. Am J Roentgenol 1994;162(Suppl): 104.

Performance of CT Colonography for Detecting Small, Diminutive, and Flat Polyps

Perry J. Pickhardt, MD[a,b,]*, David H. Kim, MD[a]

KEYWORDS

- CT colonography • Virtual colonoscopy • Colorectal polyps
- Colorectal cancer screening • Flat lesions

The main goal of colorectal screening is to reduce the incidence, morbidity, and mortality of colorectal cancer (CRC). CRC is a deadly but preventable disease, which remains a major public health issue largely because of the low rates of effective screening.[1] The recently revised screening guidelines that were created by the American Cancer Society in conjunction with the major gastroenterology and radiology societies strongly emphasize the value of CRC prevention and detection rather than CRC detection alone.[2] In particular, tests that can provide full structural evaluation of the large intestine, such as optical colonoscopy (OC) and computerized tomography colonography (CTC), are likely to be favored in the future. CTC should not be viewed as a replacement for OC but as an additional effective parallel screening option that has the potential to substantially increase adherence rates, assuming that the test is eventually widely reimbursed by third-party payers.

CTC has several potential advantages relative to OC as a screening test, as well as some disadvantages. The primary advantages include that it is generally safer, more convenient, more cost-effective, provides a limited assessment of extracolonic organs, and is equally effective as OC for detecting large colorectal polyps and

The opinions and assertions contained herein are the private views of the authors and are not to be construed as official or as reflecting the views of the Departments of the Navy or Defense.

a Department of Radiology, University of Wisconsin School of Medicine and Public Health, E3/311 Clinical Science Center, 600 Highland Avenue, Madison, WI 53792-3252, USA

b Department of Radiology, Uniformed Services University of the Health Sciences, 4301 Jones Bridge Road, Bethesda, MD 20814, USA

* Corresponding author. Department of Radiology, University of Wisconsin School of Medicine and Public Health, E3/311 Clinical Science Center, 600 Highland Avenue, Madison, WI 53792-3252.

E-mail address: pj.pickhardt@hosp.wisc.edu

cancers.[3-9] Perhaps the main drawback of CTC relates to its noninvasive nature; by itself it is a nontherapeutic test. Therefore, the determination of appropriate criteria for polypectomy referral for CTC-detected lesions is critical for clinical efficacy and cost-effectiveness considerations. There seems to be broad (albeit not universal) agreement that, in most circumstances, large polyps (defined as ≥10 mm) detected at CTC should be referred for polypectomy, whereas isolated diminutive lesions (defined as ≤5 mm) generally do not warrant colonoscopy.[5,7,9-15] The situation is less clear for small polyps (defined as 6–9 mm) detected at CTC,[2,7,14-17] because it is uncertain whether the benefits of polypectomy outweigh the risks and costs associated with the additive colonoscopy procedure. Another area of considerable controversy, not only for CTC but for CRC screening in general, is flat or nonpolypoid lesions.

This article explores the issues of small, diminutive, and flat colorectal polyps, focusing primarily on how they relate to CTC (and OC) screening. However, before delving into CTC-specific performance data, it is critical to understand and review what is known about the prevalence, histology, and natural history of polyps according to the various size categories. In particular, because advanced neoplasia represents the critical high-yield target of CRC prevention, this important subset of colorectal lesions is emphasized.

PREVALENCE, HISTOLOGY, AND NATURAL HISTORY OF POLYPS ACCORDING TO LESION SIZE

Based on a large number of clinical trials and experience, anywhere from 35% to 50% of adults more than 50 years of age may harbor at least 1 colorectal polyp.[4,5,7,18-20] This figure may increase even further with the implementation of more advanced endoscopic techniques. In most cases, the largest lesion will be diminutive. Because of the broad differences in the detection rates of diminutive lesions and their relative lack of clinical importance, polyp prevalence at the 6-mm and 10-mm size thresholds are much more reproducible and relevant values to consider. Recent colonoscopy screening studies have shown a remarkably narrow prevalence range for polyps greater than or equal to 6 mm of 13% to 16% (**Table 1**).[21] Similarly, the prevalence for large polyps is 5% to 6%, which results in about 8% of individuals in whom the largest polyp will lie within the 6- to 9-mm range. As a general rule, approximately one-third of diminutive lesions will be adenomatous (almost exclusively tubular adenomas) and two-thirds will be nonadenomatous, predominately consisting of non-neoplastic mucosal tags and hyperplastic polyps.[7,22] In polyps larger than 6 mm, the ratio of adenomatous to nonadenomatous polyps reverses, with neoplastic lesions representing approximately two-thirds of nondiminutive lesions.[4,7,22]

The ideal screening target for prevention of CRC is the advanced adenoma, which is defined as an adenoma that is large (≥10 mm) or contains histologic findings of high-grade dysplasia or a prominent villous component.[23] Although largely unproven, most experts believe that high-grade dysplasia is a more concerning feature than villous histology. The serrated polyp pathway, which is distinct from the classic adenoma-carcinoma sequence, may account for about 15% of CRC cases.[24] For this particular pathway, sessile serrated adenomas less than 10 mm without dysplasia should not be considered as histologically advanced lesions, but serrated adenomas that are large (≥10 mm) or exhibit dysplasia should also be categorized as advanced (Michael J. O'Brien, MD, personal communication, 2009). The term "advanced neoplasia" encompasses advanced (but still benign) adenomas and invasive adenocarcinoma. This term is useful for CRC screening because it combines the key features of prevention and detection.

Table 1
Relevant colorectal polyp data from modern screening cohorts

Variable	Typical Value (%)	Reported Range (%)	References
Screening prevalence of:			
All colorectal polyps ≥6 mm	14	13–16	4,5,7,18–20
Small 6- to 9-mm polyps	8	8–9	4,5,7,19,20
Large (≥10 mm) polyps	6	5–7	4,5,7,19,20
Advanced neoplasia (any polyp size)	3–4	3.3–7.1	5,7,18,20,25,92
Small 6- to 9-mm advanced adenomas	0.3	0.17–0.46	5,19,20
High-grade dysplasia in small polyps	0.05	0.048–0.064	5,20
Invasive cancer in small polyps	0.01	0–0.039	4,5,7,19,20,25
Rate of advanced histology in 6- to 9-mm adenomas	4	2.7–5.3	5,19,20,25,93
Rate of high-grade dysplasia in 6- to 9-mm adenomas	0.7	0.5–0.8	20,25
Rate of invasive cancer in 6- to 9-mm adenomas	0.1	0–0.49	4,5,7,19,20,25,93–95
Rate of invasive cancer in 1- to 2-cm adenomas	1	0.5–2.4	19,20,96

Data from Pickhardt PJ, Kim DH. Colorectal cancer screening with CT colonography: key concepts regarding polyp prevalence, size, histology, morphology, and natural history. AJR Am J Roentgenol 2009;193(1):40–6.

Although large adenomas (≥10 mm) comprise about 90% of all advanced neoplasia in the screening setting,[5,20,25] approximately 4% of 6- to 9-mm adenomas will show advanced histology, with a reported range of 2.7% to 5.3% (see **Table 1**). Assuming an 8% screening prevalence of 6- to 9-mm polyps and a 4% frequency of advanced histology, the overall screening prevalence of small advanced adenomas is approximately 0.3%, with a reported range of 0.17% to 0.56% (see **Table 1**). The presence of high-grade dysplasia in 6- to 9-mm adenomas is even more uncommon, with an overall prevalence of about 0.05% (see **Table 1**). Although the overall prevalence of diminutive polyps is many times higher than small 6- to 9-mm polyps, the prevalence of diminutive advanced neoplasia is considerably lower than that for small polyps.[20]

One striking feature of the recent screening data is the lower rate of cancer according to lesion size compared with the high-risk, symptomatic, and/or surgical cohorts in the older literature. For example, a commonly quoted historical figure for the cancer rate among small 6- to 9-mm adenomas is 0.9%.[15,26–28] However, when the recent large screening studies are tallied, the frequency of cancer decreases to 0.1% or lower, ranging from 0% to 0.5% (see **Table 1**), with most of the reported small cancers concentrated within one Korean series.[19] The percentage falls even lower if all 6- to 9-mm polyps, and not just small adenomas, are considered in the denominator. We have yet to encounter a subcentimeter invasive cancer in our combined CTC and OC experience, including more than 1000 6- to 9-mm polyps.[29] Even for large 1- to 2-cm lesions, the cancer rate seems to be only about 1% (see **Table 1**), which is considerably lower than the commonly quoted historical range of 5% to 10%, which is again based on high-risk cohorts and not screening populations.[26,27] Given that about 30% to 40% of large polyps are nonadenomatous[4,7,22] and that some large lesions detected at CTC may be false-positives,[4,30] the actual cancer risk for a 1- to 2-cm lesion detected at CTC is considerably less than 1%, lower than the frequency of significant complications at OC referral for therapeutic polypectomy.[31–34]

The natural history of small colorectal polyps has become an issue of critical importance in CRC screening. One reason for this is that CTC is an efficacious and cost-effective approach to population screening if only large polyps (≥10 mm) were considered appropriate to trigger polypectomy.[11] If all small 6- to 9-mm CTC-detected polyps were to be referred to therapeutic colonoscopy for polypectomy, the usefulness of CTC as an intermediate filter would be diminished, but likely still useful.[5,7,9] Although CTC provides an ideal tool for in vivo surveillance of small unresected polyps, there are several older studies that have followed these lesions using other colorectal examinations, including endoscopy and barium enema. Contrary to the general perception, many of the data on polyp natural history already exist from these older longitudinal trials. As a group, these longitudinal studies have repeatedly shown the benign, indolent nature of unresected subcentimeter colorectal polyps, with no study showing that leaving 6- to 9-mm polyps in place is a harmful practice.

Most longitudinal polyp surveillance studies have focused more on small 6- to 9-mm polyps,[35–40] although some have focused on diminutive[41] or large[42] lesions. In Norway, Hofstad and colleagues[37] performed serial colonoscopy on unresected subcentimeter polyps and found that only 1 (0.5%) of 189 lesions eclipsed the 10-mm threshold after a 1-year time interval. At the 3-year follow-up, most polyps in this study remained stable or regressed in size, and there was an overall tendency to net regression among the 5- to 9-mm polyps.[38] The investigators of this endoscopic trial concluded that following unresected 5- to 9-mm polyps for 3 years was a safe practice. Longitudinal studies using flexible sigmoidoscopy have also shown the stability of smaller polyps over time.[35,36,39] In one study that used serial sigmoidoscopy to follow polyps measuring up to 15 mm over a 3- to 5-year period, Knoernschild[39] reported a significant increase in polyp size in only 4% of patients. In a longitudinal study using barium enemas to follow colorectal polyps, Welin and colleagues[40] showed slow growth rates by studying 375 unresected polyps over a mean interval of 30 months. The high observed adenoma detection rates at surveillance in the National Polyp Study, in conjunction with the low observed CRC incidence, was thought to be explainable only by regression of adenomas.[43] In a high-risk cohort of patients undergoing colonoscopy surveillance following CRC surgery, Togashi and colleagues[41] followed 500 polyps 6 mm or less over an average interval of 3.6 years. They concluded that this practice was safe even in the high-risk setting. In a classic barium enema study by Stryker and colleagues,[42] the cumulative 5-year and 10-year risk of cancer related to large colorectal polyps (≥1 cm) left in place was less than 3% and 10%, respectively.

These reassuring longitudinal endoscopic and barium enema studies have done little to quell the current debate about the clinical management of small polyps detected at CTC screening.[44] Part of the problem may be a simple lack of awareness of these study results. CTC can now be used as the preferred instrument to follow unresected colorectal lesions. CTC provides superior polyp measurement capabilities compared with the other colorectal imaging examinations, including improved accuracy and reproducibility for linear size assessment.[45,46] In addition, CTC can assess polyp volume, which greatly amplifies interval changes in lesion size compared with linear measurement.

The University of Wisconsin School of Medicine and Public Health and the National Naval Medical Center (NNMC) in Bethesda, Maryland, are currently collaborating on a small-polyp natural history trial that commenced in 2004. The early interim results of CTC surveillance in 128 small colorectal polyps from the initial 100 patients has largely recapitulated the findings from the older endoscopic and barium enema trials.[47] With an average CTC follow-up interval of about 1.5 years, 12 (9.4%) of the small polyps showed interval growth, including 11 proven adenomas (1 polyp was removed but not retrieved at OC). There were no cancers that developed during this short interval, and none of the lesions grew past the 10-mm threshold. Five of the adenomas represented advanced lesions, corresponding to 4% of the total polyp cohort (ie, the expected number of advanced lesions from the entire group of 6- to 9-mm polyps). The remaining 116 polyps (90.6%) did not increase in size at CTC follow-up, and some of them had regressed. These findings suggest that interval growth can predict important histology, allowing for noninvasive identification of the small fraction of polyps for which polypectomy is clearly of benefit.

CTC DETECTION OF SMALL 6- TO 9-MM COLORECTAL POLYPS

The accuracy of CTC for detecting large polyps (≥ 10 mm) and masses (≥ 3 cm) has been well established, with most studies reporting sensitivity and specificity values of 90% or higher.[4,7,48–53] CTC performance tends to be more robust when three-dimensional (3D) polyp detection is used alongside two-dimensional (2D) evaluation, when oral contrast tagging has been applied, and when automated carbon dioxide delivery is used for colonic distention. When state-of-the-art CTC is undertaken, there is evidence to suggest that CTC sensitivity for large polyps and cancers may exceed that of OC.[5,7,54] However, there are a few notable exceptions in which the CTC sensitivity for large-polyp detection was in the 50% to 60% range,[55–57] but none of these studies used primary 3D detection, oral contrast tagging, or carbon dioxide.

The CTC performance for small 6- to 9-mm polyps is more variable (**Fig. 1**). One problem is the lack of a reliable reference standard, because the miss rate for small lesions at OC can be 10% or higher when tandem (back-to-back) colonoscopy studies are performed.[58–60] In addition, several published studies have reported by-patient results at the 6-mm and 10-mm thresholds, but not specifically for the 6- to 9-mm range. Although such results can generally be inferred, the conversion is imperfect related to the use of different polyp-matching algorithms. The patient populations are also somewhat heterogeneous, representing screening and nonscreening cohorts. For most CTC studies that have evaluated at least 100 patients, the per-patient sensitivity for small 6- to 9-mm polyps lies somewhere within the range of 50% to 95% (**Fig. 2, Table 2**).[4,7,48–53,55–57,61–65] The only outlier was the study by Cotton and colleagues,[55] in which the per-patient sensitivity was only 30%.

More recent data from the clinical CTC screening programs at the University of Wisconsin (UW) and the NNMC suggest that the performance for state-of-the-art CTC for 6- to 9-mm polyps is now approaching that for larger lesions (see **Fig. 1**). An ongoing CTC trial at NNMC continues to show sensitivity for small polyps of about 90% (Brooks Cash, personal communication, 2009). At UW, the positive predictive value of 6- to 9-mm CTC-detected polyps is more than 90%, significantly higher than results from the published clinical trials.[66] In routine clinical practice, the positive predictive value is an important quality measure, along with the overall yield of advanced neoplasia, because performance assessments by sensitivity, specificity, and accuracy cannot be measured when negative CTC cases do not go on to OC. The common CTC methodology used at UW and NNMC provide further support for primary 3D interpretation, which has also been shown to improve small-polyp detection compared with 2D detection alone in a phantom study.[67]

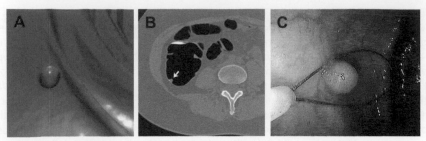

Fig. 1. Small 6-mm tubular adenoma detected at CTC screening. 3D endoluminal (*A*) and 2D transverse (*B*) CTC images show a well-circumscribed 6-mm sessile polyp (*arrow*) in the ascending colon, which proved to be a tubular adenoma after resection at same-day OC (*C*). With state-of-the-art CTC technique, the diagnostic performance for detecting small 6- to 9-mm polyps likely approaches that for larger lesions. (*From* Pickhardt PJ. The colon and rectum. In: Pickhardt PJ, Arluk GM, editors. Atlas of gastrointestinal imaging: radiologic-endoscopic correlation. Philadelphia: Saunders; 2007. p. 212; with permission.)

Even if CTC has high accuracy for detecting small polyps, it remains unclear whether all such lesions warrant immediate polypectomy. Evaluating the potential benefit (ie, preventing CRC) against the potential risks (eg, perforation, bleeding, sedation-related events) and costs (eg, OC procedure, pathology charges), it becomes clear that the conclusion will be largely driven by the input assumptions. Given the low risk (approximately 4%) that a 6- to 9-mm polyp will be an advanced adenoma and the extremely low risk (<0.1%) of CRC, deferring polypectomy may be an attractive option for individuals who have already decided to undergo a less invasive

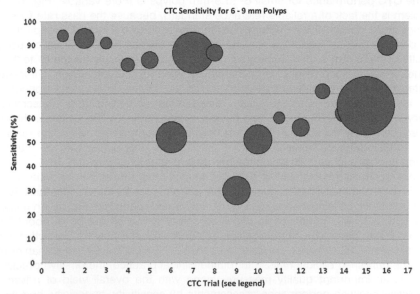

Fig. 2. Bubble graph showing CTC by-patient sensitivity for detecting 6- to 9-mm polyps for published trials that involved 100 or more patients and used OC as the reference standard. The bubble sizes correspond to the size of the patient cohorts. The studies are displayed in chronologic order, with the oldest on the left (see **Table 2**). Note the 1 outlier where the CTC sensitivity decreases to less than 50%.

Table 2
Reported per-patient sensitivities for small 6- to 9-mm polyps

Trial	Author, Year	Sensitivity	No. of Patients
1	Fenlon et al, 1999[48]	94	100
2	Yee et al, 2001[51]	93	300
3	Lefere et al, 2002[61]	91	100
4	Ginnerup Pedersen et al, 2003[97]	82	144
5	Pineau et al, 2003[50]	84	205
6	Johnson et al, 2003[56]	52	703
7	Pickhardt et al, 2003[7]	87	1233
8	Innaccone et al, 2004[98]	87	203
9	Cotton et al, 2004[55]	30	600
10	Rockey et al, 2005[57]	51	614
11	Arnesen et al, 2005[63]	60	100
12	Arnesen et al, 2007[64]	56	231
13	Jensch et al, 2008[62]	71	168
14	Kim et al, 2008[53]	62	241
15	Johnson et al, 2008[4]	65	2531
16	Graser et al, 2009[49]	90	307

screening route. To coincide with current standard of care, the current protocol at UW is to offer all patients with any CTC-detected polyp that is larger than or equal to 6 mm same-day OC for polypectomy (see **Fig. 1**). However, individuals with one or two 6- to 9-mm lesions, corresponding to a C-RADS C2 classification,[12] are also offered the option of short-term CTC follow-up in 2 to 3 years. Preliminary results with CTC surveillance (described earlier) suggest that this approach may effectively identify the small subset of lesions for which polypectomy is indicated and avoid the need for colonoscopy in most other cases. However, more data are needed before drawing firm conclusions. Given the published data establishing the risk of future advanced neoplasia related to finding multiple adenomas at the index colonoscopy,[68,69] the policy at CTC is that patients with 3 or more small polyps are referred for polypectomy. This approach corresponds with a C-RADS C3 categorization, placing 3 or more small polyps detected at CTC at the same level as 1 or more large ($\geq$ 10 mm) polyps.

Given the limited health care dollars available for expensive resources, it is critical to also consider costs alongside the anticipated health consequence for the various screening strategies. We have studied the theoretical cost-effectiveness of immediate polypectomy versus 3-year CTC surveillance for small 6- to 9-mm polyps detected at CTC screening.[17] Without any intervention, the estimated 5-year CRC death rate for patients with unresected 6- to 9-mm polyps was 0.08%, which already represents a sevenfold decrease from the 0.56% 5-year CRC death rate in the general (unscreened) population, most of whom do not harbor polyps. Therefore, for patients with 6- to 9-mm polyps detected at CTC screening, the exclusion of large polyps ($\geq$ 10 mm) and masses already confers a low CRC risk. Focusing on a concentrated cohort with only small 6- to 9-mm polyps, the death rate was further reduced to 0.03% with the CTC surveillance strategy and to 0.02% with immediate colonoscopy referral. However, for each additional cancer-related death prevented with immediate polypectomy versus CTC follow-up, 10,000 additional colonoscopy referrals would be needed, resulting in an expected 10 additional perforations and an exorbitant incremental cost-effectiveness ratio (ICER) of $372,853. We therefore concluded that the high costs, additional complications, and low incremental yield associated with immediate polypectomy of 6- to 9-mm polyps support the practice of 3-year CTC surveillance, which allows for selective noninvasive identification of small polyps at risk (as described earlier). CTC surveillance of small unresected polyps should only be undertaken in the context of a dedicated CTC program, in which a reliable mechanism for follow-up is in place and in which the patient understands the relative risks and benefits involved.

CTC DETECTION OF DIMINUTIVE (≤5 MM) COLORECTAL POLYPS

Few data exist for the performance of CTC in detecting diminutive lesions that measure 5 mm or less (**Fig. 3**). By design, most large CTC trials have not reported diminutive lesions. Without a reliable reference standard, the performance for diminutive lesions is difficult to establish. All the issues that complicate the performance evaluation for small 6- to 9-mm polyps are greatly amplified for diminutive lesions (≤5 mm). Among the studies that have attempted to assess CTC detection of diminutive polyps relative to OC, the by-polyp sensitivity has varied widely but averages to approximately 50% in systematic reviews.[70,71] One recent study carefully assessed CTC-OC correlation for diminutive adenomas using high-quality CTC and found a by-polyp sensitivity of 59% (84 of 147).[49] This value probably approaches the current best-case scenario of expected yield for diminutive lesions.

If the case can be made for the nonaggressive management of small 6- to 9-mm polyps detected at CTC, the appropriate handling of potential diminutive lesions becomes even more apparent. Even at OC, the need to remove or take biopsies of all diminutive lesions is individualized. Because of the high costs of polypectomy and pathologic assessment, as well as the limited yield in terms of important histology, some have suggested that diminutive lesions at colonoscopy could simply be ablated or resected but not sent for pathologic assessment. For several reasons, we believe it is prudent to go one step further for CTC and not report potential diminutive lesions in isolation. The likelihood of a false-positive finding is greatly increased over nondiminutive lesions (see **Fig. 3**). However, even if an isolated diminutive polyp is real, it is almost certainly just a nonneoplastic lesion (eg, hyperplastic polyp or normal mucosa) or nonadvanced tubular adenoma, neither of which has enough clinical importance to warrant polypectomy referral. The rare diminutive advanced adenoma will likely grow to a relevant size at follow-up if truly important, allowing for more selective polypectomy. The current CTC screening interval of 5 years should effectively allow for this determination. Invasive cancer in the diminutive size range is so rare that it can be assumed to be nonexistent in terms of population screening. Although the future risk related to finding multiple adenomas at OC is well established,[69] this has not been stratified by lesion size. The risk related to multiple diminutive-only lesions is unknown but probably much lower. CTC detection of at least 1 nondiminutive polyp would presumably identify most patients at increased risk, although this needs to be proven. It is also important to note that OC detection of diminutive lesions and attempted matching with CTC findings can be highly problematic, incurring additional time, costs, and complications. Therefore, a CTC study without any polyps of 6 mm or larger is considered a negative study, corresponding to C-RADS category C1.[12] However, when larger polyps are present, we often incidentally note the presence of high-confidence diminutive lesions for the endoscopist.

In terms of cost-effectiveness, the initial published analyses assumed that all CTC-detected diminutive lesions would automatically be referred to colonoscopy.[72–75] This

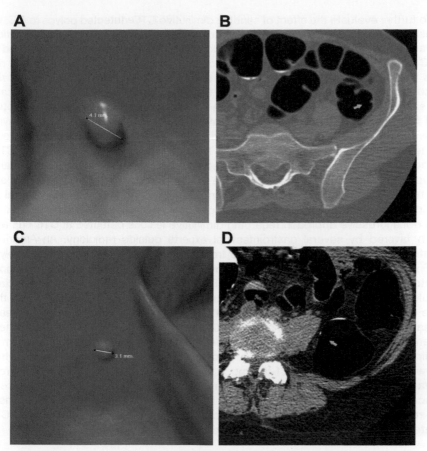

Fig. 3. Diminutive lesions at CTC screening. 3D endoluminal CTC image (*A*) shows a diminutive 4-mm lesion, which appears to be composed of soft tissue at 2D correlation (*B, arrow*). However, most diminutive lesions (*C*) will represent residual adherent stool, which will show internal tagging if oral contrast has been applied (*D, blue arrow*). Regardless of whether these lesions are true polyps or pseudolesions, we believe they should not be reported in isolation at CTC. (*From* Pickhardt PJ, Kim DH. Potential pitfalls at CTC interpretation. In: CT colonography: principles and practice of virtual colonoscopy. Philadelphia: Saunders; 2010. p. 287; with permission.)

not only fails to represent actual clinical practice but also greatly diminishes the theoretical cost-effectiveness of CTC. By using a 6-mm reporting threshold at CTC screening in a hypothetical cohort of 100,000 adults, our Markov analysis showed that CTC is a safer and more cost-effective screening option than OC.[9] CTC screening resulted in a 78% reduction in invasive endoscopic procedures compared with primary OC screening (39,374 vs 175,911), as well as more than 1000 fewer OC-related complications from perforation or bleeding. Reporting of diminutive lesions at CTC increased the CRC prevention rate by about 1%, with an ICER of more than $100,000 per life-year gained. We concluded that removal of diminutive lesions carries an unjustified burden of costs and complications relative to the minimal gains in CRC prevention.

To further evaluate the effect of sending diminutive CTC-detected polyps to OC, we constructed a decision analysis model incorporating the expected polyp distribution, advanced adenoma prevalence, CRC risk, CTC performance, and costs related to CRC screening and treatment.[11] The model conservatively assumed that CRC risk was independent of advanced adenoma size, which clearly overestimates the risk of subcentimeter polyps. For example, a 3-mm tubulovillous adenoma would carry the same cancer risk as a 3-cm villous adenoma with high-grade dysplasia. We found that the number of diminutive polyps that needed to be removed to avoid leaving behind 1 advanced adenoma was 562, and that 2352 diminutive polypectomies would be needed to prevent 1 CRC in 10 years. The ICER for removing all diminutive CTC-detected polyps was $464,407, compared with a cost saving for removal of large polyps only. We again concluded that the low likelihood of advanced neoplasia and the high costs associated with polypectomy argue against colonoscopic referral for diminutive polyps, whereas removal of large CTC-detected polyps was effective.

A nonaggressive approach regarding diminutive lesions detected at CTC has also been favored by several gastrointestinal experts outside radiology. An American Gastroenterological Association future trends report from 2004 noted that "polyps ≤ 5 mm in size do not appear to be a compelling reason for colonoscopy and poly-pectomy."[15] In an editorial from 2005, Ransohoff[13] remarked that "few clinicians would likely argue that colonoscopy is justified" for diminutive lesions, adding that "the overwhelming majority cannot possibly represent an important near-term health threat."[13] In an insightful editorial from 2001, Bond[10] remarked that "a large volume of scientific data indicates that clinicians need to shift their attention away from simply finding and harvesting all diminutive colorectal adenomas toward strategies which allow the reliable detection of the much less common, but much more dangerous advanced adenoma." Although a some gastroenterologists have suggested that colo-noscopy referral should be considered for isolated CTC-detected diminutive lesions,[44] the real controversy regarding the clinical management of polyps detected at CTC relates more to the handling of small 6- to 9-mm colorectal polyps.

CTC DETECTION OF FLAT COLORECTAL POLYPS

Colorectal polyps are generally divided into 3 major morphologic categories: sessile, pedunculated, and flat. Sessile polyps have a broad base of attachment, whereas pedunculated polyps have a defined lesion head and a polyp stalk that connects the lesion head to the adjacent colonic surface. The term "polypoid" can then refer to sessile and pedunculated polyps. Polypoid lesions account for most findings, including most advanced adenomas and cancers.[5,25] Flat lesions represent a subset of sessile polyps that, as the name implies, have a nonpolypoid or plaquelike morphology. A polyp height that is less than half its width has been commonly used as a morphologic descriptor.[76,77] However, this definition is too forgiving and could theoretically include lesions that would be more suitably labeled as sessile. For smaller flat polyps less than 1 to 2 cm, lesion elevation above the surrounding mucosal surface is typically 3 mm or less.[12] Categorization of large, superficially elevated lesions that are clearly flat in morphology but which may exceed a maximal height of 3 mm is less uniform. The term "carpet lesion," also referred to as a laterally or superficially spreading tumor, best applies to this important nonpolypoid subset that tends to be large in cross-sectional area but not bulky in appearance (**Fig. 4**).[78]

The prevalence and clinical significance of flat (nonpolypoid) lesions have been the source of recent debate. Endoscopic detection of nonpolypoid lesions may be increased by the use of advanced endoscopic techniques such as chromoendoscopy and narrow-band imaging. However, unlike the case for East Asia,[79] there is little evidence to suggest that small, flat, aggressive lesions represent a major problem in the screening population in the United States. Although a single-center Veterans Administration study by Soetikno and colleagues[77] suggested that important nonpolypoid lesions may be more common in the United States than was previously believed, a closer analysis of this work reveals that the conclusions are not well supported by the findings.[80] First, a clear distinction must be made between the flat lesions described in this study (defined as elevated lesions with a height less than half the diameter), and completely flat or depressed lesions. The investigators clearly state in this paper that "completely flat lesions are exceedingly rare" and it seems they were completely absent in this study. Furthermore, depressed lesions comprised less than 1% of all colorectal lesions (18 of 2770), only 4 of which were identified at screening. Most of these depressed lesions presumably had a raised edge, but this information was not provided. Therefore, all or nearly all of the nonpolypoid lesions in this study were elevated from the surrounding mucosa, a critical distinction that favors detection at OC and CTC. In addition, the investigators included carcinoma

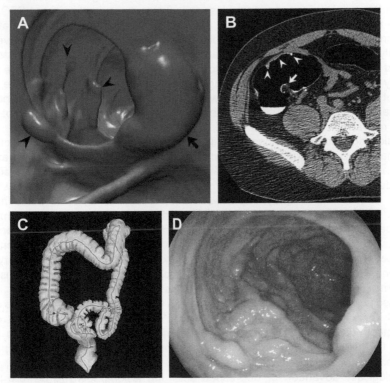

Fig. 4. Cecal carpet lesion detected at CTC screening. 3D endoluminal (*A*) and 2D transverse (*B*) CTC images show a large 4-cm laterally spreading tumor (carpet lesion) within the cecum (*arrowheads*), opposite the ileocecal valve (*arrow*). 3D colon map (*C*) shows the precise location of the lesion (*red dot*) for the endoscopist. With good CTC technique, these flat lesions can be detected with high confidence. A biopsy was taken of the lesion at OC (*D*), but could not resected endoscopically. Multiple biopsies showed tubular adenoma without high-grade dysplasia. The patient underwent laparoscopic right hemicolectomy for definitive treatment.

in situ, which is more appropriately termed "high-grade dysplasia," with invasive cancer.[81] As such, most (11 of 15) nonpolypoid cancers in this study were noninvasive advanced adenomas. The average size of advanced nonpolypoid lesions was large (1.6 cm) and similar in size to their polypoid counterparts (1.9 cm), which is also reassuring for detection at CTC (or standard OC).

By comparison, data from the National Polyp Study showed that flat adenomas were less likely to harbor high-grade dysplasia compared with sessile or pedunculated adenomas.[82] Patients with flat adenomas in this trial were not found to be at greater risk for advanced adenomas at subsequent surveillance colonoscopy. If aggressive flat lesions had somehow been missed at the index colonoscopy in the National Polyp Study, more incident cancers would presumably have developed in the course of longitudinal evaluation.[80,83]

Our own experience with flat lesions detected at CTC screening has also shown a pattern of nonaggressive lesions.[84] Of 92 flat CTC-detected lesions measuring less than 3 cm evaluated at subsequent OC, 23 (25.0%) were neoplastic, 5 (5.4%) were histologically advanced, and none was malignant. In comparison, polypoid lesions measuring less than 3 cm were more likely to be neoplastic (60.3%; 363 of 602), histologically advanced (12.1%; 73 of 602), and malignant (0.5%; 3 of 602). Most of these flat lesions measured less than 3 mm in maximal height at CTC, suggesting that this represents a suitable criterion. Of the 9 flat lesions missed at CTC but seen at colonoscopy in this screening cohort, none was histologically advanced and only 2 were neoplastic (tubular adenomas). In contrast, all 10 carpet lesions (defined as flat, laterally spreading tumors ≥3 cm) were neoplastic and 9 were histologically advanced. These findings suggest that flat lesions less than 3 cm are probably not a major concern compared with polypoid lesions of similar size, and that large carpet lesions represent the subset of polyps with flat morphology of most clinical relevance.

Considering colorectal lesions of similar (linear) size, flat lesions will be less conspicuous than polypoid lesions at CTC and OC. However, reasonable sensitivity at CTC can nonetheless be achieved with oral contrast tagging and combined 3D and 2D polyp detection methods at CTC.[76] Phantom and clinical studies have shown that the 3D endoluminal display improves the sensitivity of CTC for detecting flat lesions.[76,79,85] The 2D multiplanar images remain critical for lesion confirmation. Continued improvements in CTC interpretation and computer-aided detection software have resulted in further increases in sensitivity for detection.[86] In our recent clinical experience, more large, flat, advanced adenomas were detected at primary CTC screening compared with parallel primary OC screening, although such lesions were uncommon in either screening arm.[5] Perhaps a more legitimate concern is the increased rate of discordant findings between CTC and OC, in which flat lesions called at CTC cannot be found at subsequent OC.[66] Some of these discordant cases undoubtedly represent CTC false-positive interpretations, but we have also found several OC false-negative results where a discordant flat lesion is ultimately proved to be real on subsequent CTC and OC.

Histologically advanced or depressed small flat lesions seem to be rare in our screening population. Most flat lesions detected (or missed) at CTC are hyperplastic.[22,87] This is likely due in part to the tendency of hyperplastic polyps to flatten when the colonic lumen is distended.[88] In comparison, large serrated polyps tend to be more conspicuous at CTC in our experience. In the Mayo Clinic experience, most occult polyps at CTC (ie, missed lesions that could not be identified even retrospectively) were flat hyperplastic polyps ranging in size from 6 mm to 2.1 cm.[89] This mirrors our own clinical experience with occult lesions at CTC.[22,90] Given these collective findings, we believe that flat lesions measuring less than 3 cm remain a diagnostic challenge but do not represent a major drawback to widespread CTC screening.

Carpet lesions are an important subset of flat lesions that, despite their large surface area, can be subtle on CTC because of the paucity of raised tissue. These lesions have a strong predilection for the rectum and cecum (see **Fig. 4**).[91] Despite their large linear size, carpet lesions have a low rate of malignancy but frequently show villous features, with or without high-grade dysplasia.[78,91] Although classic carpet lesions are less conspicuous than large sessile or pedunculated polyps, they are nonetheless detectable at CTC in our experience, because of the fixed fold distortion and the raised edges that often have a rolled-up or polypoid appearance (see **Fig. 4**). Optimal preparation and distention, as well as a hybrid 3D-2D detection strategy, allow for confident detection of carpet lesions. In some cases, endoscopic mucosal resection can serve as the definitive treatment, whereas others will require more aggressive surgery.[78]

SUMMARY

With the advent of less invasive, nontherapeutic colorectal screening tests such as CTC, strict adherence to a "leave no polyp behind" approach loses its validity on clinical and economic grounds, and from a patient safety standpoint. We must remain open-minded about novel approaches to colorectal screening that will safely and effectively increase compliance rates beyond OC screening alone. All cancers presumably arise from smaller benign polyps, but this does not imply that polypectomy is indicated for every small benign lesion. The mindset of universal polypectomy has long been applied to primary OC screening, although even this may be changing because of the limited clinical yield related to diminutive polypectomy, which is also associated with significant costs and complications. An aggressive management approach to smaller polyps makes even less sense when applying safer nontherapeutic tests such as CTC that provide a filter between polyp detection and invasive therapy. More recent screening data on the low prevalence rates of important histology in small and diminutive lesions further support a nonaggressive approach. The current concepts and existing data surrounding flat (nonpolypoid) lesions also support the parallel use of CTC screening alongside primary OC screening to increase overall adherence rates.

REFERENCES

1. Jemal A, Siegel R, Ward E, et al. Cancer statistics, 2009. CA Cancer J Clin 2009; 59(4):225–49.
2. Levin B, Lieberman DA, McFarland B, et al. Screening and surveillance for the early detection of colorectal cancer and adenomatous polyps, 2008: a joint guideline from the American Cancer Society, the US Multi-Society Task Force on Colorectal Cancer, and the American College of Radiology. CA Cancer J Clin 2008;58(3):130–60.
3. Hassan C, Pickhardt P, Laghi A, et al. Computed tomographic colonography to screen for colorectal cancer, extracolonic cancer, and aortic aneurysm. Arch Intern Med 2008;168(7):696–705.
4. Johnson CD, Chen MH, Toledano AY, et al. Accuracy of CT colonography for detection of large adenomas and cancers. N Engl J Med 2008;359(12): 1207–17.

5. Kim DH, Pickhardt PJ, Taylor AJ, et al. CT colonography versus colonoscopy for the detection of advanced neoplasia. N Engl J Med 2007;357(14):1403–12.
6. Pickhardt PJ. Incidence of colonic perforation at CT colonography: review of existing data and implications for screening of asymptomatic adults. Radiology 2006;239(2):313–6.
7. Pickhardt PJ, Choi JR, Hwang I, et al. Computed tomographic virtual colonoscopy to screen for colorectal neoplasia in asymptomatic adults. N Engl J Med 2003;349(23):2191–200.
8. Pickhardt PJ, Hanson ME, Vanness DJ, et al. Unsuspected extracolonic findings at screening CT colonography: clinical and economic impact. Radiology 2008; 249(1):151–9.
9. Pickhardt PJ, Hassan C, Laghi A, et al. Cost-effectiveness of colorectal cancer screening with computed tomography colonography – the impact of not reporting diminutive lesions. Cancer 2007;109(11):2213–21.
10. Bond JH. Clinical relevance of the small colorectal polyp. Endoscopy 2001;33(5): 454–7.
11. Pickhardt PJ, Hassan C, Laghi A, et al. Small and diminutive polyps detected at screening CT colonography: a decision analysis for referral to colonoscopy. AJR Am J Roentgenol 2008;190(1):136–44.
12. Zalis ME, Barish MA, Choi JR, et al. CT colonography reporting and data system: a consensus proposal. Radiology 2005;236(1):3–9.
13. Ransohoff DF. Colonoscopy is justified for any polyp discovered during computed tomographic colonography - CON: immediate colonoscopy is not necessary in patients who have polyps smaller than 1 cm on computed tomographic colonography. Am J Gastroenterol 2005;100(9):1905–7.
14. Rockey DC, Barish M, Brill JV, et al. Standards for gastroenterologists for performing and interpreting diagnostic computed tomographic colonography. Gastroenterology 2007;133(3):1005–24.
15. Van Dam J, Cotton P, Johnson CD, et al. AGA future trends report: CT colonography. Gastroenterology 2004;127(3):970–84.
16. Pickhardt PJ. CT colonography (virtual colonoscopy) for primary colorectal screening: challenges facing clinical implementation. Abdom Imaging 2005; 30(1):1–4.
17. Pickhardt PJ, Hassan C, Laghi A, et al. Clinical management of small (6- to 9-mm) polyps detected at screening CT colonography: a cost-effectiveness analysis. AJR Am J Roentgenol 2008;191(5):1509–16.
18. Regula J, Rupinski M, Kraszewska E, et al. Colonoscopy in colorectal-cancer screening for detection of advanced neoplasia. N Engl J Med 2006;355(18): 1863–72.
19. Yoo TW, Park DI, Kim YH, et al. Clinical significance of small colorectal adenoma less than 10 mm: the KASID study. Hepatogastroenterology 2007;54(74):418–21.
20. Lieberman D, Moravec M, Holub J, et al. Polyp size and advanced histology in patients undergoing colonoscopy screening: implications for CT colonography. Gastroenterology 2008;135(4):1100–5.
21. Pickhardt PJ, Kim DH. Colorectal cancer screening with CT colonography: key concepts regarding polyp prevalence, size, histology, morphology, and natural history. AJR Am J Roentgenol 2009;193(1):40–6.
22. Pickhardt PJ, Choi JR, Hwang I, et al. Nonadenomatous polyps at CT colonography: prevalence, size distribution, and detection rates. Radiology 2004;232(3):784–90.
23. Winawer SJ, Zauber AG. The advanced adenoma as the primary target of screening. Gastrointest Endosc Clin N Am 2002;12(1):1–9, v.

24. O'Brien MJ. Hyperplastic and serrated polyps of the colorectum. Gastroenterol Clin North Am 2007;36(4):947–68.
25. Kim DH, Pickhardt PJ, Taylor AJ. Characteristics of advanced adenomas detected at CT colonographic screening: implications for appropriate polyp size thresholds for polypectomy versus surveillance. AJR Am J Roentgenol 2007;188(4):940–4.
26. Shinya H, Wolff WI. Morphology, anatomic distribution and cancer potential of colonic polyps. Ann Surg 1979;190(6):679–83.
27. Muto T, Bussey HJ, Morson BC. Evolution of cancer of colon and rectum. Cancer 1975;36(6):2251–70.
28. Matek W, Guggenmoosholzmann I, Demling L. Follow-up of patients with colorectal adenomas. Endoscopy 1985;17(5):175–81.
29. Hain KS, Pickhardt PJ, Kim DH. Rate of important histology in large and small polyps detected at CT colonography screening. Presented at Annual Meeting for the Society of Gastrointestinal Radiologists, Maui, Hawaii, March 15–20, 2009.
30. Pickhardt PJ, Taylor AJ, Kim DH, et al. Screening for colorectal neoplasia with CT colonography: initial experience from the 1st year of coverage by third-party payers. Radiology 2006;241(2):417–25.
31. Waye JD, Lewis BS, Yessayan S. Colonoscopy – a prospective report of complications. J Clin Gastroenterol 1992;15(4):347–51.
32. Silvis SE, Nebel O, Rogers G, et al. Endoscopic complications. Results of 1974 American Society for Gastrointestinal Endoscopy Survey. JAMA 1976;235(9):928–30.
33. Levin TR. Complications of colonoscopy. Ann Intern Med 2007;147(3):213–4.
34. Fruhmorgen P, Demling L. Complications of diagnostic and therapeutic colonoscopy in the Federal Republic of Germany. Results of an inquiry. Endoscopy 1979;11(2):146–50.
35. Bersentes K, Fennerty B, Sampliner RE, et al. Lack of spontaneous regression of tubular adenomas in two years of follow-up. Am J Gastroenterol 1997;92(7):1117–20.
36. Hoff G, Foerster A, Vatn MH, et al. Epidemiology of polyps in the rectum and colon – recovery and evaluation of unresected polyps 2 years after detection. Scand J Gastroenterol 1986;21(7):853–62.
37. Hofstad B, Vatn M, Larsen S, et al. Growth of colorectal polyps – recovery and evaluation of unresected polyps of less than 10 mm, 1 year after detection. Scand J Gastroenterol 1994;29(7):640–5.
38. Hofstad B, Vatn MH, Andersen SN, et al. Growth of colorectal polyps: redetection and evaluation of unresected polyps for a period of three years. Gut 1996;39(3):449–56.
39. Knoernschild HE. Growth rate and malignant potential of colonic polyps: early results. Surg Forum 1963;14:137–8.
40. Welin S, Youker J, Spratt JS Jr. The rates and patterns of growth of 375 tumors of the large intestine and rectum observed serially by double contrast enema study (Malmoe technique). Am J Roentgenol Radium Ther Nucl Med 1963;90:673–87.
41. Togashi K, Shimura K, Konishi F, et al. Prospective observation of small adenomas in patients after colorectal cancer surgery through magnification chromocolonoscopy. Dis Colon Rectum 2008;51(2):196–201.
42. Stryker SJ, Wolff BG, Culp CE, et al. Natural history of untreated colonic polyps. Gastroenterology 1987;93(5):1009–13.
43. Loeve F, Boer R, Zauber AG, et al. National Polyp Study data: evidence for regression of adenomas. Int J Cancer 2004;111(4):633–9.
44. Rex DK. Colonoscopy is justified for any polyp discovered during computed tomographic colonography - PRO: patients with polyps smaller than 1 cm on

computed tomographic colonography should be offered colonoscopy and polypectomy. Am J Gastroenterol 2005;100(9):1903–5.

45. Pickhardt PJ, Lee AD, McFarland EG, et al. Linear polyp measurement at CT colonography: in vitro and in vivo comparison of two-dimensional and three-dimensional displays. Radiology 2005;236(3):872–8.

46. Park SH, Choi EK, Lee SS, et al. Polyp measurement reliability, accuracy, and discrepancy: optical colonoscopy versus CT colonography with pig colonic specimens. Radiology 2007;244(1):157–64.

47. Pickhardt PJ, Kim DH, Cash BD, et al. The natural history of small polyps at CT colonography. Presented at Annual Meeting for the Society of Gastrointestinal Radiologists. Rancho Mirage (CA), February 17–22, 2008.

48. Fenlon HM, Nunes DP, Schroy PC, et al. A comparison of virtual and conventional colonoscopy for the detection of colorectal polyps. N Engl J Med 1999;341(20): 1496–503.

49. Graser A, Stieber P, Nagel D, et al. Comparison of CT colonography, colonoscopy, sigmoidoscopy and faecal occult blood tests for the detection of advanced adenoma in an average risk population. Gut 2009;58(2):241–8.

50. Pineau BC, Paskett ED, Chen GJ, et al. Virtual colonoscopy using oral contrast compared with colonoscopy for the detection of patients with colorectal polyps. Gastroenterology 2003;125(2):304–10.

51. Yee J, Akerkar GA, Hung RK, et al. Colorectal neoplasia: performance characteristics of CT colonography for detection in 300 patients. Radiology 2001;219(3): 685–92.

52. Iannaccone R, Laghi A, Catalano C, et al. Computed tomographic colonography without cathartic preparation for the detection of colorectal polyps. Gastroenterology 2004;127(5):1300–11.

53. Kim YS, Kim N, Kim SH, et al. The efficacy of intravenous contrast-enhanced 16-raw multidetector CT colonography for detecting patients with colorectal polyps in an asymptomatic population in Korea. J Clin Gastroenterol 2008;42(7):791–8.

54. Pickhardt PJ, Nugent PA, Mysliwiec PA, et al. Location of adenomas missed by optical colonoscopy. Ann Intern Med 2004;141(5):352–9.

55. Cotton PB, Durkalski VL, Benoit PC, et al. Computed tomographic colonography (virtual colonoscopy) – a multicenter comparison with standard colonoscopy for detection of colorectal neoplasia. JAMA 2004;291(14):1713–9.

56. Johnson CD, Harmsen WS, Wilson LA, et al. Prospective blinded evaluation of computed tomographic colonography for screen detection of colorectal polyps. Gastroenterology 2003;125(2):311–9.

57. Rockey DC, Poulson E, Niedzwiecki D, et al. Analysis of air contrast barium enema, computed tomographic colonography, and colonoscopy: prospective comparison. Lancet 2005;365(9456):305–11.

58. Heresbach D, Barrioz T, Lapalus MG, et al. Miss rate for colorectal neoplastic polyps: a prospective multicenter study of back-to-back video colonoscopies. Endoscopy 2008;40(4):284–90.

59. Kaltenbach T, Friedland S, Soetikno R. A randomised tandem colonoscopy trial of narrow band imaging versus white light examination to compare neoplasia miss rates. Gut 2008;57(10):1406–12.

60. Rex DK, Cutler CS, Lemmel GT, et al. Colonoscopic miss rates of adenomas determined by back-to-back colonoscopies. Gastroenterology 1997;112(1):24–8.

61. Lefere PA, Gryspeerdt SS, Dewyspelaere J, et al. Dietary fecal tagging as a cleansing method before CT colonography: initial results-polyp detection and patient acceptance. Radiology 2002;224(2):393–403.

62. Jensch S, De Vries AH, Peringa J, et al. CT colonography with limited bowel preparation: performance characteristics in an increased-risk population. Radiology 2008;247(1):122–32.
63. Arnesen RB, Adamsen S, Svendsen LB, et al. Missed lesions and false-positive findings on computed-tomographic colonography: a controlled prospective analysis. Endoscopy 2005;37(10):937–44.
64. Arnesen RB, Von Benzon E, Adamsen S, et al. Diagnostic performance of computed tomography colonography and colonoscopy: a prospective and validated analysis of 231 paired examinations. Acta Radiol 2007;48:831–7.
65. Pedersen BG, Christiansen TE, Bjerregaard NC, et al. Colonoscopy and multidetector-array computed-tomographic colonography: detection rates and feasibility. Endoscopy 2003;35(9):736–42.
66. Pickhardt PJ, Wise SM, Kim DH. Positive predictive value for polyps detected at screening CT colonography. European Radiology 2010. [Epub ahead of print].
67. Mang T, Schaefer-Prokop C, Schima W, et al. Comparison of axial, coronal, and primary 3D review in MDCT colonography for the detection of small polyps: a phantom study. Eur J Radiol 2009;70(1):86–93.
68. Martinez ME, Baron JA, Lieberman DA, et al. A pooled analysis of advanced colorectal neoplasia diagnoses after colonoscopic polypectomy. Gastroenterology 2009;136(3):832–41.
69. Winawer SJ, Zauber AG, Fletcher RH, et al. Guidelines for colonoscopy surveillance after polypectomy: a consensus update by the US Multi-Society Task Force on Colorectal Cancer and The American Cancer Society. Gastroenterology 2006; 130(6):1872–85.
70. Halligan S, Altman DG, Taylor SA, et al. CT colonography in the detection of colorectal polyps and cancer: systematic review meta-analysis and proposed minimum data set for study level reporting. Radiology 2006;238(3):893–904.
71. Mulhall BP, Veerappan GR, Jackson JL. Meta-analysis: computed tomographic colonography. Ann Intern Med 2005;142(8):635–50.
72. Heitman SJ, Manns BJ, Hilsden RJ, et al. Cost-effectiveness of computerized tomographic colonography versus colonoscopy for colorectal cancer screening. Can Med Assoc J 2005;173(8):877–81.
73. Ladabaum U, Song K, Fendrick AM. Colorectal neoplasia screening with virtual colonoscopy: when, at what cost, and with what national impact? Clin Gastroenterol Hepatol 2004;2(7):554–63.
74. Sonnenberg A, Delco F, Bauerfeind P. Is virtual colonoscopy a cost-effective option to screen for colorectal cancer? Am J Gastroenterol 1999;94(8): 2268–74.
75. Vijan S, Hwang I, Inadomi J, et al. The cost-effectiveness of CT colonography in screening for colorectal neoplasia. Am J Gastroenterol 2007;102(2):380–90.
76. Pickhardt PJ, Nugent PA, Choi JR, et al. Flat colorectal lesions in asymptomatic adults: implications for screening with CT virtual colonoscopy. AJR Am J Roentgenol 2004;183(5):1343–7.
77. Soetikno RM, Kaltenbach T, Rouse RV, et al. Prevalence of nonpolypoid (flat and depressed) colorectal neoplasms in asymptomatic and symptomatic adults. JAMA 2008;299(9):1027–35.
78. Tanaka S, Haruma K, Oka S, et al. Clinicopathologic features and endoscopic treatment of superficially spreading colorectal neoplasms larger than 20 mm. Gastrointest Endosc 2001;54(1):62–6.
79. Park SH, Lee SS, Choi EK, et al. Flat colorectal neoplasms: definition, importance, and visualization on CT colonography. Am J Roentgenol 2007;188(4):953–9.

80. Pickhardt PJ, Levin B, Bond JH. Screening for nonpolypoid colorectal neoplasms. JAMA 2008;299(23):2743 [author reply: 2743–4].
81. Obrien MJ, Winawer SJ, Zauber AG, et al. The national polyp study – patient and polyp characteristics associated with high-grade dysplasia in colorectal adenomas. Gastroenterology 1990;98(2):371–9.
82. O'Brien MJ, Winawer SJ, Zauber AG, et al. Flat adenomas in the national polyp study: is there increased risk for high-grade dysplasia initially or during surveillance? Clin Gastroenterol Hepatol 2004;2(10):905–11.
83. Pickhardt PJ. High-magnification chromoscopic colonoscopy: caution needs to be exercised before changing screening policy – reply. AJR Am J Roentgenol 2006;186(2):577–8.
84. Robbins J, Pickhardt PJ, Kim DH. Flat (nonpolypoid) lesions detected at CT colonography. Presented at the Annual Meeting for the Society of Gastrointestinal Radiologists, Maui, Hawaii, March 15–20, 2009.
85. Mang TG, Schaefer-Prokop C, Maier A, et al. Detectability of small and flat polyps in MDCT colonography using 2D and 3D imaging tools: results from a phantom study. AJR Am J Roentgenol 2005;185(6):1582–9.
86. Park SH, Kim SY, Lee SS, et al. Sensitivity of CT colonography for nonpolypoid colorectal lesions interpreted by human readers and with computer-aided detection. AJR Am J Roentgenol 2009;193(1):70–8.
87. Fidler JL, Johnson CD, MacCarty RL, et al. Detection of flat lesions in the colon with CT colonography. Abdom Imaging 2002;27(3):292–300.
88. Waye JD, Bilotta JJ. Rectal hyperplastic polyps – now you see them, now you don't – a differential point. Am J Gastroenterol 1990;85(12):1557–9.
89. MacCarty RL, Johnson CD, Fletcher JG, et al. Occult colorectal polyps on CT colonography: implications for surveillance. AJR Am J Roentgenol 2006;186(5): 1380–3.
90. Cornett D, Barancin C, Roeder B, et al. Findings on optical colonoscopy after positive CT colonography exam. Am J Gastroenterol 2008;103(8):2068–74.
91. Rubesin S, Saul S, Laufer I, et al. Carpet lesions of the colon. Radiographics 1985;5(4):537–52.
92. Barclay RL, Vicari JJ, Doughty AS, et al. Colonoscopic withdrawal times and adenoma detection during screening colonoscopy. N Engl J Med 2006; 355(24):2533–41.
93. Rex DK, Overhiser AJ, Chen SC, et al. Estimation of impact of American College of Radiology recommendations on CT colonography reporting for resection of high-risk adenoma findings. Am J Gastroenterol 2009;104(1):149–53.
94. Church JM. Clinical significance of small colorectal polyps. Dis Colon Rectum 2004;47(4):481–5.
95. Sprung D. Prevalence of adenocarcinoma in small adenomas. Am J Gastroenterol 2006;101:S199.
96. Odom SR, Duffy SD, Barone JE, et al. The rate of adenocarcinoma in endoscopically removed colorectal polyps. Am Surg 2005;71(12):1024–6.
97. Ginnerup Pedersen B, Christiansen TE, Bjerregaard NC, et al. Colonoscopy and multidetector-array computed-tomographic colonography: detection rates and feasibility. Endoscopy 2003;35:736–42.
98. Iannaccone R, Laghi A, Catalano C, et al. Computed tomographic colonography without cathartic preparation for the detection of colorectal polyps. Gastroenterology 2004;127:1300–11.

Debate: Diminutive Polyps Noted at CT Colonography Need Not Be Reported

Dipti K. Lenhart, MD[a], Michael E. Zalis, MD[b],*

KEYWORDS

- Colorectal polyps • CT colonography
- Diminutive polyps • Optical colonoscopy

The authors propose that radiologists should not report diminutive polyps (<6 mm in size) detected on CT colonography (CTC). This recommendation derives from 4 lines of data and reasoning: (1) the extremely low clinical significance of diminutive polyps; (2) the poor detection and characterization performance of both CTC and optical colonoscopy (OC) for these lesions; (3) the minimal, if any gain, with respect to colon cancer prevention specifically associated with their removal, and (4) the impetus to optimize use of limited medical resources and minimize overdiagnosis.

THE ADVANCED ADENOMA

The currently accepted evolution of colon cancer is via the "adenoma-carcinoma sequence," a term first coined by Jackman and Mayo in 1951,[1] and further developed and refined by pathologists including Morson, Muto, and Bussey.[2,3]

The model for progression from normal epithelium to adenoma to carcinoma is a series of genetic mutations.[4] Colonic neoplasms are thought to arise as a result of mutational activation of oncogenes (ras gene on chromosome 12p) coupled with the mutational inactivation or loss of tumor suppression genes (familial adenomatous polyposis gene on chromosome 5q, p53 gene on chromosome 17p, and DCC gene on chromosome 18q). These mutations act at several steps in the progression from

[a] Division of Abdominal Imaging and Intervention, Department of Radiology, Massachusetts General Hospital, 55 Fruit Street, White 270, Boston, MA 02114, USA
[b] Division of Abdominal Imaging and Intervention, Department of Radiology, Massachusetts General Hospital, 25 New Chardon Street, Suite 400A, Boston, MA 02114, USA
* Corresponding author. Division of Abdominal Imaging and Intervention, Department of Radiology, Massachusetts General Hospital, 25 New Chardon Street, Suite 400A, Boston, MA 02114.
E-mail address: mzalis@mgh.harvard.edu

Gastrointest Endoscopy Clin N Am 20 (2010) 227–237
doi:10.1016/j.giec.2010.02.002
1052-5157/10/$ – see front matter © 2010 Published by Elsevier Inc.
giendo.theclinics.com

normal epithelium to hyperproliferative epithelium to early, intermediate, and late adenoma, and finally to carcinoma.

The degree of dysplasia is highly correlated with risk of malignancy because on a genetic and cellular level, increasing atypia leads to a stepwise progression toward carcinoma. The presence of high-grade dysplasia is therefore a strong predictor of which adenomas will go on to become carcinomas.

There is a direct, though nonlinear, relationship between the size of an adenoma and its likelihood to harbor malignancy. In a colonoscopy series of a nonscreening population, the prevalence of carcinoma in adenomas greater than 2 cm in size was 19.4%, whereas that in adenomas of less than 1 cm was 0.07%.[5] These data reflect an upper bound for the prevalence of carcinoma, as the prevalence of carcinoma and dysplasia is observed to be lower across all size ranges in an asymptomatic screening population compared to a nonscreening cohort.[3,5–8] Other OC-based clinical series have confirmed the relationship between size and grade of dysplasia.[9,10] Accordingly, it is well established that adenoma size correlates with the degree of cellular dysplasia. Some investigators have also proposed a direct relationship between increasing villous component seen on histology and the degree of dysplasia.[8] At present, the presence of high-grade dysplasia, adenoma size, and villous characteristics are the primary characteristics used to risk-stratify a polyp with respect to its propensity to harbor or develop malignancy.

Screening studies have targeted the removal of adenomas that have the highest potential of developing into colorectal carcinoma.[11] These "advanced adenomas" are typically defined by the presence of any of the following 3 criteria: high-grade dysplasia, size 10 mm or larger, or a substantial (>25%) villous component (ie, tubulovillous or villous adenomas). Lesions demonstrating these characteristics are thought to be at high risk of developing into colorectal carcinomas compared with their less advanced counterparts.[11,12] In an asymptomatic screening population, the overall prevalence of advanced adenoma or carcinoma (collectively termed advanced neoplasia) of any size is 3% to 4%[6,13]; the prevalence of subcentimeter advanced neoplasia is only 0.3%.[14]

THE DIMINUTIVE POLYP

In CTC, polyps are stratified by size as less than 6 mm (diminutive), 6 to 9 mm (small, or sometimes referred to as 'intermediate'), and equal to or greater than 10 mm (large).[15] Because polyp histology cannot be reliably characterized in vivo, size remains the most useful characteristic to assess the carcinomatous potential of a polyp before its resection. Thus, screening guidelines are developed based on size estimates and neoplasia prevalence estimates obtained from large clinical series. Several studies have established that approximately 50% of diminutive polyps are adenomas while the other 50% are nonneoplastic.[6,16,17] The prevalence of advanced histology in diminutive polyps is quite low and the accurance of their size measurement is limited, as discussed next.

MEASUREMENT OF POLYPS BY OC AND CTC

It is worth mentioning the nature of OC and CTC measurement because prior studies providing the framework for our current thinking on polyp size and risk of malignancy rely on these size measurements, in particular OC measurements, as the reference standard.

The use of any formal measurement device is variable in both clinical and research OC practice; no single measurement method has been consistently employed to estimate size of polyps observed at OC. Measurement methods employed in research trials of colonoscopy include visual estimation, linear probe, and open biopsy forceps; the latter, for example, having been employed in the National Polyp Study.[12] Considerable variability has been reported concerning the accuracy of OC measurements, including both under- and overestimation of polyp size.[18–22] Compared with visual estimation and linear probe, Gopalswamy and colleagues demonstrated that open biopsy forceps was the least accurate polyp measurement tool, with a 12.3% mean difference from the immediate post-resection (nonprocessed specimen) reference polyp size. This gap was further accentuated in polyps less than 6 mm in size, which demonstrated a 27.9% difference from the reference polyp size.[21]

In CTC, a polyp is measured along its single largest diameter, excluding the stalk, using a software-based caliper tool deployed by all vendors of CTC interpretation software.[15] The software-based caliper tool can be used on either the 2-dimensional (2D) multiplanar displays or the 3-dimensional (3D) (endoluminal) displays now universally available for CTC interpretation software. CTC measurements are performed within the context of a calibrated reference system established by the computed tomography (CT) gantry and scan parameters. When performed in an axial plane, these measurements are precise to approximately 0.7 mm (based on the standard parameters encountered for CTC imaging: an axial 512 × 512 pixel reconstruction matrix in a 35-cm field of view).[23] Increasing use of isotropic voxel imaging, a technique available in current generation scanners, permits preservation of similar high spatial resolution and precision for all CT measurements, including 3D-rendered (endoluminal) and nonaxial plane measurements.

These technical distinctions are further borne out in recent data comparing size measurements of polyps by OC and CTC; investigators observed that mean error for 2D-CTC polyp measurements was significantly lower than that for OC.[24] In sum, CTC provides the ability to make extremely precise size measurements of colonic lesions; however, the accepted prevalence estimates for polyp dysplasia are largely based on optical colonoscopy, which as usually practiced demonstrates relatively poor size measurement accuracy for polyps in the diminutive (<6 mm) size range.

PREVALENCE OF ADVANCED ADENOMA AND CARCINOMA IN DIMINUTIVE POLYPS

In current guidelines for colon screening and surveillance, only adenomatous polyps are of concern with respect to colorectal cancer risk; hyperplastic polyps, hamartomatous/juvenile polyps, mucosal tags, and lipomas confer no increased cancer risk.

However, it should be noted that in addition to the traditional adenoma-carcinoma sequence, the microsatellite-instability pathway is postulated as an alternate pathway of carcinogenesis in which a hyperplastic polyp may progress to a sessile serrated polyp, then to a dysplastic serrated polyp (also known as a serrated adenoma), and finally to colorectal carcinoma.[25] Any malignant risk consequent to this transformation is still associated with the development of an adenomatous precursor lesion; hence, it remains valid to say that hyperplastic lesions themselves are not the target of screening. The transformation and growth rate of serrated adenomas is less well defined in comparison to corresponding data for other adenomatous lesions. However, observed pathologic data suggest that small and diminutive sessile serrated adenomas demonstrate histologic abnormalities at rates comparable to conventional small and diminutive adenomas and hence confer similar clinical risk.[25] In Church's study of small polyps,[16] he assigned serrated adenomas to the same category as tubular adenomas, assuming a similar risk for both lesions.

Correctly estimating the prevalence of different polyp histologies is complicated by the varied ways in which prevalence data has been reported. Literature concerning colon polyps has described the prevalence of advanced neoplasia in both screening and nonscreening cohorts. Prevalence data have further variously been reported as a fraction of all detected polyps versus as a fraction of adenomas only. As mentioned previously, the prevalence of advanced neoplasia is higher in nonscreening, symptomatic cohorts compared with a screening, asymptomatic population (the latter being the target population for this discussion).[3,5–8] The prevalence of advanced features would also be higher when reported as a percentage of only adenomas rather than of all detected polyps. Because neither the radiologist nor the gastroenterologist can prospectively determine which polyps are adenomas, it makes the most practical sense to evaluate the prevalence of advanced neoplasia as a fraction of *all* polyps for the purposes of determining a reporting threshold in a screening population.

In nonscreening cohorts, the rate of advanced neoplasia has been reported in the National Polyp Study as approximately 2.0% among resected diminutive adenomas,[8] and in a study by Church as 2.1% among resected diminutive polyps.[16] In a surgical series of colonic adenoma specimens, the prevalence of cancer in diminutive adenomas was reported as 1.3%.[3] These figures certainly overestimate the risk when considering a nonscreening population and when considering *all* polyps.

In contrast, Odom et al. found only 1 case of carcinoma among 2851 resected diminutive adenomas (0.04%) in a retrospective analysis of a nonscreening population.[5]

In a recent OC study of a screening cohort, Lieberman et al. found 63 advanced adenomas out of 3744 diminutive polyps (1.7%).[26] In this study, serrated adenomas were also included as advanced lesions; however, the pathology literature suggests that the risk of a serrated adenoma is similar to that of a tubular adenoma.[25] If serrated adenomas are not considered advanced adenomas, as the literature suggests, then the prevalence of advanced adenomas in the study would further decrease to 1.2%. There was 1 case of carcinoma among the 3744 diminutive polyps (0.03%).

The results reported by Kim et al. in a comparison of parallel, concurrent screening programs using CTC and OC further support the conclusion that the prevalence of advanced neoplasia in diminutive polyps is negligible.[6] These investigators prospectively evaluated the experience of 3120 CTC and 3163 OC asymptomatic screening subjects and observed that the prevalence of advanced neoplasia was similar in both arms, even though the CTC program did not report diminutive polyps of less than 6 mm. Of 2995 polyps removed, 2006 were diminutive, and of these only 4 were advanced adenomas (0.2% of all diminutive polyps). None of the polyps less than 6 mm harbored carcinoma. The 18 cases of cancer reported in the series were all in polyps 10 mm or larger. The rate of advanced adenoma for polyps 6 to 9 mm was 2.0% and for polyps 10 mm or larger was 8.6%. Combined, these data reinforce the conclusion, as has been incorporated into clinical guidelines, that the prevalence of advanced neoplasia in diminutive polyps encountered for asymptomatic colon screening is less than 1%, and that asymptomatic screening should target the identification and possible removal of advanced adenomas.

CONTRIBUTION OF VILLOUS HISTOLOGY TO ADVANCED ADENOMAS

The National Polyp Study demonstrated that adenoma size and percentage of villous component were both correlated with the presence of high-grade dysplasia.[8] The investigators stratified diminutive adenomas (<6 mm in size) into 4 histologic subtypes: 0% villous component (tubular adenomas), 1% to 25% villous component,

26% to 75% villous component, and greater than 76% villous component. This study showed a progressively increasing percentage of high-grade dysplasia with each successive histologic category: 0.7% (n = 8) of diminutive purely tubular adenomas, 4.7% (n = 2) of diminutive adenomas with 1–25% villous component, 10.0% (n = 1) of diminutive adenomas with 26–75% villous component, and 20% (n = 1) of diminutive adenomas with greater than 75% villous component demonstrated high-grade dysplasia.

This observed association between increasing villous component and high-grade dysplasia is one reason that some have used villous component as an independent risk marker of developing carcinoma. However, it is important to keep in perspective the extremely low prevalence both of high-grade dysplasia and of substantial villous histology in diminutive polyps when making this association. In the National Polyp Study, only 12 of 1270 diminutive adenomas (0.9%) demonstrated high-grade dysplasia, and only approximately 15 of 1270 demonstrated a greater than 25% villous component (1.2%). Only 2 diminutive adenomas demonstrated both high-grade dysplasia and substantial villous histology (0.2%).[8] As a fraction of *all polyps encountered*, these prevalence data would be even lower.

The traditional definition of advanced adenomas has included all polyps with 25% or greater villous component, and it is not clear from the literature why this categorization is so inclusive when the National Polyp Study data demonstrate that adenomas with 25% villous component and adenomas with 75% villous component demonstrate different prevalences of high-grade dysplasia.[8] These data have led to recent debate in the pathology literature suggesting that the cancer risk ascribed to a polyp based on the presence of villous features is significant only when villous features comprise nearly all of the adenoma.[27]

Further obscuring the assessment of clinical significance of villous features in diminutive lesions is the considerable interobserver variability among pathologists in determining both the presence and percentage of villous features within a polyp. Using the National Polyp Study data, the authors analyzed interobserver variability using kappa statistics among the central study pathologists and the pathologists at the respective institutions where the polyps were originally obtained. All the pathologists used predefined World Health Organization criteria for villous features and high-grade dysplasia. There was a correlation of greater than 90% among pathologists with respect to determination of high-grade dysplasia; however, there was substantially less agreement with respect to the determination of the presence or absence of villous component, despite the presence of preestablished criteria (O'Brien MJ [Department of Pathology, Boston Medical Center, Boston, MA], personal communication, October 8, 2009).

A similar comparison was undertaken in the Multicenter Study on Colorectal Adenomas,[28] in which 4 gastrointestinal pathologists reviewed and classified 100 polyps. The histologic classification of adenomas was significantly different among all 4 pathologists, with median kappa values of 0.50, 0.15, and 0.36 for the diagnosis of tubular, tubulovillous, and villous adenomas, respectively. Along similar lines, in a Danish study comparing the interobserver variability among 3 pathologists in their evaluation of adenomas, the investigators observed only a 61% agreement among the 3 pathologists in characterizing adenoma histology in terms of villous component.[29] Finally, a study comparing the accuracy of community pathologists to a reference-standard consensus demonstrated that tubular adenoma was incorrectly upgraded to tubulovillous or villous adenoma in 35% of readings.[30]

In summary, there is a lack of concordance in interpreting the presence and degree of villous change and few data establishing that tubulovillous histology in a diminutive adenoma independently confers a clinically significant risk. It may be prudent to reconsider whether diminutive lesions with tubulovillous features and no observed high-grade dysplasia should be included as advanced adenomas.

The accurate clinical categorization of these lesions is important because it underlies the assumed clinical impetus to report or resect diminutive lesions, the vast majority of which demonstrate benign histology by any criteria. If only those lesions that contain high-grade dysplasia or carcinoma, regardless of villous histology, are included in the designation of an advanced lesion, then the percentage of advanced adenomas among diminutive lesions would be reduced by nearly half, further challenging the prudence of reporting diminutive lesions. For example, in Church's nonscreening OC study, inclusion of only those lesions with high-grade dysplasia or carcinoma would decrease the prevalence of advanced adenomas from 2.1% to 0.9% of all diminutive polyps, and in the National Polyp Study from 2.0% to 0.9% of all diminutive adenomas.[8,16] When considering the more applicable screening study by Lieberman et al. the prevalence of advanced adenoma would decrease from 1.2% to 0.05% (2 cases of high-grade dysplasia or carcinoma among 3744 diminutive polyps).[26]

In the authors' view, the combination of: (1) low prevalence of high-grade dysplasia and substantial villous component in diminutive polyps; (2) poor measurement characteristics of diminutive polyps; (3) low interobserver agreement for the presence and percentage of villous histology; and (4) limited outcome data highlighting the clinical risk of diminutive tubulovillous polyps without high-grade dysplasia all suggest that the classification of tiny tubulovillous polyps as "high-risk" based on the presence of villous component alone represents an overestimation of risk.

GROWTH OF POLYPS

Several prior studies have attempted to evaluate the natural history of polyps when left in situ. An early barium study from the Mayo Clinic followed polyps 10 mm or larger detected on barium enema for at least 12 months (mean 69 months).[31] In these large polyps, the investigators determined the cumulative risk of malignancy at 5, 10, and 20 years after detection to be 2.5%, 8%, and 24%, respectively. However, they did not collect data on small or diminutive polyps.

An early sigmoidoscopy study followed 213 patients with polyps ranging from 2 to 15 mm in size.[32] On the initial sigmoidoscopy, a permanent mark was tattooed at the base of each polyp to facilitate future reexamination. During the 3- to 5-year follow-up period, 4% of polyps increased in size, 70% demonstrated stability, 8% decreased in size, and 18% regressed completely. Only 2 polyps demonstrated malignancy on follow-up, both of which were larger than 6 mm.

Hoff et al. performed a prospective colonoscopic study in which they followed 194 polyps less than 5 mm in 102 individuals.[33] At the end of a 2-year period, they redetected 143 of the previously unresected polyps (74% redetection rate) and found 57 new polyps, of which 42 (21%) were adenomas. None of the new or redetected adenomas demonstrated advanced histology. There was an average growth of only 0.4 mm in 2 years for all redetected polyps (not including the polyps that had completely regressed), and none of the polyps reached a size of 5 mm. If a growth rate of 0.2 mm per year were inferred, than the doubling time of the average diminutive polyp measuring 2.7 mm would be greater than 10 years.

Another study by Hofstad et al. prospectively evaluated polyps less than 10 mm in size for a 3-year period with annual colonoscopy for redetection.[34] Of all adenomas, 25% were unchanged in size, 40% demonstrated growth, and 35% either completely regressed or diminished in size at 3 years. The mean growth of adenomas less than

5 mm in size was approximately 0.5 mm over 3 years; these data were reported for adenomas only and would be expected to be even lower when considering all polyps.

A recent study by Kim et al., included a subset of 158 patients with 1 or 2 small polyps 6 to 9 mm in size who elected for short-term CTC surveillance rather than immediate polypectomy. Fifty-four of these patients who returned for follow-up surveillance during the study period had 70 small polyps detected initially, of which 67 polyps (96%) remained stable or decreased in size (and were measuring using the more precise size measurement tools available to CTC). The remaining 3 polyps grew at least 1 mm (but remained <10 mm in size); on removal, none of these demonstrated advanced features.[6]

Several lines of data, including both endoscopic and CTC studies, suggest that many lesions, especially those less than 6 mm, are quiescent or in fact regress over time. Of the small fraction that do grow, the low observed growth rate suggests ample opportunity within the context of regular screening to detect lesions that reach a size at which the prevalence of advanced histologic abnormalities would merit intervention.

DETECTION PERFORMANCE OF OC

It is a common assumption that all existing polyps in a patient are removed on a colonoscopic survey; however, only those polyps that are seen are removed. Several polyps may be left behind as the OC miss rate is not negligible. Two studies used back-to-back colonoscopies to determine the colonoscopy miss rate.[35,36] One study by Rex et al. found a 27% miss rate for diminutive adenomas less than 6 mm, 13% for small 6- to 9-mm adenomas, and 6% for adenomas 10 mm or larger, with an overall miss rate of 24% for all adenomas.[36] This same study found a 28% miss rate for all nonadenomatous polyps. Another study by Hixson et al. determined the miss rate to be 14.7% for polyps less than 10 mm.[35]

The studies using back-to-back colonoscopy assumed colonoscopy to be its own reference standard. Using OC with segmental unblinding of CTC results as a reference standard, Pickhardt et al. demonstrated that 21 of 210 adenomas were missed by OC, yielding a 10% miss rate of colonoscopy for all adenomas 6 mm or larger.[37]

These studies suggest that in the course of current clinical practice, a substantial fraction of polyps, most of which are diminutive in size, are left behind in patients simply because they are not detected by OC.

DETECTION PERFORMANCE OF CT COLONOGRAPHY

In the study by Yee et al. evaluating the performance characteristics of CTC, 301 diminutive polyps were detected on optical colonoscopy, of which 178 were also seen on CTC, yielding a sensitivity of 60% for diminutive polyps.[38] There were 64 false-positive polyps detected on CTC (but not confirmed on OC), yielding a positive predictive value for diminutive polyps of CTC of 74%. These data suggest that only 74% of diminutive polyps that are prospectively called on CTC will be true polyps, and conversely that 26% will not be true lesions. Fecal material or normal mucosal projections can mimic tiny polyps, reducing the specificity of CTC findings.

When we combine the 74% CTC positive predictive value for all diminutive lesions with a 73% likelihood that a colonoscopist will detect a diminutive lesion (based on the 27% OC miss rate described by Rex et al.) referred from CTC,[36] this leads to the conclusion that only approximately 50% of diminutive lesions originally detected by CTC would be correctly classified and subsequently detected by follow-up OC. This low system performance is fortuitous, given the exceedingly low prevalence of significant histologic abnormalities among diminutive polyps (whose villous histology is often difficult to reliably grade) and the nonzero (approximately 0.4%) rate of complications associated with optical colonoscopy.[39] The risk for complication from OC is arguably greater than the prevalence of advanced neoplasia among diminutive polyps.

COST-EFFECTIVENESS

To assess the cost-effectiveness of different screening strategies, Pickhardt et al. applied a mathematical Markov model on a hypothetical cohort of 100,000 screening patients.[40] The first strategy assumed a no-size threshold in reporting polyps detected on CTC, whereas the second strategy assumed a minimum 6-mm size threshold for reporting polyps. The model assumed that 2940 cases of colorectal cancer would occur without screening. Using a no-size threshold of reporting, 1110 cases (37.3%) would be prevented compared with 1073 cases (36.5%) using a 6-mm threshold. The difference in reduction between the 2 techniques was only 0.8%, at a much greater cost to society if using the no-threshold strategy. The cost per life-year gained was $7138 for no-threshold reporting versus $4361 for a 6-mm threshold, a difference of $2777 per life-year gained. The OC referral rate with no-threshold reporting was over 1.5 times that for a 6-mm threshold. The associated complications of OC, including anesthesia complications, bowel perforation and bleeding, were doubled in a no-threshold strategy compared with a 6-mm threshold.

Zauber et al.[41] in an analysis commissioned by the Agency for Health Care Research and Quality (AHRQ), recently studied competitive colon screening strategies in 3 models that included polyp reporting by CTC beginning at a 6-mm size threshold. The base case scenario for this study assumed 100% subject adherence with optical colonoscopy, a rate of adherence that, to the authors' knowledge, has never been observed in any study of OC-based population screening. Not surprisingly, given this assumption in the base case scenario, OC dominated CTC. Subsequently in the same study, however, the investigators performed a sensitivity analysis in which they relaxed the 100% screening adherence assumption and reanalyzed the data using more realistic projections of OC and CTC adherence rates. Under these more realistic assumptions, screening by CTC at a 6-mm reporting threshold was comparably cost-effective to OC screening with respect to colon cancer mortality reduction.

SHOULD WE REPORT DIMINUTIVE POLYPS IF WE ALSO DETECT NONDIMINUTIVE POLYPS?

If the radiologist detects and reports a polyp of a size larger than 6 mm, the question arises as to whether synchronous diminutive polyps in the same patient should also be reported. In the context of regular screening, these diminutive polyps pose negligible risk for the development of colorectal cancer. Although the patient will already be undergoing a colonoscopy, the removal of diminutive lesions confers almost no added cancer prevention benefit while exposing patients to a nonzero risk of bowel perforation and bleeding. Moreover, the low detection performance of both CTC and OC for diminutive lesions still applies in this circumstance, potentially leading to wasted effort on the part of the endoscopist searching for false-positive diminutive pseudolesions. In the authors' view, the data support the policy that a single, consistent standard be employed in interpretation of CTC and that diminutive lesions should not be separately reported.

USE OF COLONOSCOPY

The current recommendation for postpolypectomy surveillance is at 3 years in a patient at high risk of developing metachronous advanced adenoma (ie, a patient with >2 adenomas of any size, ≥1 cm adenoma, adenoma with substantial villous histology or high-grade dysplasia, or family history of cancer) and at 5 years for a low-risk patient. Surveillance is not recommended for a hyperplastic polyp.[12,42]

Despite these established guidelines, use of colonoscopy by both gastroenterologists and surgeons exceeds these recommendations. In a survey conducted by the National Cancer Institute to assess the prevailing perception of appropriate postpolypectomy surveillance,[43] more than 50% of gastroenterologists reported that they would initiate a surveillance colonoscopy at 3 years or sooner after having removed a single small (<1 cm) adenoma, despite the recommended surveillance interval of 5 years for such a lesion. For high-risk patients, nearly half of gastroenterologists recommended surveillance at 1 to 3 years, though the recommended interval is at 3 years. For hyperplastic lesions for which no surveillance is advocated, 24% of gastroenterologists and 54% of general surgeons reported that they would recommend surveillance.

Excess reporting of diminutive lesions would contribute to the observed tendency toward overuse of limited and expensive endoscopy resources. Moreover, in the context of regular screening intervals, which are assumed for all screening strategies including CTC, if a diminutive lesion were to enlarge to 6 mm, it would likely be identified on future studies and appropriately reported at that time. Whereas the positive predictive value of CTC for diminutive lesions is only 74%,[38] the positive predictive value of CTC for adenomas larger than 6 mm is approximately 90%.[44]

SUMMARY

Colorectal polyps less than 6 mm in size pose a negligible risk to the development of colorectal carcinoma. The sensitivity and specificity for detection of diminutive lesions on all available examinations including CTC and OC is relatively low. In the context of regular screening, the low clinical significance of diminutive polyps, their slow to negligible growth, and the low detection performance of CTC and OC for these lesions, would contribute to wasted health care resource and excess morbidity if each diminutive polyp were referred for potential resection. Respect for patient safety, attention to proper use of resources, and appropriate focus on larger, clinically significant polyps lead to the conclusion that colonic polyps of less than 6 mm should not be separately reported.

REFERENCES

1. Jackman RJ, Mayo CW. The adenoma-carcinoma sequence in cancer of the colon. Surg Gynecol Obstet 1951;93(3):327–30.
2. Morson B. President's address. The polyp-cancer sequence in the large bowel. Proc R Soc Med 1974;6734(6 Pt 1):451–7.
3. Muto T, Bussey HJ, Morson BC. The evolution of cancer of the colon and rectum. Cancer 1975;36(6):2251–70.
4. Fearon ER, Vogelstein B. A genetic model for colorectal tumorigenesis. Cell 1990; 61(5):759–67.
5. Odom SR, Duffy SD, Barone JE, et al. The rate of adenocarcinoma in endoscopically removed colorectal polyps. Am Surg 2005;71(12):1024–6.
6. Kim DH, Pickhardt PJ, Kim DH, et al. CT colonography versus colonoscopy for the detection of advanced neoplasia. N Engl J Med 2007;357(14):1403–12.
7. Lieberman DA, Holub JL, Moravec MD, et al. Prevalence of colon polyps detected by colonoscopy screening in asymptomatic black and white patients. JAMA 2008; 300(12):1417–22.

8. O'Brien MJ, Winawer SJ, Zauber AG, et al. The National Polyp Study. Patient and polyp characteristics associated with high-grade dysplasia in colorectal adenomas. Gastroenterology 1990;98(2):371–9.

9. Shinya H, Wolff WI. Morphology, anatomic distribution and cancer potential of colonic polyps. Ann Surg 1979;190(6):679–83.

10. Konishi F, Morson BC. Pathology of colorectal adenomas: a colonoscopic survey. J Clin Pathol 1982;35(8):830–41.

11. Bond JH. Polyp guideline: diagnosis, treatment, and surveillance for patients with colorectal polyps. Practice Parameters Committee of the American College of Gastroenterology. Am J Gastroenterol 2000;95(11):3053–63.

12. Winawer SJ, Zauber AG, O'Brien MJ, et al. Randomized comparison of surveillance intervals after colonoscopic removal of newly diagnosed adenomatous polyps. The National Polyp Study Workgroup. N Engl J Med 1993;328(13):901–6.

13. Pickhardt PJ, Kim DH. Advanced vs. "high risk" adenomas: identifying the relevant target for CT colonography screening. Am J Gastroenterol 2009;104(6):1599–600 [author reply: 1600].

14. Pickhardt PJ, Kim DH. Colorectal cancer screening with CT colonography: key concepts regarding polyp prevalence, size, histology, morphology, and natural history. AJR Am J Roentgenol 2009;193(1):40–6.

15. Zalis ME, Barish MA, Choi JR, et al. CT colonography reporting and data system: a consensus proposal. Radiology 2005;236(1):3–9.

16. Church JM. Clinical significance of small colorectal polyps. Dis Colon Rectum 2004;47(4):481–5.

17. Gottlieb LS, Winawer SJ, Sternberg S, et al. National Polyp Study: the diminutive colonic polyp. (Abstract submitted to A/S/G/E 1984). Gastrointest Endosc 1984;30(2):143.

18. Fennerty MB, Davidson J, Emerson SS, et al. Are endoscopic measurements of colonic polyps reliable? Am J Gastroenterol 1993;88(4):496–500.

19. Margulies C, Krevsky B, Catalano MF. How accurate are endoscopic estimates of size? Gastrointest Endosc 1994;40(2 Pt 1):174–7.

20. Schwartz E, Catalano MF, Krevsky B. Endoscopic estimation of size: improved accuracy by directed teaching. Gastrointest Endosc 1995;42(4):292–5.

21. Gopalswamy N, Shenoy VN, Choudhry U, et al. Is in vivo measurement of size of polyps during colonoscopy accurate? Gastrointest Endosc 1997;46(6):497–502.

22. Morales TG, Sampliner RE, Garewal HS, et al. The difference in colon polyp size before and after removal. Gastrointest Endosc 1996;43(1):25–8.

23. Bushberg JT, Seibert JA, Leidholdt EM, et al. The essential physics of medical imaging. Article 10. Baltimore (MD): Williams and Wilkins; 2008. p. 268.

24. Park SH, Choi EK, Lee SS, et al. Linear polyp measurement at CT colonography: 3D endoluminal measurement with optimized surface-rendering threshold value and automated measurement.

25. O'Brien MJ. Hyperplastic and serrated polyps of the colorectum. Gastroenterol Clin North Am 2007;36(4):947–68, viii.

26. Lieberman D, Moravec M, Holub J, et al. Polyp size and advanced histology in patients undergoing colonoscopy screening: implications for CT colonography. Gastroenterology 2008;135(4):1100–5.

27. Srivastava A, Redston M, Farraye FA, et al. Hyperplastic/serrated polyposis in inflammatory bowel disease: a case series of a previously undescribed entity. Am J Surg Pathol 2008;32(2):296–303.

28. Costantini M, Sciallero S, Giannini A, et al. Interobserver agreement in the histologic diagnosis of colorectal polyps. the experience of the multicenter adenoma colorectal study (SMAC). J Clin Epidemiol 2003;56(3):209–14.

29. Jensen P, Krogsgaard MR, Christiansen J, et al. Observer variability in the assessment of type and dysplasia of colorectal adenomas, analyzed using kappa statistics. Dis Colon Rectum 1995;38(2):195–8.
30. Rex DK, Alikhan M, Cummings O, et al. Accuracy of pathologic interpretation of colorectal polyps by general pathologists in community practice. Gastrointest Endosc 1999;50(4):468–74.
31. Stryker SJ, Wolff BG, Culp CE, et al. Natural history of untreated colonic polyps. Gastroenterology 1987;93(5):1009–13.
32. Knoernschild HE. Growth rate and malignant potential of colonic polyps: early results. Surg Forum 1963;14:137–8.
33. Hoff G, Foerster A, Vatn MH, et al. Epidemiology of polyps in the rectum and colon. Recovery and evaluation of unresected polyps 2 years after detection. Scand J Gastroenterol 1986;21(7):853–62.
34. Hofstad B, Vatn MH, Andersen SN, et al. Growth of colorectal polyps: redetection and evaluation of unresected polyps for a period of three years. Gut 1996;39(3):449–56.
35. Hixson LJ, Fennerty MB, Sampliner RE, et al. Prospective blinded trial of the colonoscopic miss-rate of large colorectal polyps. Gastrointest Endosc 1991;37(2):125–7.
36. Rex DK, Cutler CS, Lemmel GT, et al. Colonoscopic miss rates of adenomas determined by back-to-back colonoscopies. Gastroenterology 1997;112(1):24–8.
37. Pickhardt PJ, Nugent PA, Mysliwiec PA, et al. Location of adenomas missed by optical colonoscopy. Ann Intern Med 2004;141(5):352–9.
38. Yee J, Akerkar GA, Hung RK, et al. Colorectal neoplasia: performance characteristics of CT colonography for detection in 300 patients. Radiology 2001;219(3):685–92.
39. Podolsky DK. Going the distance—the case for true colorectal-cancer screening. N Engl J Med 2000;343(3):207–8.
40. Pickhardt PJ, Hassan C, Laghi A, et al. Cost-effectiveness of colorectal cancer screening with computed tomography colonography: the impact of not reporting diminutive lesions. Cancer 2007;109(11):2213–21.
41. Zauber AG, Knudsen AM, Rutter CM, et al. Cost-effectiveness of CT colonography to screen for colorectal cancer. Report to AHRQ from the Cancer Intervention and Surveillance Modeling Network (CISNET) for MISCAN, SimCRC, and CRC-SPIN Models. 2008. Available at: http://www.cms.hhs.gov/determinationprocess/downloads/id58TA.pdf. Accessed February 11, 2010.
42. Bond JH. Virtual colonoscopy—promising, but not ready for widespread use. N Engl J Med 1999;341(20):1540–2.
43. Mysliwiec PA, Brown ML, Klabunde CN, et al. Are physicians doing too much colonoscopy? A national survey of colorectal surveillance after polypectomy. Ann Intern Med 2004;141(4):264–71.
44. Pickhardt PJ, Taylor AJ, Kim DH, et al. Screening for colorectal neoplasia with CT colonography: initial experience from the 1st year of coverage by third-party payers. Radiology 2006;241(2):417–25.

Debate: Small (6–9 mm) and Diminutive (1–5 mm) Polyps Noted on CTC: How Should They Be Managed?

David Lieberman, MD

KEYWORDS

- Colon polyps • Colonoscopy • Colon imaging
- CT colonography

THE DILEMMA

Structural examinations of the colon have evolved over time. Until the 1960s, full colon visualization could only be achieved with barium enema. With the advent of colonoscopy, direct visualization with polyp detection and removal were possible. Since 2000, new diagnostic technologies have emerged that enable visualization, but not removal, of polyps. Capsule endoscopy is new, and still under development.[1] This discussion focuses on detection by computed tomographic colonography (CTC) of diminutive (1–5 mm) and small (6–9 mm) polyps.

These technologies create a dilemma: if polyps are visualized, do they need to be reported and do they need to be removed? Although there is clear consensus that polyps 10 mm or larger need to be removed, there is still controversy surrounding the appropriate reporting and management of small 1- to 5-mm and 6- to 9-mm polyps.

BACKGROUND
Likelihood of Detection of Diminutive and Small Polyps

CTC

From 2003 to 2007, CTC technology was evolving with the development of hardware (64-slice computed tomography [CT] scanners) and software for 2-dimensional and 3-dimensional imaging of the colon.[2–4] A large multicenter study was published in 2008 using modern technology and fully trained radiologists, which compared CTC to optical colonoscopy.[5] The investigators did not report findings less than 5 mm. Sensitivity for detection of polyps 6 to 9 mm in size was 65.3%. In a recent study

Division of Gastroenterology and Hepatology, Oregon Health and Science University, 3181 South West Sam Jackson Park Road, Portland, OR 97239, USA
E-mail address: lieberma@ohsu.edu

Gastrointest Endoscopy Clin N Am 20 (2010) 239–243
doi:10.1016/j.giec.2010.02.012
1052-5157/10/$ – see front matter © 2010 Elsevier Inc. All rights reserved.

that used advanced adenoma as the end point (defined as >20% villous or high-grade dysplasia), CTC sensitivity for advanced lesions 6 to 9 mm in size was 56.7%.[6]

Most experts believe that CTC is not accurate for detection of 1- to 5-mm lesions. These lesions are often barely polypoid (resulting in false-negative examinations) or may be confused with residual stool (resulting in false-positive examinations). One large study reported that CTC detected only 50 of 654 (7.6%) 1- to 5-mm polyps.[3] Therefore, most studies do not include diminutive polyps in their analysis.

Colonoscopy

Colonoscopy is the gold standard for detection of polyps in the colon, but it is far from perfect. In tandem colonoscopy studies, patients had a colonoscopy by one endoscopist who noted all polyps, and then a second endoscopist who removed all polyps. Although polyps 10 mm or larger were rarely missed, small polyps of less than 10 mm were commonly missed. Hixson and colleagues[7] reported missing 14.7% of polyps under 10 mm; Rex and colleagues[8] reported missing 27% of polyps 1 to 5 mm, and 13% of polyps 6 to 9 mm in size. These studies may underestimate the miss-rate because lesions missed by the first examiner could also be missed by the second.

With the advent of CTC, colonoscopy could be compared with another modality by using a method of segmental unblinding. CTC was performed, followed by colonoscopy. After each segment of colon was examined, the CTC results were revealed to the endoscopist. If a polyp was seen on CTC, but not colonoscopy, the segment was reexamined. If a polyp was then found on the second look, it was considered a missed lesion at colonoscopy. Using this methodology, polyps 10 mm or larger were missed in 2% to 12% of colonoscopies performed by expert endoscopists who knew that their performance was being assessed.[2–4]

Likelihood that Diminutive and Small Polyps are Neoplastic or have Advanced Features

Only 35% to 50% of small (1–5 mm) polyps will be neoplastic; 60% to 70% of polyps 6–9 mm will be neoplastic (**Table 1**). Among lesions that are adenomatous, several studies have analyzed polyps for advanced features, defined as villous histology, high-grade dysplasia, or cancer in screening cohorts. For adenomas 1 to 5 mm, advanced features were found in 2.7% to 3.4% of adenomas 1 to 5 mm in size, and in 8.2% to 9.7% of adenomas 6 to 9 mm in size.[9,10]

In the analysis by Lieberman and colleagues,[9] the rate of advanced histology based on largest polyp size was determined. This analysis included polyps that were nonneoplastic. In patients whose largest was polyp 1 to 5 mm, the rate of advanced histology was 1.7%; if the largest polyp was 6 to 9 mm, the rate of advanced histology was 6.6%. Advanced histology was found in 30.6% of polyps 10 mm or larger.

Table 1 Likelihood of polyp neoplasia based on polyp size		
	1–5 mm (% Neoplastic)	**6–9 mm (% Neoplastic)**
Pickhardt et al[2]	n = 966; 35.6%	n = 262; 60.7%
Johnson et al[4]		n = 392; 62.8% (5–9 mm)
Rockey et al[5]		n = 158; 61.4%
Lieberman et al[9]	n = 3744; 50%	n = 1198; 67.7%

Would Histologic Features or the Number of Neoplastic Polyps Help Inform a Surveillance Strategy for Patients?

Surveillance guidelines[11] recommend a 3-year surveillance interval if patients have polyps with advanced histology or have 3 or more adenomas of any size. These data are based on evidence that such patients have a higher risk of developing advanced neoplasia during a surveillance period.[11,12] Lacking histology or an accurate recording of the number of polyps, it would be difficult to recommend an appropriate surveillance strategy.

THE LARGEST POLYP IS 6 TO 9 MM: MANAGEMENT

Both CTC and colonoscopy may miss some polyps in this size range, as noted earlier. If the largest polyp is 6 to 9 mm, almost 7% of patients will have at least one polyp with advanced histologic features, which will rarely include invasive cancer or high-grade dysplasia. The number needed to colonoscope in order to identify one patient with advanced histology is 15.[9] However, there may be additional benefit to detection and removal of nonadvanced adenomas. Sixty percent to 70% of polyps in this size range are neoplastic without advanced features. There is evidence that detection and removal may reduce the incidence of colorectal cancer.[13] The number needed to colonoscope in order to detect one patient with any neoplasia would be 1.6. Recent colorectal cancer screening guidelines have recommended that all patients with polyps 6 to 9 mm in size should be offered colonoscopy[14] so that these polyps can be removed.

THE LARGEST POLYP IS 1 TO 5 MM: MANAGEMENT

The greatest controversy surrounds the reporting and management of patients whose largest polyp is 1 to 5 mm. In a per-patient analysis, 1- to 5-mm polyps are the only finding in 28.5% of patients who received screening with colonoscopy.[9] In a per-polyp analysis, polyps of this size accounted for 74% of the polyps found in 1233 adults[2]; this is a common clinical situation. Fifty percent or fewer of these polyps will be neoplastic, and advanced features will be rare. These lesions are commonly missed with both CTC and colonoscopy.

Should 1- to 5-mm Polyps be Reported?

Conventional practice of colonoscopy includes the reporting of all polypoid lesions. However, it is likely that many small polyps are overlooked, or seen but not reported. This scenario may be particularly true for clusters of small polyps in the rectum, which are most likely to be hyperplastic. Therefore, it is likely that many endoscopists may not report all small polyps at colonoscopy.

CTC is not accurate for detection of 1- to 5-mm polyps.[3] Lesions of this size are often flat and probably not seen with CTC. In addition, false-positive findings caused by residual stool affect the overall accuracy and positive predictive value. The viewpoint of most radiologists is that polyps of this size should not be reported, because the finding will not be reliable. Reporting could result in futile attempts to find small polyps at colonoscopy.

The "nonreporting" position implies that if patients have polyps of this size, they are clinically inconsequential. As noted above, the risk of advanced histology in 1- to 5-mm polyps is very small. However, clinical significance for determination of surveillance interval is based on the number of adenomas. Patients with 3 or more adenomas (of any size) are at increased risk for advanced adenomas during surveillance.[11] The studies did not stratify by polyp size, so most of the studies included both large and small adenomas in the analysis. If a patient has *only* small adenomas (3 or more), the risk of subsequent advanced neoplasia is uncertain. Based on current guidelines, the author would recommend a 3-year surveillance interval for individuals with 3 or more adenomas, irrespective of size. Failure to report small polyps could result in possible "undersurveillance."

There are other potential consequences of "nonreporting." It is not clear whether patients with small polyps seen at CTC should have follow-up earlier than patients with no polyps. There may be medicolegal consequences of nonreporting, but there are many precedents in radiology for not reporting clinically insignificant findings.

Risk of Leaving Small Polyps In Situ

Few natural history studies have been performed, all involving small cohorts of a few hundred patients.[15–18] If the largest polyp was 1 to 5 mm, the risk of advanced features was less than 2%. If the polyp was an adenoma, the likelihood of any growth over 1 to 2 years was less than 50%. Based on the little evidence that exists, leaving small polyps in situ for 3 years would have a very low risk of serious progression. If findings were reported, and if patients had follow-up imaging with CTC, it may be possible to improve our understanding of the natural history.

THE AUTHOR'S OPINION

I believe that CTC reports should include the finding of 1- to 5-mm polyps, if they can be identified with "high" reliability. If 1- to 5-mm polyps are the only finding, clinicians may opt to follow the patient without colonoscopy, and repeat the CTC at 3 to 5 years, knowing that the likelihood of serious histology and progression in this time period is very small. Such an approach would enable studies of natural history to determine an evidence-based approach to small polyps. This approach may be an especially reasonable one in older patients or individuals with significant comorbidities or on anti-coagulation therapy. In these individuals, the primary goal of the screening examination would be exclusion of obvious serious pathology. In younger healthy individuals, patients may prefer to have a clearing colonoscopy.

One important consequence of reporting 1- to 5-mm polyps is the effect on the cost of a CTC screening program. If rates of referral to colonoscopy are high (>25%), the test is unlikely to be cost-effective relative to screening with colonoscopy, unless the cost of CTC is very low. Future studies that define the natural history of 1- to 9-mm polyps will provide important evidence to support the safety of noninvasive follow-up of small polyps. CTC provides an ideal method for such studies.

REFERENCES

1. Van Gossum A, Munoz Navas M, Fernandez-Urien I, et al. Capsule endoscopy versus colonoscopy for the detection of polyps and cancer. N Engl J Med 2009;361:264–70.
2. Pickhardt PJ, Choie R, Hwang I, et al. Computed tomographic virtual colonoscopy to screen for colorectal neoplasia in asymptomatic adults. N Engl J Med 2003;349:2191–200.
3. Cotton PB, Durkalski VL, Pineau BC, et al. Computed tomographic colonography (virtual colonoscopy): a multicenter comparison with standard colonoscopy for detection of colorectal neoplasms. JAMA 2004;291:1713–9.

4. Rockey DC, Paulson E, Niedzwiecki D, et al. Analysis of air contrast barium enema, computed tomographic colonography and colonoscopy: prospective comparison. Lancet 2005;365:305–11.

5. Johnson CD, Chen MH, Toledano AY, et al. Accuracy of CT colonography for detection of large adenomas and cancers. N Engl J Med 2008;359:1207–17.

6. Regge D, Laudi C, Galatola G, et al. Diagnostic accuracy of computed tomographic colonography for the detection of advanced neoplasia in individuals at increased risk of colorectal cancer. JAMA 2009;301:2453–61.

7. Hixson LJ, Fennerty MB, Sampliner RE, et al. Prospective blinded trial of the colonoscopic miss-rate of large colorectal polyps. Gastrointest Endosc 1991;37: 125–7.

8. Rex DK, Cutler CS, Lemmel GT, et al. Colonoscopic miss rates of adenomas determined by back-to-back colonoscopies. Gastroenterology 1997;112:24–8.

9. Lieberman DA, Moravec M, Holub J, et al. Polyp size and advanced histology in patients undergoing colonoscopy screening: implications for CT colonography. Gastroenterology 2008;135:1100–5.

10. Butterly LF, Chase MP, Pohl H, et al. Prevalence of clinically important histology in small adenomas. Clin Gastroenterol Hepatol 2006;4:343–8.

11. Winawer SJ, Zauber AG, Fletcher RH, et al. Guidelines for colonoscopy surveillance after polypectomy: a consensus update by the US Multi-Society Task Force on colorectal cancer and the American Cancer Society. Gastroenterology 2006; 130:1872–85.

12. Lieberman DA, Weiss DG, Harford WV, et al. Five year colon surveillance after screening colonoscopy. Gastroenterology 2007;133:1077–85.

13. Winawer SJ, Zauber AG, Ho MN, et al. Prevention of colorectal cancer by colonoscopic polypectomy. N Engl J Med 1993;329:1977–81.

14. Levin B, Lieberman DA, McFarland B, et al. Screening and surveillance for early detection of colorectal cancer and adenomatous polyps, 2008: a joint guideline from the American Cancer Society, the US Multi-Society Task Force on Colorectal Cancer, and the American College of Radiology. Gastroenterology 2008;134: 1570–95.

15. Hoff G, Forerster A, Vatn MH, et al. Epidemiology of polyps in the rectum and colon. Scand J Gastroenterol 1986;21:853–62.

16. Hofstad B, Vatn MH, Andersen SN, et al. Growth of colorectal polyps: redetection and evaluation of unresected polyps for a period of three years. Gut 1996;39: 449–56.

17. Bersantes K, Fennerty MB, Sampliner RE, et al. Lack of spontaneous regression of tubular adenomas in two years of follow-up. Am J Gastroenterol 1997;92: 1117–20.

18. Togashi K, Shimura K, Konoshi F, et al. Prospective observation of small adenomas in patients after colorectal cancer surgery through magnification chromocolonoscopy. Dis Colon Rectum 2008;51:196–201.

Improving the Accuracy of CTC Interpretation: Computer-Aided Detection

Ronald M. Summers, MD, PhD

KEYWORDS

- CT colonography • Computer-aided detection
- Observer performance • Colonic polyps

Computer-aided detection (CAD) for computed tomographic colonography (CTC) was introduced in the late 1990s. CAD has developed rapidly and early clinical trials of CAD are beginning to appear in the literature. This article presents a brief overview of the current clinical status of CTC CAD. The article concludes with a description of some advanced computerized display technologies that assist CTC readings and may play an important role in improving the diagnostic efficacy of CTC.

RATIONALE FOR CAD

It has been shown that perceptual error reduces the sensitivity of CTC by 14% for polyps 1 cm in size or larger.[1] Given the multitude of images in a CTC study, the causes of perceptual error are not mysterious. Depending on the reconstruction interval, there can be 1200 images or more to interpret. For example, images in the prone and supine positions must be interpreted. Some investigators examine the colon antegrade and retrograde, and in lung and soft tissue windows. Three-dimensional virtual endoscopic views may also be needed for problem solving. Average interpretation times ranging from 15 to 25 minutes per study have been reported in the literature.[2,3]

Interpretive errors can lead to substantial reductions in the sensitivity of polyp detection.[4] Polyps can be missed if they are located between or behind haustral folds,

Grant support: The intramural research program of the National Institutes of Health Clinical Center supported this work.

Potential financial interest: The author has pending and/or awarded patents and receives royalty income from iCAD Medical. His laboratory received free research software from Viatronix and receives research support from iCAD Medical.

Imaging Biomarkers and Computer-Aided Diagnosis Laboratory, Radiology and Imaging Sciences, National Institutes of Health Clinical Center, Building 10, Room 1C368X MSC 1182, Bethesda, MD 20892-1182, USA

E-mail address: rms@nih.gov

in areas of poor bowel preparation or inadequate distention or because of inconspicuousness caused by flat shape. Factors affecting the ability to perceive abnormalities on large two-dimensional CT data sets and three-dimensional endoluminal fly-through images require further study.[5]

EFFECT OF READER FATIGUE

There is as yet little or no information about the effect of reader fatigue on the diagnostic efficacy of CTC interpretation. Anecdotally, radiologists report an upper limit on the number of CTC cases they can interpret per day, typically less than 10. Because interpretation of the CTC data is complex and requires manipulation of different types of images and sustained concentration, it is likely that fatigue is an issue. In addition, without addressing the lengthy interpretive process, it is unlikely that costs for CTC can be substantially reduced. It is therefore likely that CAD implementations that reduce fatigue will be beneficial for improving accuracy and reducing costs. Although some benefits of CAD in improving radiologist performance have been proved, it has not yet been shown that these benefits accrue because of a reduction in fatigue. However, fatigue and perceptual errors are closely intertwined. More research is needed in this area.

Performance of 1 Reader Versus 2 Readers (Single vs Double Reading) Without CAD

Double reading of medical images has been shown to increase sensitivity in certain settings, for example in interpretation of mammograms.[6] There has been relatively little work on double reading of CTC. In a study using 3 readers, Johnson and colleagues[7] found that the per patient and per polyp sensitivities tended to be higher and the specificity lower with double reading than for some single readings. However, there was considerable variability in the sensitivities of the 3 readers for polyp detection. In part, a hope is that CAD will provide a similar benefit to that of double reading but without the additional cost of the second human interpreter.

PRINCIPLES OF CAD

The purpose of CAD is to locate possible polyps automatically and annotate the images or present a list of image locations. The radiologist reviews the output of the CAD and makes the final diagnosis.

The main function of the CAD software is to identify sites with features characteristic of polyps.[8–12] Examples of useful features for CAD include surface shape and CT attenuation. Once these features are identified, the CAD software classifies sites of detection as potential polyps or false-positive diagnoses. A suitable CAD system has high sensitivity for detection of clinically significant polyps (those more than a size threshold, eg, 0.5 or 1.0 cm) and a low number of false-positive detections. All current CTC CAD systems produce on average at least 1 false-positive detection per CTC examination. Hence, review of the CAD marks by a trained reader is still required to prevent unnecessary referrals for colonoscopic polypectomy.

Once potential polyps are detected by CAD, they must be shown to the radiologist who makes the final diagnosis. There are several ways to do this. One way is to label sites directly on CTC images to show the radiologist where the potential polyps may be found.[13] These labels can be turned on or off so that they do not obscure the original images. To save time, the radiologist can jump directly to the labeled images. Labels can be applied to the two-dimensional cross-sectional and three-dimensional endoluminal images.

COMMON FALSE-POSITIVES

The most common CAD false-positives are on the ileocecal valve, thick haustral folds, residual fecal matter, and the rectal tube.[14–16] It is possible to reduce the numbers of these false-positives through various techniques. For example, the ileocecal valve can be identified because it tends to be large and contain fat leading to lower CT attenuation than that of polyps.[17,18] The rectal tube can be identified by its location in the rectum and by detecting its hollow channel.[19,20]

False-positives caused by residual fecal matter and thick haustral folds can be more difficult to eliminate. High-quality bowel preparation and adequate colonic distention can reduce these problems.[21–24]

REASONS FOR FALSE-NEGATIVES

The most common reasons for CAD false-negatives are flat polyps, inadequate colonic distention, residual fecal matter, adhering contrast medium, polyp at air-fluid boundary, and small polyp size.[14,15,25]

A flat polyp has a low elevation above the surface of the adjacent colonic mucosa. Flatter polyps are less conspicuous to radiologists and the CAD software.[26,27] Hyperplastic polyps tend to be flatter than adenomatous polyps making them less conspicuous and more difficult to diagnose.[28,29] The poorer sensitivity of CTC for detecting hyperplastic polyps may be beneficial by avoiding unnecessary colonoscopy and polypectomy for these lesions, which have lower malignant potential.[30]

Inadequate colonic distention can be prevented by careful technique and the use of carbon dioxide insufflators.[23,24] Quality assessment software can identify poor colonic distention in real time and allow correction before the patient leaves the examination room.[21,22]

Residual fecal matter and fluid can cover polyps and obscure them. Fecal and fluid tagging with barium- and iodine-based contrast materials enables visualization of such polyps.[2]

The CT attenuation of polyps adjacent to endoluminal contrast material can be artificially increased. This phenomenon, known as pseudoenhancement, can prevent polyp detection because the inflated CT values may greatly exceed typical soft tissue attenuation values. Software corrections can greatly improve the sensitivity for detecting such polyps, particularly those submerged under contrast-enhanced fluid.[31–33]

Contrast material can adhere to some polyps.[34] CAD software must be able to identify such polyps. Software that identifies polyps with adherent contrast material is under development.[35]

Polyps at the air-fluid boundary can be difficult to detect whether or not the fluid is tagged with contrast material. Software that improves electronic fluid subtraction at the air-fluid boundary may enable detection of such polyps.[36,37]

CAD performance tends to decrease for smaller polyps.[14] Polyps from 6 to 9 mm in size are of particular interest because patient management (surveillance vs immediate polypectomy) may depend on whether polyp size is at the high or low end of this range.[38] Even with the use of modern thin-section CT scanners, it is likely that CAD sensitivity for 6- and 7-mm polyps is substantially less than that of 8- and 9-mm polyps although these size subcategories are usually not reported separately.

CURRENT STATUS OF CTC CAD

CTC CAD is at an advanced stage of development.[39] Several small clinical trials have been published. Several commercial and precommercial CAD systems have been developed and have undergone or are undergoing regulatory review. In stand-alone CAD trials in the computer laboratory, as opposed to observer studies in which the performance of radiologists with CAD assistance is evaluated, the baseline sensitivities for detecting large ($\geq$10 mm) polyps are as high as 85% to 100% with less than 10 false-positives per patient.[10,12,14,40–42] These sensitivities reach or exceed those achieved by radiologists.

CAD has not yet been developed to handle the problem of extracolonic findings.[43–46] The multiplicity of potential sites and types of extracolonic findings makes it particularly difficult to develop a CAD system to detect them all.

STAND-ALONE CAD TRIALS: BASELINE PERFORMANCE OF CAD IN THE LABORATORY

In 2005, Summers and colleagues[14] published the results of a large stand-alone CAD trial. The investigators trained their CAD system on CTC data sets of 394 patients and tested 792 data sets, both sets taken from the Department of Defense screening CTC data set reported earlier by Pickhardt and colleagues.[2] The reference standard was segmentally unblinded optical colonoscopy. For the test set, per polyp and per patient sensitivities for CAD were both 89.3% (25 of 28 polyps) for detecting identifiable adenomatous polyps at least 1 cm in size. The false-positive rate was 2.1 per patient. The CAD system detected 1 cancer originally missed by the colonoscopists. At 8-mm and 10-mm adenoma size thresholds, the per patient sensitivities of CAD (85.4% and 89.3%, respectively) were not significantly different from those of optical colonoscopy before segmental unblinding.

Halligan and colleagues[47] published an external validation of a CAD system for CTC. External validation refers to the assessment of CAD applied to data different from that on which the CAD software was trained. The results of the external validation provide information about the generalizability of the CAD to different patient populations. The per polyp sensitivity of their CAD system was 94% for detecting polyps 6 mm or larger, indicating good generalizability. The false-positive rates ranged from 14 to 43 depending on the settings of a sphericity filter.

Summers and colleagues[15] reported an external validation study of their CAD system. Their CAD system had per polyp sensitivities of 91.5% for adenomas 10 mm or larger and 82.1% for adenomas 6 to 9 mm. The per patient sensitivities were 97.6% and 82.4%, respectively. The mean and median false-positive rates were 9.6 and 7.0 per patient, respectively.

Van Ravesteijn and colleagues[48] reported CAD sensitivities for polyps 6 mm or larger ranging from 85% to 100% with between 4 and 6 false-positives per scan. They applied their CAD system to 4 different data sets. They also performed a cross-center external evaluation and found that the trained CAD system generalized to data from different medical centers and with different patient preparations.

Lee and colleagues[25] reported the sensitivity of 3 different CAD systems for detecting simulated polyps in an anthropomorphic colonic phantom. For polyps 6 mm or larger, the differences in the per polyp sensitivities amongst the 3 CAD systems were not statistically significant. Sensitivities were lowest for flat polyps, intermediate for sessile polyps, and greatest for pedunculated polyps. The false-positive rates ranged from 2.6 to 4.6 per scan and were not statistically different but the distribution of causes of false-positives did differ amongst the 3 CAD systems.

EFFECT OF CAD ON OBSERVER PERFORMANCE: CAD AS A FIRST, CONCURRENT, OR SECOND READER

The stand-alone performance of CAD software in the laboratory described in the previous section describes the theoretic best performance achievable. However, when used in the clinic, CAD software rarely achieves its full potential. To assess the likely clinical benefit of CAD, researchers conduct observer performance experiments in which radiologists use CAD to read unknown cases. The experiments are typically conducted in a simulated clinical setting and to date have not been prospective clinical trials.

Radiologists may use CAD in 1 of 3 ways: as a first, concurrent, or second reader (**Fig. 1**). It is not yet clear how well the 3 methods compare with one another and this may depend on the particular CAD implementation. Therefore, the observations in this section should be regarded as preliminary.

In the first reader paradigm, the radiologist only reviews the CAD results and does not review the entire colon. This method has the potential advantage of reduced interpretation time and high specificity (because the choice of false-positives is limited to the CAD findings) but the potential disadvantage of lower sensitivity relative to the concurrent and second reader paradigms. At present, radiologists are naturally reluctant to use the first reader paradigm because only the computer reviews the entire CTC data set.

In the concurrent reader paradigm, the CAD marks are visible during the radiologist's primary interpretation of the images. The radiologist evaluates the CAD marks as they appear in the image. The potential advantages of this method are improved sensitivity and reduced interpretation time. These advantages may not actually be realized because the CAD marks could distract the radiologist from other findings in the vicinity of a mark, leading to "satisfaction of search" errors.[49] The radiologist could also mischaracterize CAD false-positives, leading to decreased specificity as well.

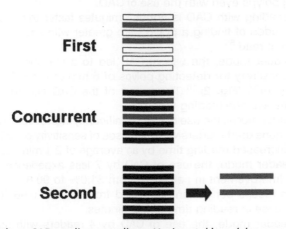

Fig. 1. Simplified three CAD reading paradigms. Horizontal bars (*clear, gray, solid*) represent CTC images. Clear bar indicates image has no CAD marks and is not reviewed by reader. Gray bar indicates image has CAD marks and is reviewed by reader. Black bar indicates image has no CAD marks and is reviewed by reader. In first reader mode, reader only reviews images with CAD marks. In concurrent reader mode, CAD marks are present during the reader's first pass through all the images. In second reader mode, all images are reviewed first without CAD marks, then reader reviews only images with CAD marks to arrive at final diagnosis.

In the second reader paradigm, the radiologist reviews the images, arrives at a preliminary diagnosis, reviews the CAD findings, and revises the preliminary diagnosis to arrive at a final diagnosis. Because CAD is not perfect, the radiologist should not disregard polyp candidates they identified that were not found by CAD. The potential advantage of this technique is sensitivity higher than either the first or concurrent reader paradigms. The disadvantages are the longest interpretation times and potentially reduced specificity compared with either the first or concurrent reads.

Although a CAD system may be marketed as being optimized for 1 of these 3 reading methods, it is quite possible that radiologists will adapt their reading style to another reading method based on personal choice and experience.

Several research publications have recently evaluated the performance of radiologists assisted by CAD. These publications are preliminary works with small numbers of cases and readers. Some of the relevant findings include:

1. Two-dimensional reading with the use of CAD may be quicker than three-dimensional reading without CAD, with similar sensitivity.[50]
2. CAD false-positives tend to be easily dismissed by expert radiologists.[51] Most polyps missed by expert readers were detected by CAD, potentially leading to increased sensitivity if correctly characterized by the readers.
3. Three-dimensional viewing slightly increased reader accuracy in classifying CAD polyp candidates as true- or false-positives.[52] Factors significantly associated with reader accuracy included polyp size and quality of the examination.
4. CAD in the first reader mode had similar sensitivity for detecting polyps and patients with polyps compared with that of reading without the aid of CAD.[53] The use of CAD decreased observer variability and reduced the time required to detect the first polyp by about half a minute.
5. For nonexpert readers, when CAD is used as a concurrent reader, CAD improves the sensitivity of the readers particularly for detecting polyps of 9 mm or less, and reduces interpretation times.[54] However, nonexpert readers had poor sensitivity for detecting polyps even with the use of CAD.
6. Concurrent reading with CAD is about 3 minutes faster than second read with CAD but the odds of finding a polyp were greater with second read compared with concurrent read.[55]
7. In second reader mode, the use of CAD led to a statistically significant 15% increase in sensitivity for detecting polyps of 6 mm or more, but it reduced the specificity by 14% (**Fig. 2**).[16] The review of the CAD findings added about 3 minutes to the average reading time.
8. In second reader mode, the use of CAD significantly improved sensitivity for polyp detection by nonexpert readers with increases of sensitivity of 15% to 20%.[56] The use of CAD increased reading time by an average of 2.1 minutes.
9. In second reader mode, the use of CAD by 7 less experienced readers led to a significant improvement in sensitivity from 81.0% to 90.8%.[57] The number of false-positive results per patient increased from 0.70 to 0.96. The use of CAD led to an increase in reading time of 3.6 minutes.
10. In second reader mode, the use of CAD by 4 readers with some experience reading CTC led to detection of a few more positive patients than CTC without CAD but the improvement in per patient sensitivity was not statistically significant for patients with polyps 6 mm or larger or for patients with polyps 10 mm or larger.[58] Specificity was nearly unchanged with CAD compared to without CAD.
11. Increasing numbers of CAD false-positive marks may not adversely affect specificity although the effect on sensitivity is unknown.[59] An increased number of CAD

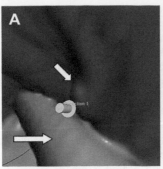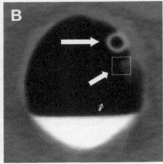

Fig. 2. Rectal 7-mm adenomatous polyp (*short white arrow*) initially missed by 4 readers but found by 3 of the readers after the use of CAD in the second reader mode. CAD prompts (*pink indicator in A, rectangle in B*) and rectal tube (*long white arrows*) are indicated. The polyp may have been missed initially because it was partially hidden behind the rectal tube. (*Reprinted from* Petrick N, Haider M, Summers RM, et al. CT colonography and computer-aided detection as a second reader: observer performance study. Radiology 2008;246(1):148–56.)

marks did lengthen reading times in the second reader mode, adding about half a minute to the time for review of the CAD output when there were more than 15 false-positive CAD marks per data set.

CHALLENGES AHEAD

Although CTC CAD research is producing exciting results, there are many challenges ahead.[60] The major advances are expected to be in the areas of increased sensitivity for smaller polyps, decreased false-positive rates, electronic stool subtraction for the uncleansed colon, and matching of detections on the supine and prone examinations.[61–64] The availability of larger databases of proven cases will contribute to these developments.

The major clinical challenge will be to evaluate the effect of CAD in an actual clinical interpretive setting. Studies will need to show that CAD improves clinical sensitivity without placing an undue burden through reduced specificity or increased interpretation time. Appropriate training in how to use CAD may be a key to its success. The economics also need to be addressed, as CAD software may be expensive and the use of CAD is as yet not reimbursed. In an economic analysis, CAD may improve the colorectal cancer prevention rate and may be cost-effective for CTC screening.[65]

INNOVATIVE DISPLAYS FOR CTC

Since its inception, CTC has been closely associated with innovative display methodologies.[66–68] For example, in 1994 Vining and colleagues[69] introduced virtual colonoscopy using surface reconstructions to model the interior of the colon. Many radiologists primarily use two-dimensional image display to interpret CTC, but some research indicates that three-dimensional virtual colonoscopy displays may lead to improved sensitivity for detecting polyps although this has been somewhat controversial.[70]

Although three-dimensional virtual colonoscopy displays seem natural because of their similar appearances compared with optical colonoscopy displays, endoluminal visualization methods have some limitations. For example, polyps can be hidden behind haustral folds during endoluminal inspection.[71] Novel displays such as

Mercator map and stereographic projections have been proposed to address the problem of unseen regions.[67] Modification of the three-dimensional viewing angle may also improve sensitivity and reduce the number of unseen regions.[67,72]

One type of innovative display is called virtual dissection, virtual pathology, or "filet" view.[73–75] These displays use computer software to virtually cut open the colon so that it can be inspected as if it were a pathologic specimen. The virtual dissection technique allows the physician to see the colon laid out flat without the need to navigate its various bends and blind spots. However, the virtual dissection display is susceptible to distortion. Modifications of this technique have been developed to reduce the distortion.[76] In addition, CAD has been integrated into some virtual dissection displays.[77,78] In one study, virtual dissection with CAD used in the first reader mode had sensitivity exceeding 94% for detecting polyps 1 cm or larger; the effect on specificity however was unclear.

Another promising display technology is the virtual unfolded cube display.[79] In this display, a radiologist sees a 360° view of the colon and can inspect forward, side, and rear views of the colon simultaneously. The virtual unfolded cube display may improve detection of polyps hidden behind haustral folds.

A novel display has been proposed that uses the location of the 3 tenia coli for circumferential coregistration of supine and prone CTC scans. This display brings the CTC scans into rotational alignment enabling improved matching of findings on the supine and prone three-dimensional endoluminal images.[80]

SUMMARY

Preliminary results in CTC CAD are encouraging. There is evidence that high sensitivity and a low number of false-positive detections per examination are achievable. The application of CAD to clinical practice is likely to help less experienced radiologists by improving their sensitivity for detecting polyps but may not reduce reading times. Novel displays may improve diagnostic accuracy and can be combined with CAD. With advances in computer technology and larger image databases, CAD performance is likely to improve rapidly and will hopefully benefit patients in the near future.

ACKNOWLEDGMENTS

I thank Sandy Napel, PhD, for critical review of the manuscript and helpful discussions.

REFERENCES

1. Fletcher JG, Johnson CD, Welch TJ, et al. Optimization of CT colonography technique: prospective trial in 180 patients. Radiology 2000;216(3):704–11.
2. Pickhardt PJ, Choi JR, Hwang I, et al. Computed tomographic virtual colonoscopy to screen for colorectal neoplasia in asymptomatic adults. N Engl J Med 2003;349(23):2191–200.
3. Johnson CD, Chen MH, Toledano AY, et al. Accuracy of CT colonography for detection of large adenomas and cancers. N Engl J Med 2008;359(12):1207–17.
4. Doshi T, Rusinak D, Halvorsen RA, et al. CT colonography: false-negative interpretations. Radiology 2007;244(1):165–73.
5. Summers RM. How perceptual factors affect the use and accuracy of CAD for interpretation of CT images. In: Samei E, Krupinski E, editors. The handbook of medical image perception and techniques. Cambridge: Cambridge University Press; 2009. p. 313–21.

6. Shaw CM, Flanagan FL, Fenlon HM, et al. Consensus review of discordant findings maximizes cancer detection rate in double-reader screening mammography: Irish National Breast Screening Program experience. Radiology 2009; 250(2):354–62.

7. Johnson CD, MacCarty RL, Welch TJ, et al. Comparison of the relative sensitivity of CT colonography and double-contrast barium enema for screen detection of colorectal polyps. Clin Gastroenterol Hepatol 2004;2(4):314–21.

8. Summers RM, Beaulieu CF, Pusanik LM, et al. Automated polyp detector for CT colonography: feasibility study. Radiology 2000;216(1):284–90.

9. Yoshida H, Nappi J. Three-dimensional computer-aided diagnosis scheme for detection of colonic polyps. IEEE Trans Med Imaging 2001;20(12):1261–74.

10. Paik DS, Beaulieu CF, Rubin GD, et al. Surface normal overlap: a computer-aided detection algorithm, with application to colonic polyps and lung nodules in helical CT. IEEE Trans Med Imaging 2004;23(6):661–75.

11. Sundaram P, Zomorodian A, Beaulieu C, et al. Colon polyp detection using smoothed shape operators: preliminary results. Med Image Anal 2008;12(2): 99–119.

12. Wang Z, Liang Z, Li L, et al. Reduction of false positives by internal features for polyp detection in CT-based virtual colonoscopy. Med Phys 2005;32(12): 3602–16.

13. Summers RM, Pusanik LM, Malley JD, et al. Method of labeling colonic polyps at CT colonography using computer-assisted detection. Presented at Computer Assisted Radiology and Surgery (CARS). San Francisco (CA), June 28–July 1, 2000.

14. Summers RM, Yao J, Pickhardt PJ, et al. Computed tomographic virtual colonoscopy computer-aided polyp detection in a screening population. Gastroenterology 2005;129(6):1832–44.

15. Summers RM, Handwerker LR, Pickhardt PJ, et al. Performance of a previously validated CT colonography computer-aided detection system in a new patient population. AJR Am J Roentgenol 2008;191(1):168–74.

16. Petrick N, Haider M, Summers RM, et al. CT colonography and computer-aided detection as a second reader: observer performance study. Radiology 2008; 246(1):148–56.

17. Summers RM, Yao J, Johnson CD. CT colonography with computer-aided detection: automated recognition of ileocecal valve to reduce number of false-positive detections. Radiology 2004;233(1):266–72.

18. O'Connor SD, Summers RM, Yao J, et al. CT colonography with computer-aided polyp detection: volume and attenuation thresholds to reduce false-positive findings owing to the ileocecal valve. Radiology 2006;241(2):426–32.

19. Iordanescu G, Summers RM. Reduction of false positives on the rectal tube in computer-aided detection for CT colonography. Med Phys 2004;31(10): 2855–62.

20. Suzuki K, Yoshida H, Nappi J, et al. Massive-training artificial neural network (MTANN) for reduction of false positives in computer-aided detection of polyps: suppression of rectal tubes. Med Phys 2006;33(10):3814–24.

21. Deshpande KK, Summers RM, Van Uitert RL, et al. Quality assessment for CT colonography: validation of automated measurement of colonic distention and residual fluid. AJR Am J Roentgenol 2007;189(6):1457–63.

22. Van Uitert RL, Summers RM, White JM, et al. Temporal and multiinstitutional quality assessment of CT colonography. AJR Am J Roentgenol 2008;191(5): 1503–8.

23. Shinners TJ, Pickhardt PJ, Taylor AJ, et al. Patient-controlled room air insufflation versus automated carbon dioxide delivery for CT colonography. AJR Am J Roentgenol 2006;186(6):1491–6.

24. Burling D, Taylor SA, Halligan S, et al. Automated insufflation of carbon dioxide for MDCT colonography: distension and patient experience compared with manual insufflation. AJR Am J Roentgenol 2006;186(1):96–103.

25. Lee MW, Kim SH, Park HS, et al. An anthropomorphic phantom study of computer-aided detection performance for polyp detection on CT colonography: a comparison of commercially and academically available systems. AJR Am J Roentgenol 2009;193(2):445–54.

26. Summers RM, Frentz SM, Liu J, et al. Conspicuity of colorectal polyps at CT colonography: visual assessment, CAD performance, and the important role of polyp height. Acad Radiol 2009;16(1):4–14.

27. Park SH, Ha HK, Kim AY, et al. Flat polyps of the colon: detection with 16-MDCT colonography–preliminary results. AJR Am J Roentgenol 2006;186(6):1611–7.

28. Summers RM, Liu J, Yao J, et al. Automated measurement of colorectal polyp height at CT colonography: hyperplastic polyps are flatter than adenomatous polyps. AJR Am J Roentgenol 2009;193(5):1305–10.

29. Pickhardt PJ, Choi JR, Hwang I, et al. Nonadenomatous polyps at CT colonography: prevalence, size distribution, and detection rates. Radiology 2004;232(3):784–90.

30. East JE, Saunders BP, Jass JR. Sporadic and syndromic hyperplastic polyps and serrated adenomas of the colon: classification, molecular genetics, natural history, and clinical management. Gastroenterol Clin North Am 2008;37(1):25–46, v.

31. Nappi J, Yoshida H. Adaptive correction of the pseudo-enhancement of CT attenuation for fecal-tagging CT colonography. Med Image Anal 2008;12(4):413–26.

32. Liu J, Yao J, Summers RM. Scale-based scatter correction for computer-aided polyp detection in CT colonography. Med Phys 2008;35(12):5664–71.

33. Tsagaan B, Nappi J, Yoshida H. Nonlinear regression-based method for pseudoenhancement correction in CT colonography. Med Phys 2009;36(8):3596–606.

34. O'Connor SD, Summers RM, Choi JR, et al. Oral contrast adherence to polyps on CT colonography. J Comput Assist Tomogr 2006;30(1):51–7.

35. Liu J, Chang Y, Summers RM. Automated detection of adherent contrast phenomenon on colonic polyps on CT colonography. Presented at RSNA. Chicago, November 29 to December 4, 2009.

36. Franaszek M, Summers RM, Pickhardt PJ, et al. Hybrid segmentation of colon filled with air and opacified fluid for CT colonography. IEEE Trans Med Imaging 2006;25(3):358–68.

37. Wang S, Li L, Cohen H, et al. An EM approach to MAP solution of segmenting tissue mixture percentages with application to CT-based virtual colonoscopy. Med Phys 2008;35(12):5787–98.

38. Pickhardt PJ. By-patient performance characteristics of CT colonography: importance of polyp size threshold data. Radiology 2003;229(1):291–3 [author reply: 293; discussion: 293].

39. Summers RM, Yoshida H. Future directions: computer-aided diagnosis. In: Dachman AH, editor. Atlas of virtual colonoscopy. New York: Springer; 2003. p. 55–62.

40. Yoshida H, Nappi J, MacEneaney P, et al. Computer-aided diagnosis scheme for detection of polyps at CT colonography. Radiographics 2002;22(4):963–79.

41. Kiss G, Van Cleynenbreugel J, Suetens P, et al. Computer aided diagnosis for CT colonography via slope density functions. Medical Image Computing and Computer-Assisted Intervention (MICCAI) 2003;2878(Pt 1):746–53.

42. Bogoni L, Cathier P, Dundar M, et al. Computer-aided detection (CAD) for CT colonography: a tool to address a growing need. Br J Radiol 2005;78(Spec No 1): S57–62.

43. Hara AK, Johnson CD, MacCarty RL, et al. Incidental extracolonic findings at CT colonography. Radiology 2000;215(2):353–7.

44. Gluecker TM, Johnson CD, Wilson LA, et al. Extracolonic findings at CT colonography: evaluation of prevalence and cost in a screening population. Gastroenterology 2003;124(4):911–6.

45. Pickhardt PJ, Taylor AJ. Extracolonic findings identified in asymptomatic adults at screening CT colonography. AJR Am J Roentgenol 2006;186(3): 718–28.

46. Xiong T, McEvoy K, Morton DG, et al. Resources and costs associated with incidental extracolonic findings from CT colonography: a study in a symptomatic population. Br J Radiol 2006;79(948):948–61.

47. Halligan S, Taylor SA, Dehmeshki J, et al. Computer-assisted detection for CT colonography: external validation. Clin Radiol 2006;61(9):758–63 [discussion: 764–5].

48. van Ravesteijn VF, van Wijk C, Truyen R, et al. Computer aided detection of polyps in CT colonography using logistic regression. IEEE Trans Med Imaging 2009;29(1):120–31.

49. Berbaum KS, Franken EA Jr, Dorfman DD, et al. Satisfaction of search in diagnostic radiology. Invest Radiol 1990;25(2):133–40.

50. Taylor SA, Halligan S, Slater A, et al. Polyp detection with CT colonography: primary 3D endoluminal analysis versus primary 2D transverse analysis with computer-assisted reader software. Radiology 2006;239(3):759–67.

51. Taylor SA, Halligan S, Burling D, et al. Computer-assisted reader software versus expert reviewers for polyp detection on CT colonography. AJR Am J Roentgenol 2006;186(3):696–702.

52. Shi R, Schraedley-Desmond P, Napel S, et al. CT colonography: influence of 3D viewing and polyp candidate features on interpretation with computer-aided detection. Radiology 2006;239(3):768–76.

53. Mani A, Napel S, Paik DS, et al. Computed tomography colonography – feasibility of computer-aided polyp detection in a "first reader" paradigm. J Comput Assist Tomogr 2004;28(3):318–26.

54. Halligan S, Altman DG, Mallett S, et al. Computed tomographic colonography: assessment of radiologist performance with and without computer-aided detection. Gastroenterology 2006;131(6):1690–9.

55. Taylor SA, Charman SC, Lefere P, et al. CT colonography (CTC): investigation of the optimum reader paradigm using computer aided detection (CAD) software. Radiology 2008;246(2):463–71.

56. Mang T, Peloschek P, Plank C, et al. Effect of computer-aided detection as a second reader in multidetector-row CT colonography. Eur Radiol 2007;17(10): 2598–607.

57. Baker ME, Bogoni L, Obuchowski NA, et al. Computer-aided detection of colorectal polyps: can it improve sensitivity of less-experienced readers? Preliminary findings. Radiology 2007;245(1):140–9.

58. de Vries AH, Jensch S, Liedenbaum MH, et al. Does a computer-aided detection algorithm in a second read paradigm enhance the performance of experienced

computed tomography colonography readers in a population of increased risk? Eur Radiol 2009;19(4):941–50.

59. Taylor SA, Greenhalgh R, Ilangovan R, et al. CT colonography and computer-aided detection: effect of false-positive results on reader specificity and reading efficiency in a low-prevalence screening population. Radiology 2008;247(1):133–40.

60. Summers RM. Challenges for computer-aided diagnosis for CT colonography. Abdom Imaging 2002;27:268–74.

61. Cai W, Zalis ME, Nappi J, et al. Structure-analysis method for electronic cleansing in cathartic and noncathartic CT colonography. Med Phys 2008;35(7):3259–77.

62. Nappi J, Yoshida H. Virtual tagging for laxative-free CT colonography: pilot evaluation. Med Phys 2009;36(5):1830–8.

63. Wang S, Van Uitert RL, Summers RM. Automated matching of supine and prone colonic polyps based on PCA and SVMs. Presented at Progress in Biomedical Optics and Imaging – Proceedings of SPIE. February 17–21, 2008.

64. Nappi J, Okamura A, Frimmel H, et al. Region-based supine-prone correspondence for the reduction of false-positive CAD polyp candidates in CT colonography. Acad Radiol 2005;12(6):695–707.

65. Regge D, Hassan C, Pickhardt PJ, et al. Impact of computer-aided detection on the cost-effectiveness of CT colonography. Radiology 2009;250(2):488–97.

66. Beaulieu CF, Jeffrey RB, Karadi G, et al. Visualization modes for CT colonography: blinded comparison of axial CT, virtual endoscopy, and panoramic-view volume rendering. Radiology 1998;209P:296–7.

67. Paik DS, Beaulieu CF, Jeffrey RB Jr, et al. Visualization modes for CT colonography using cylindrical and planar map projections. J Comput Assist Tomogr 2000; 24(2):179–88.

68. Beaulieu CF, Jeffrey RB Jr, Karadi C, et al. Display modes for CT colonography. Part II. Blinded comparison of axial CT and virtual endoscopic and panoramic endoscopic volume-rendered studies. Radiology 1999;212(1):203–12.

69. Vining DJ, Teigen EL, Stelts D, et al. Virtual colonoscopy: a 60-second colon examination. Radiology 1995;197(P):281.

70. Pickhardt PJ, Lee AD, Taylor AJ, et al. Primary 2D versus primary 3D polyp detection at screening CT colonography. AJR Am J Roentgenol 2007;189(6):1451–6.

71. Pickhardt PJ, Nugent PA, Mysliwiec PA, et al. Location of adenomas missed by optical colonoscopy. Ann Intern Med 2004;141(5):352–9.

72. East JE, Saunders BP, Boone D, et al. Uni- and bidirectional wide angle CT colonography: effect on missed areas, surface visualization, viewing time and polyp conspicuity. Eur Radiol 2008;18(9):1910–7.

73. Hoppe H, Quattropani C, Spreng A, et al. Virtual colon dissection with CT colonography compared with axial interpretation and conventional colonoscopy: preliminary results. AJR Am J Roentgenol 2004;182(5):1151–8.

74. Haker S, Angenent S, Tannenbaum A, et al. Nondistorting flattening maps and the 3-D visualization of colon CT images. IEEE Trans Med Imaging 2000;19(7):665–70.

75. Wang G, McFarland EG, Brown BP, et al. GI tract unraveling with curved cross sections. IEEE Trans Med Imaging 1998;17(2):318–22.

76. Kim SH, Lee JM, Eun HW, et al. Two- versus three-dimensional colon evaluation with recently developed virtual dissection software for CT colonography. Radiology 2007;244(3):852–64.

77. Johnson KT, Fletcher JG, Johnson CD. Computer-aided detection (CAD) using 360 degree virtual dissection: can CAD in a first reviewer paradigm be a reliable

substitute for primary 2D or 3D search? AJR Am J Roentgenol 2007;189(4): W172–6.

78. Hock D, Ouhadi R, Materne R, et al. Virtual dissection CT colonography: evaluation of learning curves and reading times with and without computer-aided detection. Radiology 2008;248(3):860–8.

79. Vos FM, van Gelder RE, Serlie IW, et al. Three-dimensional display modes for CT colonography: conventional 3D virtual colonoscopy versus unfolded cube projection. Radiology 2003;228(3):878–85.

80. Huang A, Roy DA, Summers RM, et al. Teniae coli-based circumferential localization system for CT colonography: feasibility study. Radiology 2007;243(2):551–60.

Radiologists Should Read CT Colonography

David H. Kim, MD*, Perry J. Pickhardt, MD

KEYWORDS

• CT colonography • Virtual colonoscopy • Interpretation

The debate regarding computed tomographic colonography (CTC) interpretation has elicited strong opinions and statements. Who is qualified to read CTC has become a central issue between radiologists and gastroenterologists in recent years, particularly with the maturation of CTC into an effective colorectal cancer screening modality.[1] In general, radiologists have an inherent advantage from prior imaging training, particularly in computed tomography (CT), whereas gastroenterologists are better versed in clinical topics surrounding the issue of colorectal cancer screening and hold unique experiences from colonoscopy. Although there are several important attributes of a quality CTC reader, it is clearly apparent to experienced CTC readers that the core of interpretation rests on a skill set rooted in the principles of cross-sectional imaging. Without a firm grasp of cross-sectional skills, evaluation of a CTC examination cannot be done. Any attempt to do so is inherently flawed and will ultimately lead to poor quality. This view forms the foundation of the argument that "radiologists should read CTC" or perhaps more correctly stated, "are better qualified to interpret CTC." In arguing this position, this article explores the components necessitating effective CTC interpretation, illustrating the need for cross-sectional imaging skills and exposing the common misconception regarding the role of the 3-dimensional (3D) endoluminal image. The issue of evaluation of extracolonic findings with CTC interpretation is also discussed. Once these concepts have been defined, the authors discuss whether radiologists or gastroenterologists would better be able to fulfill the requirements to provide quality interpretation.

COMPONENTS OF CTC INTERPRETATION

Despite the moniker of virtual colonoscopy, CTC is not truly virtual endoscopy. The postprocessing of CTC data can create images (ie, the 3D endoluminal view) that

Financial disclosures: D.H.K. and P.J.P. are consultants for Viatronix and Medicsight. They are co-founders of VirtuoCTC.

Department of Radiology, University of Wisconsin School of Medicine and Public Health, E3/311 600 Highland Avenue, Madison, WI 53792-3252, USA

* Corresponding author.

E-mail address: dkim@uwhealth.org

Gastrointest Endoscopy Clin N Am 20 (2010) 259–269

doi:10.1016/j.giec.2010.02.005

giendo.theclinics.com

simulate colonoscopy (**Fig. 1**); however, the interpretative skill set for CTC significantly differs from that of endoscopy. CTC is a low-dose, noncontrast CT examination. CTC has been optimized for luminal pathology where the bowel has been cleansed, any residual stool tagged, and the colon distended. The acquired thin section 2-dimensional (2D) CT images (typically 500 in each series; both supine and prone series are obtained) are then directly evaluated much in the same fashion as a standard CT examination as well as being postprocessed into various 3D series for additional evaluation.

There are 2 basic tasks in CTC interpretation. The first involves that of detection, where a list of potential polyps is generated. It is important to realize that many of these polyp candidates are not true soft tissue polyps but instead represent colonic folds or stool (tagged or untagged) (**Fig. 2**). The second task involves evaluating these polyp candidates to winnow down the list to the few true soft tissue polyps. The specific steps to accomplish these 2 tasks are different, dependent on the particular interpretative approach employed (primary 2D or primary 3D). However, both strategies require a solid foundation in cross-sectional imaging. Although there are proponents for one approach over another, data from the ACRIN 6664 study suggest that the best CTC readers employ both strategies as needed for a given examination.[2]

A primary 2D approach is so named for the use of the source 2D images during the polyp detection task. Image review is similar to the method of routine CT evaluation. Here, the 2D CT images (typically in the axial plane) are viewed in stack mode. By scrolling through the dataset, possible polyp candidates are identified as focal soft tissue protrusions into the colonic lumen that persist between the supine and prone series. The need for a strong cross-sectional skill set is obvious. It is important to realize that there are elements of characterization intertwined with detection with a primary 2D approach. Here, the assessment of the internal soft tissue make-up of the polyp candidate is undertaken during the detection phase. A suspected polyp is then confirmed at 3D where the 3D series is viewed to confirm morphology.[3] In other words, the soft tissue structure represents a focal polypoid structure and does not elongate out into a colonic fold (**Fig. 3**). Thus, detection is by the 2D series and confirmation (of morphology) is at 3D.

The alternative method of CTC interpretation is a primary 3D approach.[4] The basis of this strategy involves the use of a postprocessed series, which converts the CT data

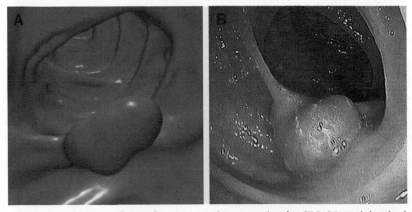

Fig. 1. A 73-year-old man who underwent routine screening by CTC. 3D endoluminal view (*A*) mirrors the optical image (*B*), demonstrating a large lobulated polyp. Pathology was positive for a tubulovillous adenoma.

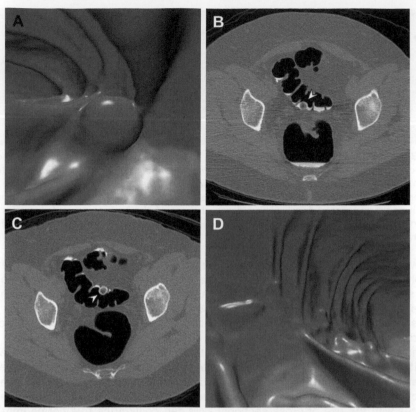

Fig. 2. Pseudopolyp related to stool. 3D endoluminal view (*A*) demonstrates a large sessile polyp in the sigmoid colon. Supine 2D transverse CTC image (*B*) shows that this polyp actually represents an untagged stool ball (*arrowhead*), which is mobile with prone positioning (*C*). 3D endoluminal CTC view (*D*) in another patient with a poor bowel preparation shows many potential polyps that simply represent pseudopolyps related to stool.

into a 3D perspective. This strategy has only been possible in recent years because of the marked advances in underlying computer hardware and software. Likely in part to the similarity of appearance to the optical colonoscopic image, a common misperception has arisen wherein it is thought that CTC interpretation can be accomplished by viewing the "virtual endoscopic" images alone without any assessment of the 2D images. In other words, the 3D postprocessing of the CT source data can compensate for a lack of 2D interpretative skills and knowledge of underlying cross-sectional principles. As is discussed below, such is not the case. Cross-sectional skills are crucial for this approach.

In the primary 3D approach, the postprocessed 3D image series (such as the endoluminal fly through) is used to detect potential polyps. Thus, morphology is used as the sole marker for detection without input from other factors such as internal composition. This approach has been cited as one of the significant factors accounting for improved polyp detection rates.[5] The rationale is that the postprocessing of the source data allows for easy recognition of focal polypoid structures from the colonic haustra. As opposed to a 2D approach for which the mental translation of a 3D structure from 2D data can be tedious or difficult, it is done here automatically by the computer,

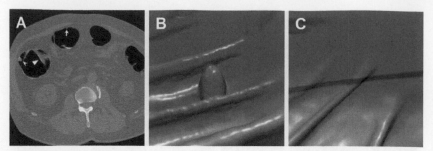

Fig. 3. Primary 2D approach to interpretation. 2D transverse CTC image (*A*) is used for polyp detection whereby a true soft tissue polyp (*arrowhead*) must be distinguished from colonic folds. This task is easy when the fold (*triangle*) elongates out in the transverse plane but becomes more difficult when seen in cross section (*arrow*). 3D endoluminal CTC view (*B*) confirms the suspected focal polypoid morphology of the true polyp and discounts the colonic fold in cross section (*C*). The red line in *C* denotes the level and orientation of the 2D transverse slice of *A*.

allowing for an easier detection pattern for the CTC reader. Perceptual errors where a polyp is mistaken for a fold are less likely at a primary 3D approach (**Fig. 4**). Although this strategy is more likely to capture a true soft tissue polyp, it generates a much larger number of pseudopolyps. Because the internal lesion composition is not considered at this step, any structure with a polypoid morphology will be reconstructed to mimic a true polyp (**Fig. 5**).

Thus, the second task of CTC interpretation (ie, polyp confirmation) holds even greater importance with a primary 3D interpretative schema and ultimately determines whether a quality interpretation results. Although 3D tools such as translucency rendering can suggest whether a polyp is of soft tissue density, only the 2D images with the use of cross-sectional skills can confirm the true polyps from the large list of polyp candidates generated by this approach. If a reader cannot perform this step competently, too many false positives will result and an unacceptably high number of CTC examinations will be erroneously referred to therapeutic colonoscopy.

Although a complete listing and description of the required cross-sectional skills for characterization is beyond the scope of this paper, it is helpful to cover the basic skills

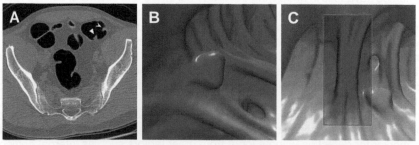

Fig. 4. Perceptual errors at primary 2D interpretation. 2D transverse CTC image (*A*) shows the difficulty of perceiving a true polyp by this strategy. The true polyp (*arrowhead*) can mimic a fold (*triangle*) and the detection algorithm requires sustained mental effort to maintain sensitivities. Contrast this to a primary 3D approach where the focal polypoid morphology of the true polyp (*B*) seen in *A* is easily distinguished from the colonic fold (highlighted area in *C*) in *A*.

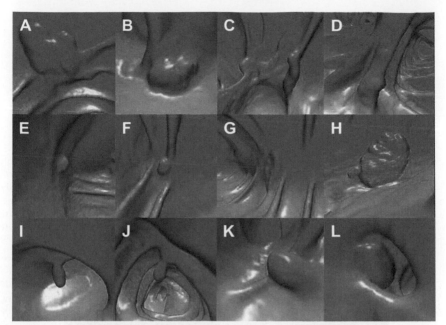

Fig. 5. 3D appearance of polyps and stool. A collage of images shows that morphology alone cannot separate out a polyp from residual stool. Use of 3D endoluminal images alone leads to unacceptably high false-positive rates. The vast majority of suspected polyps will turn out to simply represent stool. The true polyps in the collage are: (*A*) serrated adenoma with high-grade dysplasia, (*C*) carpet lesion, (*E*) subcentimeter tubular adenoma, (*G*) large hyperplastic polyp, (*I*) pedunculated tubulovillous adenoma, and (*K*) large sessile tubulovillous adenoma; while (*B, D, F, H, L*) represent stool and (*J*) a drop of contrast.

used in the determination of a classic polyp in order to gain a sense of the these requirements. Once detected, a potential polyp is confirmed at CTC by demonstrating 2 criteria on the 2D series. First, the candidate is fixed in location between the supine and prone series (**Fig. 6**). A strong grasp of cross-sectional anatomy is required to make this determination. Often, the colon shifts in location between the supine and prone series, particularly those portions on an elongated mesentery. The reader must use the few internal colonic landmarks (eg, counting haustra from a definable point such as a diverticulum) and the relationship to the extracolonic structures to convince himself or herself that the polyp candidate is either fixed in location (ie, a polyp) or moves (ie, stool). Second, the internal make-up of the polyp candidate should be a homogeneous soft tissue density to distinguish from untagged or partially tagged stool (see **Fig. 6**). Again, a solid basis in cross-sectional principles is required to make this determination, as artifacts such as beam hardening or volume averaging must be taken into account for a given 2D appearance of the polyp candidate, otherwise leading to incorrect interpretations (**Fig. 7**).

INCIDENTAL EXTRACOLONIC FINDINGS AND INTERPRETATION

Although the focus of CTC interpretation is on the colon, it is important to realize that this CT examination unavoidably images the entire abdomen and pelvis, although is somewhat limited due to the low-dose, noncontrast nature of the examination.

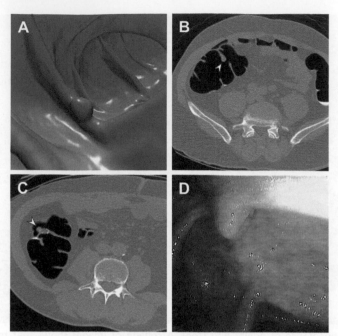

Fig. 6. Confirmation of suspected 3D polyp. A 56-year-old man with a possible polyp in the ascending colon on screening CTC (*A*). 2D transverse supine (*B*) and prone (*C*) views are required for confirmation. In addition to demonstrating a homogeneous soft tissue attenuation, the polyp (*arrowhead*) must be in the same location within the colon between the different patient positions. Note that this can be a difficult determination as the underlying colon shifts in position for this true polyp, which was also seen at colonoscopy (*D*). Pathology revealed a tubular adenoma.

Diagnostic algorithms for incidental extracolonic findings certainly need to be carefully thought out to minimize unnecessary workup, but inevitably, significant unsuspected diagnoses will be uncovered outside of the colon. Screening series have shown rates of 2% to 3% for such diagnoses, which include asymptomatic extracolonic cancers and vascular aneurysms.[6,7] Uncovering these unsuspected entities should presumably result in an additional positive effect on this screening population. Indeed, modeling studies have shown substantial gains in life years by CTC screening strategies over colonoscopy-based screening because of the coincident ability of CTC to detect aortic aneurysms.[8]

Should an individual who interprets CTC be required to evaluate these areas outside of the colon? An argument has been raised that the purpose of CTC is colorectal screening and the extracolonic findings are outside the purview of the examination. Consequently, these areas could be ignored (or even "blacked out" by electronic means). Such an exclusion is arbitrary at best but, more importantly, given the significant extracolonic diagnoses that could be uncovered, the approach would not be ethical. Unlike colonoscopy where only the colorectum can be evaluated, CTC is a CT examination that examines the entire abdomen and pelvis.

An argument has also been forwarded that the 2 portions of the examinations can be separated and interpreted by different readers. This argument reflects the uneasiness with the cross-sectional ability of a reader and the idea that the colonic evaluation can be accomplished without a strong cross-sectional skill set. As discussed above, the

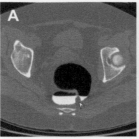
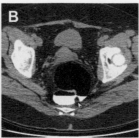
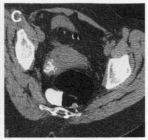

Fig. 7. Confounding artifacts. 2D transverse CTC images with polyp (*A*) and soft tissue (*B*) windows suggest that the polyp may be fatty in nature. Decubitus view (*C*), however, demonstrates conflicting information where it is more of soft tissue attenuation. It is important to realize that beam hardening related to the contrast pool can cause reconstruction artifacts that lead to this appearance, and not to mistake this true soft tissue polyp for a lipoma.

colonic interpretation requires these skills even with a primary 3D approach. In the authors' experience, a reader who is uncomfortable with the extracolonic evaluation likely does not hold the requisite skills to read the colonic portion of this CT examination either. In addition, fragmenting this interpretation unnecessarily increases complexity and introduces the possibility of error. Many processes overlap between the colonic and extracolonic. For example, it is not uncommon for extracolonic processes to be present as colonic "lesions" on the 3D display (**Fig. 8**). When separated, who becomes responsible for such processes? When a single reader interprets the entire CTC examination, such questions are moot and an unnecessary source of possible error is eliminated.

WHO SHOULD INTERPRET CTC: RADIOLOGIST OR GASTROENTEROLOGIST?

Now armed with this background, let us consider the question of who is best suited to interpret this examination. The answer to this debate should rest on the ability to provide accurate, quality interpretations; and, as shown earlier, such interpretation is fundamentally dependent on a well-grounded cross-sectional skill set. This singular powerful argument is the reason why radiologists should interpret CTC. It trumps all other arguments that may favor gastroenterologist-driven interpretations. Gastroenterologists may claim they would provide better interpretations resulting from their greater understanding of colorectal risk factors and potential modifiers, familiarity with the underlying disease process, more encompassing perspective (given their knowledge base in related gastroenterological entities), and their procedural experiences in colonoscopy and endoscopic ultrasound. As the process of interpretation has been examined, it should be obvious that these reasons only peripherally affect CTC interpretation, compared with the need for a solid basis in cross-sectional anatomy and principles.

Who holds these skills and knowledge base? Radiologists have a large advantage due to their training. A typical radiologist has developed these necessary skills over a 4-year residency (and possibly an additional 1-year fellowship). He or she has interpreted many thousands of cross-sectional studies divided between the head, neck, body (chest/abdomen/pelvis), and extremities during residency. He or she has undergone formal training in radiation physics. The radiologist has gained extensive experience over an extended period of several years. This experience allows for a solid

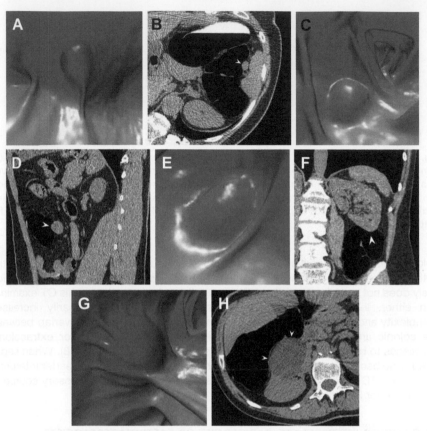

Fig. 8. Extracolonic structures presenting as polyps at CTC. 3D endoluminal CTC views suggest sizeable colonic polyps (*A, C, E, G*), which simply represent extracolonic structures impressing on the colon. 2D transverse CTC image (*B*) shows that *A* represents a splenule (*arrowhead*), 2D sagittal image (*D*) shows that *C* is a collapsed small bowel loop (*arrowhead*), 2D coronal image (*F*) shows that *E* represents the inferior pole of the left kidney, and 2D transverse image (*H*) shows that *G* represents a large renal cyst (*arrowheads*). (*From* Pickhardt PJ, Kim DH. CT colonography: principles and practice of virtual colonoscopy. Philadelphia: Saunders; 2010. p. 329, 330, 388; with permission.)

grounding in cross-sectional principles and as well experiential learning in discovering the exceptions and nuances to the rule. Radiologists learn to manipulate CT scanning parameters, such as decreasing slice thickness or altering tube current (mA) for a variety of different clinical settings. Thus, a radiologist is well equipped to anticipate the effect of these changes and consequently, the effect of various artifacts such as beam hardening or volume averaging on the image appearance and, potentially, on interpretation (see **Fig. 7**).

Even with this solid skill set base, however, additional training is required. There is growing evidence that experience with pathology-proven cases alone is not enough to guarantee good performance.[9,10] An interpretative learning curve is seen with CTC, foe which CTC-specific skills need to be acquired.[11] There is growing consensus that dedicated training is needed to increase accuracy.[12,13] With dedicated training (and perhaps competency exams), excellent performance can be attained as seen in the various multicenter CTC trials; trials where the CTC examinations were interpreted by radiologists.[4,14]

Despite this marked advantage, it is important to realize that radiologists must become knowledgeable about the larger context of colorectal screening—clinical issues where gastroenterologists currently excel. Although cross-sectional skills are at the core of accurate interpretation, it is necessary for radiologists to become well versed on the disease entity and the implications for a detected polyp to provide the best overall care for a CTC screening patient. What are the risks from an identified polyp relative to size and what are the appropriate options? Much like mammography, the radiologist must take an active role in the future management of a patient dependent on the examination results. In the authors' opinion, acquiring this knowledge and accepting the added responsibility is a far easier task for a radiologist than is acquiring the required cross-sectional skill set for a gastroenterologist with no previous imaging training.

Let us examine the situation for Gastroenterology. Gastroenterologists' interpretations are hindered by the lack of formal cross-sectional training. Current American Gastroenterological Association (AGA) guidelines call for interpretation of 75 pathology-proven CTC cases and a proctored 6-week experience with a qualified CTC reader to gain the necessary skills.[15] Can a physician acquire the necessary cross-sectional skills and additional specific CTC skills with this abbreviated experience? Given the scope of knowledge required to acquire a solid grounding in cross-sectional principles and anatomy, the authors would argue that such training would not adequately prepare a gastroenterologist. An additional 25 cases (American College of Radiology guidelines suggest a 50-case experience for radiologists[16]) and a 6 week experience does not equate with the multiple years of training undertaken by a radiologist.

Gastroenterologists have argued otherwise, pointing to studies that suggest adequate CTC interpretation performance rates with sensitivities in the 86% to 90% at the large polyp threshold, comparable to radiologists.[17,18] Gastroenterologists argue that the experiences from colonoscopy can compensate for the abbreviated training. As discussed in the previous sections, the reason why this is incorrect should be apparent. Colonoscopic skills only superficially aid in CTC interpretation. The post-processed 3D endoluminal series do allow for a search pattern similar to colonoscopy and certainly colonoscopic skills help to detect these polyp candidates, thus maintaining appropriate sensitivity. However, this is typically at the expense of very poor specificities. The colonoscopic skills do not translate into differentiating the often numerous residual stool pseudopolyps from the few true soft tissue polyps. Young and colleagues[18] demonstrated lower but comparable sensitivities of 83.6% at an 8-mm polyp threshold for a group of gastroenterologist readers (vs 93.9% value for radiologists) but at the cost of low specificity at 78%. The specificity for radiologists in the study at the same size threshold was 92.2%. As discussed previously, the low specificity is likely a reflection of the lack of cross-sectional skills. Herein lies a fundamental issue regarding an accurate, quality CTC interpretation: sensitivity alone does not equate with quality. The real determinants of quality rest on an appropriately high specificity for a given sensitivity. Although an argument may be made that the most important aspect for screening is high sensitivity (even at the expense of increased false positives), it holds less weight if one group (ie, radiologists) can interpret the examination with higher specificity at the same sensitivity level. Again, specificity is wholly dependent on a firm grasp of cross-sectional principles. With decreased specificity, false-positive rates are increased and patients are sent unnecessarily for therapeutic colonoscopy. This is one of the important but hidden costs of poor quality, where medical resources are consumed and healthy screening patients are exposed to potential complications that should have been avoided if a quality CTC interpretation had been done.

Computer-aided detection (CAD) has been touted as an equalizer that may help nonradiologist interpretation of CTC. These devices, however, tend to increase sensitivity at the expense of decreased specificity by presenting additional polyp candidates to the reader. Again, without a cross-sectional skill set, accurate confirmation of a potential polyp suffers. Petrick and colleagues[19] demonstrated an average increase of sensitivity of about 15% with a corresponding decrease of specificity of 14% with the use of CAD. No increase in reader performance as demonstrated by increased area under the receiver operating characteristic curve occurred.

Can a gastroenterologist obtain the necessary cross-sectional skills to become a quality CTC reader? Certainly so, but this requires an extended, dedicated effort, likely much more than outlined in the present AGA guidelines. It requires training and experience to acquire skills that radiologists obtain through a 4-year residency and through additional training for CTC-specific skills. Given the highly specialized endoscopic skills obtained during a multiyear gastroenterology fellowship, one wonders if such efforts by gastroenterology would be better served by using these important skills to increase the numbers of screening colonoscopies and to therapeutically remove the large polyps referred by CTC.

SUMMARY

The debate of who should interpret CTC is marked by strong opinions and statements. Ultimately, quality should be the final arbiter of who should read this examination. The basis for accurate quality examinations resides on a firm grasp of cross-sectional anatomy and principles. Without this skill set, interpretation is doomed to failure, regardless whether a primary 2D or 3D approach is used. As CTC is a CT examination first, the entire abdomen and pelvis must also be evaluated. The extracolonic structures cannot be ignored, as significant unsuspected diagnoses will be uncovered. From prior training and skill set, radiologists are well suited in obtaining the CTC-specific skills needed to interpret this examination with quality. Gastroenterologists are at a disadvantage due to their lack of baseline cross-sectional skills, and would need extended effort to provide a similar level of performance. Thus, it is more logical for radiology than gastroenterology to interpret this screening examination. Given the large population that needs to be screened, physicians from both groups will be needed to increase screening examinations of both types, with radiologists interpreting CTC and gastroenterologists performing colonoscopy.

REFERENCES

1. Levin B, Lieberman DA, McFarland B, et al. Screening and surveillance for the early detection of colorectal cancer and adenomatous polyps, 2008: a joint guideline from the American Cancer Society, the US Multi-Society Task Force on Colorectal Cancer, and the American College of Radiology. Gastroenterology 2008;134(5):1570–95.
2. Hara AK, Blevins M, Chen M, et al. National CT colonography trial (ACRIN 6664): do reader preferences affect performance at CT colonography? Radiological Society of North America Annual Meeting. Chicago (IL), November 30–December 5, 2008; A278.
3. Dachman AH, Kuniyoshi JK, Boyle CM, et al. CT colonography with three-dimensional problem solving for detection of colonic polyps. Am J Roentgenol 1998; 171(4):989–95.

4. Pickhardt PJ, Choi JR, Hwang I, et al. Computed tomographic virtual colono-scopy to screen for colorectal neoplasia in asymptomatic adults. N Engl J Med 2003;349(23):2191–200.
5. Pickhardt PJ, Lee AD, Taylor AJ, et al. Primary 2D versus primary 3D polyp detection at screening CT colonography. Am J Roentgenol 2007;189(6):1451–6.
6. Pickhardt PJ, Hanson ME, Vanness DJ, et al. Unsuspected extracolonic findings at screening CT colonography: clinical and economic impact. Radiology 2008; 249:151–9.
7. Kim DH, Pickhardt PJ, Taylor AJ, et al. CT colonography versus colonoscopy for the detection of advanced neoplasia. N Engl J Med 2007;357(14):1403–12.
8. Hassan C, Pickhardt PJ, Kim DH. Computed tomographic colonography to screen for colorectal cancer, extracolonic cancer, and aortic aneurysm: model simulation with cost-effectiveness analysis. Arch Intern Med 2008;168(7): 696–705.
9. Burling D, Halligan S, Atchley J, et al. CT colonography: interpretative performance in a non-academic environment. Clin Radiol 2007;62(5):424–9.
10. Taylor SA, Halligan S, Burling D, et al. CT colonography: effect of experience and training on reader performance. Eur Radiol 2004;14(6):1025–33.
11. Spinzi G, Belloni G, Martegani A, et al. Computed tomographic colonography and conventional colonoscopy for colon diseases: a prospective, blinded study. Am J Gastroenterol 2001;96(2):394–400.
12. Fletcher JA, Herman BA, Chen M, et al. ACRIN 6664: Living on the high plateau—can training and testing be used to ensure high performance at CT colonography? Radiological Society of North America Annual Meeting. Chicago (IL), November 30–December 5, 2008; A280.
13. Soto JA, Barish MA, Yee J. Reader training in CT colonography: how much is enough? Radiology 2005;237(1):26–7.
14. Johnson CD, Chen MH, Toledano AY, et al. Accuracy of CT colonography for detection of large adenomas and cancers. N Engl J Med 2008;359(12):1207–17.
15. Rockey DC, Barish M, Brill JV, et al. Standards for gastroenterologists for performing and interpreting diagnostic computed tomographic colonography. Gastroenterology 2007;133(3):1005–24.
16. American College of Radiology. ACR practice guideline for the performance of computed tomography (CT) colonography in adults. ACR Practice Guideline 2009, in press.
17. Dachman AH, Kelly KB, Zintsmaster MP, et al. Formative evaluation of standardized training for CT colonographic image interpretation by novice readers. Radiology 2008;249(1):167–77.
18. Young PE, Ray QP, Hwang I, et al. Gastroenterologists' interpretation of CTC: a pilot study demonstrating feasibility and similar accuracy compared with radiologists' interpretation. Am J Gastroenterol 2009;104(12):2926–31.
19. Petrick N, Haider M, Summers RM, et al. CT colonography with computer-aided detection as a second reader: observer performance study. Radiology 2008; 246(1):148–56.

Gastroenterologists Should Read CT Colonography

Steve Carpenter, MD

KEYWORDS

- CT colonography • Optical colonoscopy
- Colon cancer screening

Screening for colorectal neoplasms has become the standard of care in advanced medical settings worldwide. Identifying asymptomatic colorectal neoplastic lesions has been shown to reduce colorectal cancer incidence and the overall cost of medical care. Clinicians have several alternatives at their disposal as they consider screening for their respective patient population. Many different organizations have spent considerable time weighing the evidence to establish appropriate evidence-based guidelines directing clinicians how to appropriately manage screening; 2 important methods to consider are optical colonoscopy and computed tomographic colonography (CTC).[1]

The purpose of this article is to make the case that gastroenterologists should read CTC. By virtue of their training, there is no question that radiologists may provide this service competently. Gastroenterologists are well trained to detect and remove colonic abnormalities using optical colonoscopy. In training and practice, gastroenterologists develop considerable experience in colonic pathology and anatomic variation. Given this experience in three-dimensional intracolonic imaging, gastroenterologists are also well suited to interpret intracolonic images obtained via CTC. Furthermore, gastroenterologists work within a patient care infrastructure that provides a personal relationship with patients, and leads patients effectively and efficiently through their options for effective colorectal cancer screening. Central to the argument that gastroenterologists read CTC is the benefit of experience with three-dimensional video-assisted colonic imaging and the physician-patient relationship.

OPTICAL COLONOSCOPY

Clinicians use optical colonoscopy as a primary means to screen the entire colon not only for cancer but also for precancerous adenomatous lesions. Most adenomas may

Department of Internal Medicine, Mercer University School of Medicine, Memorial University Medical Center, 4700 Waters Avenue, Savannah, GA 31404, USA
E-mail address: carpest1@memorialhealth.com

Gastrointest Endoscopy Clin N Am 20 (2010) 271–277
doi:10.1016/j.giec.2010.02.006
1052-5157/10/$ – see front matter © 2010 Published by Elsevier Inc.

giendo.theclinics.com

be removed at the time of optical colonoscopy. The size, location, shape, and pathologic nature of polyps may be determined during this single clinical encounter, providing the patient and clinician with valuable information to guide the future colorectal cancer screening strategy. Often, the clinician doing the endoscopic procedure has an established relationship with the patient and may provide recommendations regarding care at a subsequent clinical encounter. Established Centers of Digestive Health, worldwide, have proved to be successful in driving the colorectal cancer effort.

Clearly, many patients and health care providers are comfortable with this protocol of patient care; however, optical colonoscopy does have its disadvantages. The procedure requires adequate colon cleansing to allow for complete mucosal evaluation, and many patients state that the arduous task of colonic preparation is a major drawback to the entire process. Often, colonoscopy requires moderate conscious sedation, requiring the clinician to reflect on the patient's overall underlying medical condition: "Can my patient tolerate this degree of sedation?" From the patient's perspective, moderate conscious sedation provides them with a comfortable medical procedure but also requires that the patient have access to reliable transportation from the medical setting. As a result, the patients not only have to absent themselves from their daily responsibilities, but their transporter must also take time from their routines to ensure safe passage home. This is a significant issue to consider when reviewing the overall cost of the colorectal cancer screening effort. During the insertion procedural phase and, if need be, polypectomy, perforation of the colon may occur. Although this is a relatively rare complication, it can and does occur in the care of asymptomatic patients. In addition, bleeding even after the most simple of polypectomies may occur and thus may require hospitalization or even administration of blood products. Because of the potential for colonic perforation, postpolypectomy bleeding, and other complications, adequately trained medical personnel must carefully discuss these possibilities to obtain meaningful informed consent from all patients before the procedure. There is simply no substitute for an excellent patient-physician relationship.

Optical colonoscopy is not a perfect screening modality. Several tandem colonoscopy studies demonstrate that, for many reasons, adenomatous colon polyps may be missed during the procedure. Polyps may be behind folds, obscured by colonic debris, or simply not seen by the endoscopist. This issue has prompted considerable focus by gastrointestinal societies on quality parameters such as adenoma detection rate, cecal intubation rate, and colonoscopic withdrawal times. Many endoscopy centers have initiated routine documentation of these important quality measures and, collectively, we hope these developments can improve the overall colorectal cancer screening effort. Several studies demonstrate that adequate training and experience translate into improved quality; but we require additional experienced endoscopists. As the age of our patients increases and the population grows, we need to train more endoscopists with a firm grasp on the limitations of endoscopy and their role in the overall improvement of quality colorectal cancer screening.

CT COLONOGRAPHY

CT colonography (CTC) is a promising colorectal screening tool, and several key factors make this method of colorectal cancer screening attractive to clinicians and patients. The procedure does not require moderate conscious sedation. Therefore, patients may provide their own transportation and return to work immediately following the examination, assuming the patient does not require further evaluation. As the colon is imaged digitally, the risk of procedurally related complications, such as perforation and bleeding, is reduced. Improvements in CT technology over the years have resulted in continuous improvement in image quality and data acquisition time, and so in as little as 10 minutes, patients may have their procedure completed and be on the way back to society. Most importantly, CTC has resulted in increased patient awareness of the colorectal cancer screening effort. As CTC has received considerable attention in the lay press, more patients realize the value of cancer screening and may participate in the process; anything that increases overall patient awareness and acceptance of the process of cancer screening is beneficial.

Despite these advantages, CT colonoscopy has its own problems. Many patients are disappointed to discover that CTC requires adequate colon preparation for optimal colonic imaging. In fact, the preparation is more complicated as contrast and fecal tagging agents are necessary to adequately differentiate stool from polyps. Trained medical personnel are required to describe the importance and nature of preparation to patients. Current screening recommendations suggest that some patients might have 5 or more CT examinations during their lifetime if CT is the primary colorectal cancer screening modality. Radiation exposure is inherent to the procedure, leading to increased concern about this degree of cumulative radiation exposure, but radiology societies have largely dismissed this issue.[2] As a medical community, we do not fully understand the effects of medical radiation in a screening effort and long-term studies are needed. If a polyp is identified via CTC, most patients require optical colonoscopy for polyp removal. Some have suggested that small polyps may be followed with CT at shortened screening intervals. Although some patients may be comfortable with repeated CT examinations to follow a lesion, those in primary care know other patients will have concern about the safety of this watch-and-wait approach.

DISCUSSION

During CTC, extracolonic information is acquired.[3] A standardized CT colonography reporting and data system (CRADS) has been developed and is useful for CTC report uniformity.[4] Findings of major clinical relevance, categorized as E4 findings, arise in approximately 4% to 10% of CTC examinations. Examples of E4 findings include renal cell carcinoma, ovarian carcinoma, and an abdominal aortic aneurysm of worrisome size. Indeterminate extracolonic abnormalities are categorized as E3 findings in the CRADS system and are identified in approximately 30% of CTC examinations. Examples of E3 findings include suspicious renal and liver cysts. Findings of low clinical importance, such as simple liver and renal cysts, are placed in category E2. The frequency of E3 findings may be expected to increase, particularly if radiologists are liability averse. Furthermore, in a liability-concerned environment, some radiologists may be inclined to hedge on E2 abnormalities of low clinical importance, thereby increasing the percentage of E3 findings reported. Repeating scans to follow indeterminate findings will increase the overall cost of colorectal cancer screening. This is an important consideration when analyzing CTC from a cost efficacy perspective. Individual CT reports often suggest that E3 findings be followed at the discretion of the patient and referring physician. In the author's clinical experience, patients tend to worry about any of these extracolonic findings. Time and patience is required to discuss even simple E2 findings with patients. In some cases, these discussions heighten the individual patient's health care-related anxiety. An excellent doctor-patient relationship is useful in lessening this degree of anxiety and proves invaluable in many respects. For CTC to be clinically and cost effective, it is imperative that radiologists take great care in the nature of CTC extracolonic reporting and be prudent with E2 and E3 findings. Likewise, primary care physicians or gastroenterologists must communicate meaningfully with patients.

Appropriately trained radiologists should interpret extracolonic findings identified at CT colonoscopy. Although interpretation of extracolonic CT images is thoroughly covered in gastroenterology training and practicing gastroenterologists review multiple CT images within a given work day, gastroenterologists do not have the expertise or privilege to provide an official interpretation of extracolonic CT data. In CTC centers, 1 prime goal is to provide the patient with the opportunity for a same-day optical colonoscopy. Within 20 or 30 minutes, a gastroenterologist reading CTC can provide an immediate intracolonic interpretation as the patient waits. There is no acute need for the extracolonic interpretation. CTC centers run by gastroenterologists can send CT images digitally and thus outsource the reading of extracolonic images. Gastroenterologists who provide CTC within their own center therefore have the opportunity to identify excellent radiologists who deliver high-quality interpretations. Small centers can even send CTC images to major university centers. Several high-quality radiologists have developed their own corporations to provide this service, allowing colorectal cancer screening centers to track the quality of extracolonic interpretations and change to an alternate vendor if necessary to ensure high-quality patient care. Extracolonic findings require careful evidence-based management. Colon cancer screenings centered in 1 locale provide patients with the opportunity to review and discuss colonic and extracolonic findings with 1 clinician in 1 sitting. Appropriate evidence-based management of all findings may be coordinated in this fashion.

All members of the population should receive some form of testing to improve colorectal cancer screening outcomes. Unfortunately, this is not yet the case. There are many reasons for this lack of adherence, but some patients remain concerned about endoscopy. CTC presents patients with an alternative, as we have no perfect screening modality. Before making a decision, it is desirable that each patient has an understanding of the positive and negative attributes of available methods. Communication about the alternatives requires patience and time. A formal consultative visit can prove immensely beneficial. Although primary care physicians are perfectly suited to provide this service during routine visits, because of issues of time and the complexity of primary care, a thorough discussion is often not possible. Physicians who carefully follow the topic of colorectal screening realize that the data are far from static. Many primary care physicians are not fully versed about the sensitivity and specificity of optical colonoscopy and CTC in asymptomatic patients or the proper surveillance intervals for adenomas. Many patients are interested in discussing the data and options, and gastroenterologists are in a prime position to provide this expertise.

With regard to the interpretation of colonic findings obtained during CTC, gastroenterologists have a wealth of experience with optical colonoscopy. Reading CTC fly-through images is intuitive to endoscopists. Standards for gastroenterologists performing and interpreting diagnostic CTC have been established and training programs organized by professional gastrointestinal organizations are effective in orienting endoscopists to this new technology.[5] Although courses can be helpful for introduction, there is no substitute for hands-on experience; this can be achieved via mentored leader programs. Ideally, personal hands-on experience is obtained in centers providing CTC and optical colonoscopy services. Gastroenterologists may interpret colonic CTC images proficiently with accuracy similar to that of radiologists.[6] Interpreting physicians must have adequate training and experience to ensure highly accurate readings. Experience and level of training directly correlate with accuracy. Colonoscopists with considerable experience with endoscopic imaging find CTC colonic interpretation intuitive; however, there is a learning curve to acquire proficiency with the software used for CTC. Several vendors have created excellent CTC software and revision of these platforms continues. Gastroenterologists interested in CTC proficiency should select 1 software platform and learn it well. Development of expertise in CTC requires a substantial time commitment.

It is reasonable to consider that CTC may become part of the gastrointestinal core curriculum for fellowship training.[7] It is important that current gastroenterology fellows develop a basic familiarity with the indications, interpretation, and limitations of CTC. More in-depth training in CTC may become a reality where resources are available, requiring cooperation with departments of radiology. Some have suggested a new track within traditional gastroenterology training, wherein imaging becomes the focus and fellows would concentrate on technologies such as wireless capsule endoscopy and CTC. A comprehensive training curriculum would need to be established and training standards for current fellows developed.

Established gastroenterologists who gravitate toward CTC and have an interest in interpretation must first demonstrate expertise and then make a personal commitment toward maintenance of proficiency. Radiologists require a meaningful physician peer review program for accreditation. Currently, there exists no infrastructure in gastroenterology societies for this quality control process. Randomly selected CTC studies would need to be reviewed on a regularly scheduled basis, requiring repeat reading of completed studies. Although members of one's own organization might feasibly perform this task, this method of peer review might not result in meaningful critique. Therefore, review networks will need to be organized and the results must be readily available, with reviewers able to correlate the interpretation and original report with corresponding endoscopic and pathologic findings. Some recommend that a national database be developed in the infancy of CTC so that CTC, endoscopic, and pathologic findings might be correlated and meaningfully studied. Policies and procedures must be in place to resolve discrepant peer review findings providing the means for CTC centers to achieve quality outcomes improvement.[8] For gastroenterologists to participate on a wide-scale basis in CTC interpretation, gastroenterology societies must either partner with other societies to develop appropriate peer review, quality, and safety policies and procedures, or they must initiate the process independently. Many questions remain about this process of peer review. Although this is a substantial hurdle for gastroenterology to overcome, available data confirm that gastroenterologists have the expertise to proficiently interpret CTC images, meaningfully participate in this colorectal cancer screening approach, and provide patients with colorectal cancer screening by a variety of methods within a single center.

As physicians we need to identify and eliminate barriers that interfere with patient adherence to colorectal screening. Patients will benefit from a single center approach to colorectal cancer screening with a strong emphasis on providing the option of same-day optical colonoscopy should a mucosal abnormality be identified on CTC. Occasionally, because of technical or anatomic issues, optical colonoscopy may not provide complete colonic imaging. Having CTC immediately available is optimal from a patient convenience perspective, but offering the option of same-day CTC and optical colonoscopy will require a coordinated scheduling effort to ensure adequate time is preserved for endoscopy to provide definitive therapy for those with abnormal colonic findings on CTC. Same-day optical colonoscopy will require prompt interpretation of CTC data and immediate referral for optical colonoscopy. It is unlikely that patients will embrace an approach wherein optical colonoscopy follows CTC by more than 1 or 2 hours. Furthermore, studies on the quality of colonic preparation imply that if optical colonoscopy occurs greater than 4 hours after CTC, we can

CT Colonography: Perforation Rates and Potential Radiation Risks

Berrington de Gonzalez A, DPhil[a],*,
Kwang Pyo Kim, PhD[b], Judy Yee, MD[c]

KEYWORDS

- Computed tomography • Colorectal cancer • Screening
- Radiation • Risk • Perforation • Colonography

Colorectal cancer is a common cancer that can be detected in advance by screening.[1] Unfortunately screening uptake is relatively low, partly because the acceptability of the available screening tools, such as optical colonoscopy and fecal occult blood testing, is low.[2] Computed tomographic colonography (CTC) has emerged as a potential screening tool that may provide good efficacy combined with greater acceptability.[1] Despite the evidence that it can be as sensitive as optical colonoscopy for large polyp and cancer detection, it is not yet recommended as a routine screening tool by all organizations in the United States. The American Cancer Society recently added CTC to its list of recommended screening tools for colorectal cancer.[1] However, concerns were raised by the US Preventive Services Task Force[3] and Medicare[4] about the potential harms, including perforation rates, radiation doses, and the risk of radiation-related cancer. In this article, the authors review the current evidence for these potential harms from CTC and compare them to the potential harms from the alternatives, including colonoscopy and double-contrast barium enema. The related issue of the consequences of identifying extracolonic findings, including anxiety and additional testing, (see article by Yee and colleagues elsewhere in this issue for further exploration of this topic).[5]

This research was supported by the Intramural Research Program of the National Institutes of Health and the National Cancer Institute.

[a] Division of Cancer Epidemiology & Genetics, Radiation Epidemiology Branch, National Cancer Institute, 6120 Executive Boulevard, Bethesda, MD 20892, USA
[b] Department of Nuclear Engineering, Kyung Hee University, 1 Seocheon-dong, Giheung-gu, Yongin-si, Gyeonggi-do, Republic of Korea
[c] University of California, San Francisco, Veterans Affairs Medical Center, 4150 Clement Street, San Francisco, CA 94121, USA
* Corresponding author.
E-mail address: berringtona@mail.nih.gov

Gastrointest Endoscopy Clin N Am 20 (2010) 279–291
doi:10.1016/j.giec.2010.02.003
1052-5157/10/$ – see front matter. Published by Elsevier Inc.

COLONIC PERFORATION

Perforation of the colon is an exceedingly uncommon complication of CTC. An advantage of CTC is that unlike colonoscopy, it does not require the insertion and maneuvering of an endoscope to the cecum. Instead, the patient undergoes gas insufflation of the colon using a small rectal tube, which is considered to be safer than colonoscopy. In addition, patients are sedated for their colonoscopy procedure, whereas patients who undergo CTC are able to avoid the cardiopulmonary risks of sedation because they remain awake during the scanning and are also able to be immediately assessed for any signs and symptoms of overdistention of the colon or possible perforation.

The first reports of colonic perforation related to CTC were published in 2004, about 10 years after the introduction of the technique. Perforation generally occurred in patients who had known colonic pathology. Kamar and colleagues[6] reported a case of rectal perforation in a patient with a large obstructive rectosigmoid carcinoma. An intrarectal balloon had been inflated in the patient, and the perforation was thought to be related to manual overinflation of the rectum with room air in the presence of an obstructing mass. Two other instances of perforation related to CTC occurred in patients with active inflammatory bowel disease. Coady-Fariborzian and colleagues[7] reported a patient with long-standing steroid-dependent ulcerative colitis who developed cecal perforation during CTC. Triester and colleagues[8] reported colonic perforation during CTC in a patient with active fibrostenosing Crohn disease. The patient had multiple strictures in the rectum and sigmoid colon and at an ileoascending colon anastomosis, which placed her at high risk for possible perforation.

A national survey performed at 50 sites in the United Kingdom evaluated adverse events of CTC in 17,067 patients who had symptoms of possible colorectal cancer.[9] There were 9 perforations reported occurring at 6 centers for an overall perforation rate of 0.05%. However, for 5 of the 9 patients, perforations had identifiable causes, such as insufflation of a rectal stump; forced placement of a rectal catheter; ulcerative colitis; obstructive sigmoid carcinoma; and perforation before CTC, which was thought to be related to the bowel preparation. Four of 9 patients were entirely asymptomatic, and extraluminal gas was noted on the computed tomographic (CT) scan between 6 hours and 4 hours after the procedure. All 4 patients had already returned home, did not have any clinical symptoms of perforation when contacted, and were treated conservatively. Thus, the symptomatic perforation rate from this study was 0.03%. The investigators note that the symptomatic perforation rate is the clinically relevant perforation rate that should be used for comparison with other types of colon studies because CTC inherently detects even tiny amounts of free air that would otherwise not be detected by other examinations such as colonoscopy, sigmoidoscopy, or barium enema.

A retrospective study assessed the risk of perforation from CTC in 11,870 patients at 11 centers in Israel.[10] There were 7 cases of colon perforation occurring at 5 sites, yielding a total perforation rate of 0.06%. Four cases of perforation occurred in patients referred for CTC after incomplete colonoscopy. The mean age of patients in this study was high at 78 years. All studies were performed after room air insufflation, and an intrarectal balloon was inflated in 6 of 7 cases of perforation. Surgery was performed in 4 of 7 patients with colon perforation, and 3 patients were treated conservatively for a symptomatic perforation rate of 0.03%. Risk factors for perforation that were determined in this study included severe diverticulosis in 3 patients, obstructive carcinoma in 1 patient, and left inguinal hernia trapping sigmoid colon in 4 patients with some diseases occurring concomitantly.

The largest study to date was a survey of 16 medical centers across 5 countries (Working Group on Virtual Colonoscopy) conducted to evaluate the symptomatic perforation rate and the overall significant complication rate of CTC.[11] A total of 21,923 CTC examinations were included, with about half of the cases performed for screening and the other half being diagnostic cases. Two perforations were reported in patients undergoing diagnostic CTC. Manual room air insufflation was used in the 2 patients. One patient had a known annular sigmoid carcinoma and was symptomatic before the CTC. One patient was asymptomatic and did not require hospitalization or any treatment for the perforation. The overall perforation rate was 0.009% (2 of 21,923), and the symptomatic perforation rate was determined to be 0.005% (1 of 21,923). It was concluded that the safety profile for CTC is favorable, particularly for screening purposes.

In comparing the published series of perforations occurring during CTC, the symptomatic perforation rate has been found to range from 0.005% to 0.03%.[9–11] These rates impart a significantly more favorable safety profile for CTC compared with colonoscopy. Most patients who have perforations during CTC have had conditions that likely contributed to or exacerbated barotrauma to the bowel wall during insufflation of the colon. Obstructive or occlusive lesions, such as those from carcinoma, diverticulosis, benign inflammatory stricture, and left inguinal hernia containing sigmoid colon, have been found to be associated with perforation. Specific attention is recommended to the left groin in patients with known preexisting left inguinal hernia during the insufflation process of CTC.[12,13] Insufflation is discontinued if there is increase in size of the hernia sac. Active inflammatory bowel diseases, such as ulcerative colitis, with weakening of the bowel wall can increase the risk for perforation. Other causes of weakening of the colon wall such as a colonoscopic biopsy or polypectomy may increase the likelihood of perforation during CTC. In some sites, performing CTC is postponed in this situation until 1 to 2 weeks after the biopsy.[12,14] The inflation of a balloon-tipped catheter may increase the likelihood of rectal perforations, and the catheter is recommended to be used with caution by appropriately trained personnel. There are also reports of colonic perforation during CTC in patients without known colonic disease.[15,16] These perforations occurred in elderly patients who were managed conservatively with antibiotic treatment.

Colonic perforation is a known risk of conventional colonoscopy screening and occurs in 0.06% to 0.19% of cases. The perforation rate is approximately 0.1% for diagnostic colonoscopy and 0.2% for therapeutic colonoscopy in larger series.[17–23] Thus, perforation rates for diagnostic colonoscopy are significantly higher than for CTC. However, positive findings from CTC screening typically require a subsequent colonoscopy, and, therefore, the total perforation rate for the combination of procedures is somewhat higher than the rate for the CTC alone. Mechanical trauma caused by the colonoscope is thought to be the primary cause of perforation. The sigmoid colon is a common site for perforation during colonoscopy. Diverticulosis typically occurs in the sigmoid, which is also often redundant and tortuous and which may be more fixed if pelvic adhesions are present. High pneumatic pressure during insufflation of the colon can contribute to an increased risk for perforation during colonoscopy. The risk of perforation also increases during a therapeutic colonoscopy when polypectomy is performed. Colonoscopic biopsy, particularly when deep, is also a risk factor for perforation of the colon. The reported mortality rate for colonoscopy ranges from 0% to 0.07%.[17–23] To date there have been no deaths associated with the performance of CTC.

The double-contrast barium enema has been reported to have a risk of perforation ranging between 0.004% and 0.2%.[24,25] The complications related to colon perforation caused by barium enema are thought to be more clinically significant than those that occur during CTC. In one study, 10% of patients who suffered colon perforation from barium enema died of barium peritonitis.[25] Perforations occurring as a result of barium enema are typically due to trauma from insertion of the rectal tube or overinflation of the intrarectal retention balloon.[26,27] Perforation during barium enema may also occur if the procedure is performed in patients with a weakened colon wall, such as caused by ischemia, steroid use, or a deep colonic biopsy. Similar to CTC, to decrease the likelihood of perforation during barium enema, it is recommended to wait for at least 1 week after biopsy.[16]

RADIATION DOSE AND CANCER RISK

Several recent studies have raised concerns about the radiation-related cancer risks from CT scans.[28,29] The typical radiation doses from CTC, the sensitivity and specificity of low-dose CTC, the potential radiation-related cancer risks from the screening, and the follow-up examinations for extracolonic findings are discussed.

Radiation Dose

Most medical examinations that involve ionizing radiation only expose certain parts of the body to radiation,which is referred to as partial body exposure. Absorbed organ doses and effective doses are the key quantities used to summarize doses from such partial body exposures. Here the authors briefly describe these quantities, estimation methods, and sample dose estimates for CTC screening.

The amount of radiation energy that is absorbed per gram of tissue is called the absorbed dose.[30] It is measured in grays (Gy) whereby 1 Gy corresponds to 1 joule of energy absorbed per kilogram. The biologic effect per unit of absorbed dose depends on the particular tissue that is exposed, as some tissues have been shown to be more sensitive to radiation than others. For example, a dose given to the breast is more likely to cause cancer than the same dose given to the rectum.[30] To compare doses from different tests involving partial body exposure, the effective dose is typically used. The effective dose is a weighted average of the absorbed doses to each exposed organ with weights that reflect the relative radiosensitivity of each organ.[31]

Radiation dose from CT scanning depends on patient size, CT scanner model, and protocol. For the same CT scanner and the same protocol, patients with smaller body size (eg, pediatric patients) receive higher radiation doses because there is less tissue to attenuate the radiation before it reaches a particular organ. Even for the same CT scanner model, the protocol used may vary between hospitals or technicians. The operational factors specified in the protocol include number of scans, scan length, image thickness, degree of overlap between adjacent x-ray beams (pitch or table feed), tube current-time product (mAs), and tube potential (kVp).[32]

There are several operational factors that typically result in higher doses. Repeated CT scanning, such as multiphase examinations, increases the radiation dose. For example, 2 sets of images are obtained during CTC, with the patient first in the supine position and then in the prone position, and so the radiation dose is typically doubled. Radiation dose also increases rapidly with the beam potential (kVp): as a rule of thumb, by a power of 2.5.[33] A longer scan length results in radiation exposure to a greater anatomic region and hence a higher radiation dose. Thinner images provide better image resolution and improved visibility of small objects. However, beam intensity needs to be increased to reduce the noise in these thinner images, which concurrently increases the radiation dose. CT scan images can be obtained in contiguity, as well as with an overlap, or a gap between x-ray beams. The degree of the overlap or the gap between the beams is expressed by pitch. A pitch of less than 1 indicates overlapped beam exposure. Therefore, radiation dose is inversely proportional to pitch. Tube current-time product (mAs) is the product of tube current (mA) and gantry rotation time (sec), and radiation dose is linearly proportional to mAs. In general, the key factors that are modified to reduce the radiation exposure from a CT scan are the tube current and the beam potential.

Because there are multiple factors in the CT protocol that influence radiation exposure in different directions, special software programs have been developed to estimate organ-specific and effective doses from CT scans for a user-defined input involving CT scan parameters and scanner type (eg, CT Expo[34] and ImPACT[35]). These programs use preestablished organ dose databases generated by radiation transport computer simulations, which simulate radiation interactions in the human body.[36–39] The patient is assumed to be a "standard man," who is defined as measuring 170 cm in height and 70 kg in weight. These programs are useful for comparing doses across protocols or scanners but cannot be used to estimate the dose to a specific individual.

Since the introduction of CTC using single-detector CT scanners, there has been the development of multidetector CT scanners with incorporation of low-dose CT techniques. The 2009 American College of Radiology practice guideline for the performance of CTC in adults specifies that screening studies that are performed in individuals without signs or symptoms of colorectal cancer should be performed using a low-dose, nonenhanced multidetector CT technique.[40] The use of technique charts or automatic exposure control is suggested so that patient size may be accounted for. The CT protocol used also varies depending on the clinical indication for the test. Although there are parameters that may be specific to particular CT scanners, in general for a tube potential of 120 kVp, an effective mAs of between 50 and 80 is recommended when performing screening CTC (low-dose CTC). If diagnostic CTC is being performed in a patient with symptoms of possible colorectal carcinoma, intravenous contrast may be necessary and CT acquisition parameters may typically require higher mAs. The performance characteristics of low-dose CTC are reviewed in detail below.

Sensitivity and Specificity of Low-Dose CTC

Early studies have shown that tube current may be decreased to reduce radiation exposure without compromising polyp detection on CTC. This detection is possible because of the inherent large difference in density between the air-filled lumen and the soft tissue attenuation of colonic polyps.[41] In one such study, CTC was performed using single-detector CT in 2 patient groups. In the first group, 8 patients with 31 polyps were scanned using 140 mA, 5-mm collimation, pitch of 1.3, and 3-mm reconstruction interval. In the second group, 10 patients with 30 polyps were scanned using 70 mA, 5-mm collimation, pitch of 1, and 1-mm reconstruction interval. There was 100% sensitivity for detection of polyps of size 5 mm and larger for both groups. The radiation dose for dual position CTC at 70 mA was determined to be 50% lower than the dose for a standard CT scan of the abdomen and pelvis and similar to the radiation dose for a barium enema.

A study evaluating multidetector CTC at various radiation dose levels was performed in 50 patients at high risk for the development of colorectal carcinoma and showed no compromise in polyp detection ability with lower-dose protocols.[42] Patients were scanned using 120 kVp and 100 mAs. Two low-dose CT scans were then obtained by simulating 50 mAs and 30 mAs. Although there was overall decreased image quality at 30 mAs, the per-patient sensitivity for the detection of polyps measuring 5 mm and larger was 90% at all dose levels. Similarly, the per-polyp sensitivity for detecting polyps measuring 5 mm and larger ranged between 85% and 92% for all doses.

Low-dose thin-section multidetector CTC, followed by conventional colonoscopy, was performed in 105 patients who had symptoms of possible colorectal cancer.[43] CT scan parameters included 120 kVp, 50 mAs, and thin sections with 1.25-mm reconstructions at a 1.0-mm interval. The per-lesion sensitivities for detection of polyps of size 6 to 9 mm and 10 mm and larger were 70% and 93%, respectively. Overall specificity was excellent at 98%. The effective doses for dual position CTC were 5.0 mSv for men and 7.8 mSv for women. This study demonstrated that low-dose multidetector CTC has excellent sensitivity and specificity for the detection of large polyps.

Most recently, low-dose CTC technique has also been evaluated successfully in average-risk patients without symptoms of colorectal disease. A performance trial using the newest 64-slice multidetector CT was conducted in 307 subjects who underwent CTC for screening.[44] Patients were scanned using a tube voltage of 120 kVp and a tube current of 70 mAs in the supine position, which was decreased to 30 mAs in the prone position. A new dose-modulation technique was used to adapt the tube current automatically to patient anatomy. The calculated mean radiation dose to patients was 4.5 mSv for the entire examination, which is significantly reduced from earlier studies. The sensitivity and specificity of CTC for the detection of adenomatous polyps larger than 5 mm were 91% and 93%, respectively, and for adenomatous polyps larger than 10 mm were 92% and 98%, respectively.

Several studies have evaluated the potential for decreasing the radiation dose for CTC even further. A pilot study reported excellent results with very low-dose CTC in 27 patients with symptoms of possible colorectal cancer.[45] Multidetector CT was performed with 140 kVp and 10 mAs. All 9 cancers were identified, and there was 100% sensitivity for polyps 10 mm and larger (3 of 3) as well as for polyps between 6 and 9 mm (3 of 3). Total radiation dose for dual position CTC was 1.7 mSv for men and 2.3 mSv for women, which was a 40% to 70% decrease in radiation dose compared with prior studies. A follow-up study using the same lower-dose CTC protocol was performed in 158 patients and revealed similar excellent results.[46] CTC performed with 10 mAs resulted in 100% sensitivity for carcinomas (22 of 22), 100% sensitivity for large polyps (13 of 13), and 83% sensitivity for small polyps (20 of 24). There was 97% specificity, and the positive and negative predictive values were 94% and 98%, respectively. The simulated effective doses for combined supine and prone acquisitions were 1.8 mSv in men and 2.4 mSv in women. CTC using effective mAs of 10 was performed in 88 patients who underwent 2 sequential colonoscopies with results of the second colonoscopy serving as the reference standard for determination of the performance of the CTC and the first colonoscopy.[47] The per-polyp sensitivities for lesions 6 mm and larger for CTC and the initial colonoscopy were 86% and 84%, respectively. The initial colonoscopy missed 16 polyps, 6 of which were identified by low-dose CT. The per-patient sensitivities for polyps of size 6 mm and larger for CTC and the first colonoscopy were 84% and 90%, respectively, with specificities of 82% and 100%, respectively.

An alternative approach that has been proposed for dose reduction is to scan patients in only 1 position. However, it is not clear if scanning in 1 position will provide adequate colonic cleansing and distention, given that dual position scanning typically allows for shifting of residual material in the colon and improved distention.[48] In a study evaluating low-dose CTC, 137 patients were scanned only in the supine position.[49] CT scan parameters included 120 kVp and effective mAs of 10. The effective dose using this type of protocol was 0.7 mSv for men and 1 mSv for women. The sensitivities for detection of polyps larger than 10 mm, between 5 and 9.9 mm, and less than 5 mm in size were 78.6%, 85.7%, and 57%, respectively, with the specificity for each size group at 100%, 92.8%, and 85.9%, respectively. It was concluded that low-dose CTC is feasible with substantial radiation dose reduction, but additional studies are required to evaluate whether there is a compromise in small poly detection ability when scanning in 1 position. Current standard practice consists of scanning patients in supine and in prone positions.[40]

There have been other efforts to determine whether radiation dose could be lowered even more. A pilot study was performed in 15 patients who were scanned using different mAs levels ranging between 0.4 mAs and 100 mAs correlating with doses ranging from 0.05 mSv to 12 mSv.[50] Sensitivity was 80% to 100% for the detection of large polyps (>10 mm) for all mAs and dose levels. The mean sensitivity for identifying polyps of size 5 mm and larger was 74% across all mAs and dose levels except for the lowest level of 0.4 mAs. The number of false-positive results decreased as the mAs decreased for 5-mm and larger lesions. This decrease was thought to be due to increased noise and smoothing algorithms applied to the lowest-dose images. Continued investigation is needed to explore the clinical value of very low–dose CTC.

A recent international survey of 34 institutions aimed to evaluate what protocols were actually being used in practice at present.[51] Based on the institutions' protocols, the estimated effective dose for CTC screening ranged from 2.6 mSv to 14.7 mSv per examination and the median dose was 5.6 mSv. The largest source of variation in the protocols was the mAs, which varied from 25 to 100 mAs for the supine scan. These survey results suggest that low-dose protocols are being used in many different countries, but there is still wide variation in practice. The effective dose from a double-contrast barium enema is of a similar magnitude to that from CTC, but also highly variable. A recent literature review found that the average dose per procedure was 8 mSv but with a range of 2 to 18 mSv.[52]

Radiation-Related Cancer Risk

Despite the fact that low-dose protocols are being used routinely and have shown excellent sensitivity and specificity for lesion detection, there are still concerns about the potential cancer risks. Numerous epidemiologic studies have established that radiation can cause most types of cancer and that there is unlikely to be a threshold below which there is no risk.[30] The study of the Japanese atomic bomb survivors in Nagasaki and Hiroshima, known as the Life Span Study, is the most important study of the long-term effects of radiation exposure. The key strengths are its large size (N ≈ 120,000), long-term follow-up (>50 years), and the fact that the population was not selected because of a specific disease or an occupation and therefore includes a wide range of ages of healthy men and women who were exposed to a broad range of radiation doses (0–4 Gy). A common misconception about the Life Span Study is that it is a study of high-dose radiation exposures. The median dose in the exposed population is 250 mGy, and about 25% of the population had exposures in the range of 5 to 100 mGy.[53] For solid cancers the risk is approximately linear in dose, whereas for leukemia the dose-response is curvilinear so that the risk per unit dose is lower at lower dose levels. There is also evidence of a significantly increased cancer risk in the 0- to 150-mGy dose range, and the magnitude of the risk per unit dose is similar to the risk across the whole dose range. Risks are generally found to be higher if exposure occurs at younger ages, and after exposure there seems to be a lifelong elevation in cancer risk.

Other populations that have been studied for the long-term effects of radiation include those exposed for medical reasons (both therapeutic and diagnostic), and occupational groups such as radiologists and nuclear power workers.[30] These studies also contribute important information on the risks from repeated low-dose radiation exposures, as opposed to the acute single exposure that was received in the Japanese atomic bombing. Although they provide additional evidence of significantly elevated cancer risks for low doses of radiation (<100 mGy), most studies do not have adequate power to enable precise risk estimates at these low dose levels, especially taking into account factors such as age at exposure and site of cancer.[54] Therefore, risks from low doses are generally estimated by extrapolating models based on the results from the whole range of exposures received in the Life Span Study. Such risk projection methods based on existing data can provide a much more timely estimate of the long-term risk of radiation-related cancer.

A recent committee for the National Research Council (the Biological Effects of Ionizing Radiation [BEIR] VII committee) developed detailed models for estimating the lifetime risk of radiation-related cancer for the US population.[30] These risk models are based primarily on the most recent follow-up of the Japanese atomic bomb survivors because for most cancer sites, they remain the most detailed models available for estimating the risks by sex, age, and time since exposure.[53] These risk models, with minor modifications (mainly the addition of cancers of several sites, such as pancreatic, rectal, kidney, esophageal, oral, and brain cancers), combined with the organ-specific dose estimates (described later in this article) have been used to estimate the lifetime risk of radiation-related cancer after CTC screening.

Whereas effective dose estimates are useful for comparing doses from different protocols, cancer risk estimation is best performed with organ dose estimates. Because there are no recently published estimates of organ-specific doses from CTC in the United States, the authors used CT-Expo[34] and a CTC screening protocol from the recent American College of Radiology Imaging Network (ACRIN) trial for the LightSpeed 64-slice scanner (GE Healthcare, Waukesha, WI, USA) (120 kVp, 50 mAs, pitch of 1, and image thickness of 1.25 mm[55]) to estimate organ doses for a typical screening examination in the United States. Organ dose estimates varied from 14 mGy to the stomach to 2 mGy to the lung for men and from 15 mGy to the kidney to 1 mGy to the breast for women. The effective dose per screening examination was 8 mSv for a man and 9 mSv for a woman. The scanner that the authors used for these calculations is one that is commonly used in the United States, and the protocol is in line with the recommendations for CTC screening from the American College of Radiology.[40]

The authors estimated that a single CTC screen at age 60 years would result in a lifetime risk of radiation-related cancer of approximately 0.05% (ie, 5 cancers per 10,000 individuals screened). The risks were similar for men and women. For a single screen at age 50 years, the risks were slightly higher (0.06%) and at age 70 years were lower (0.03%), primarily because of the longer versus shorter life expectancy. If an individual undergoes multiple screens, for example, screening every 5 years from age 60 to 75 years, then the total risk would be approximately 0.016% (2 × 0.05% + 2 × 0.03%). Because the effective dose estimates for barium enema are broadly similar to those for CTC, the radiation-related cancer risks will also be similar.

Previous estimates of the radiation-related cancer risk from CTC screening were approximately twice as high, even though they were based on similar organ doses (0.14% for a single screen at age 50 years compared with 0.06%).[56] The difference between these risk estimates was mostly due to the assumptions underlying the radiation risk models. The previous study used the BEIR V committee's risk models from a report published in 1990.[57] The main change between the 2 reports was the assumption of how risks are transported from the Japanese to the US population. The BEIR VII report provides an in-depth description of the new data and justification for these alternative assumptions.[30] Most other national and international committees that provide risk projection estimates currently use similar methods to those used in the BEIR VII report (eg, United Nations Scientific Committee on the Effects of Atomic Radiation [UNSCEAR][58]). There are several uncertainties and assumptions that go into the estimation, and it is not unreasonable to assume that the risks may vary by a factor of 2.[30] Therefore, the previous estimates of 0.14% for a screen at age 50 years could be taken as approximate upper bounds for the potential risk.

Unlike colonoscopy, the whole abdomen is visible during CTC screening. Potential abnormalities outside of the colon can therefore be picked up. Many US screening studies have collected data on the number of patients who had clinically significant extracolonic findings that required further imaging. The proportion of patients who had follow-up CT scans to investigate these findings was generally in the range of 5% to 10%[59–61]; in one small study it was 24%.[62] The most common follow-up scan was a CT scan of the abdomen. Abdomen/pelvis and chest CT scans were also performed. The dose from an abdomen/pelvis CT scan performed with and without contrast is about 20 mSv,[52] which results in a radiation risk that is about twice as high as the risk from CTC. However, because only a small proportion (eg, 10%) of the screening population will receive these additional scans, it is unlikely that these scans will increase the average risk to the whole screening population by more than 20%.

SUMMARY

Although several organizations have raised concerns about the safety of CTC, the current evidence suggests that the risks are likely to be small. The data on colonic perforation suggest that the rate is low (0.005%–0.03%), especially compared with colonoscopy (0.06%–0.19%). Also, because no sedation is required the cardiopulmonary risks are avoided. Current CTC technique uses low-dose parameters. The 2009 American College of Radiology practice guidelines specifically recommend the use of low-dose technique for screening CTC. Studies have been performed showing that with the use of multidetector CT scanners the ability to detect polyps of size 6 mm and larger is maintained with low-dose techniques. New dose-modulation techniques that are now available may be used to help reduce radiation dose further. For a typical low-dose US protocol, the effective dose estimate was 8 mSv for men and 9 mSv for women. Based on these doses, the risk of radiation-related cancer is about 0.05% from a single screening at age 60 years. Risks from follow-up scans are unlikely to increase the total risk to the population undergoing screening by more than 20%. Radiation doses and hence risks from double-contrast barium enema are likely to be similar in magnitude.

The potential benefits from CTC screening are likely to be high because of the ability to prevent colon cancer cases as well as deaths.[1] When further quantitative data on the magnitude of these benefits become available, a full risk-benefit analysis can be conducted. Given that the risks are relatively small, it seems likely that the benefits from CTC screening will exceed these risks for most individuals.

REFERENCES

1. Levin B, Lieberman DA, McFarland B, et al. American Cancer Society Colorectal Cancer Advisory Group, US Multi-Society Task Force, American College of Radiology Colon Cancer Committee. Screening and surveillance for the early

detection of colorectal cancer and adenomatous polyps, 2008: a joint guideline from the American Cancer Society, the US Multi-Society Task Force on Colorectal Cancer, and the American College of Radiology. CA Cancer J Clin 2008;58(3): 130–60.

2. Schenck AP, Peacock SC, Klabunde CN, et al. Trends in colorectal cancer test use in the medicare population, 1998–2005. Am J Prev Med 2009;37(1):1–7.

3. U.S. Preventive Services Task Force. Screening for colorectal cancer: U.S. Preventive Services Task Force recommendation statement. Ann Intern Med 2008;149(9):627–37.

4. Decision memo for screening computed tomography (CTC) for colorectal cancer (CAG-00396N). Centers for Medicare and Medicaid Services (CMS). 2009. Available at: https://www.cms.hhs.gov/mcd/viewdecisionmemo.asp?from2= viewdecisionmemo.asp&id=220&. Accessed May 15, 2009.

5. Yee J. Extra-colonic findings on CT colonography. Gastrointest Endosc, in press.

6. Kamar M, Portnoy O, Bar-Dayan A, et al. Actual colonic perforation in virtual colonoscopy: report of a case. Dis Colon Rectum 2004;47:1242–6.

7. Coady-Fariborzian L, Angel LP, Procaccino JA. Perforated colon secondary to virtual colonoscopy: report of a case. Dis Colon Rectum 2004;47:1247–9.

8. Triester SL, Hara AK, Young-Fadok TM, et al. Colonic perforation after Computed Tomographic Colonography in a patient with fibrostenosing Crohn's disease. Am J Gastroenterol 2006;101:189–92.

9. Burling D, Halligan S, Slater A, et al. Potentially adverse events at CT colonography in symptomatic patients: national survey of the United Kingdom. Radiology 2006;239(2):464–71.

10. Sosna J, Blachar A, Amitai M, et al. Colonic perforation at CT colonography: assessment of risk in a multicenter large cohort. Radiology 2006;239:457–63.

11. Pickhardt PJ. Incidence of colonic perforation at CT colonography: review of existing data and implications for screening of asymptomatic adults. Radiology 2006;239:313–6.

12. Sosna J, Sella T, Bar-Ziv J, et al. Perforation of the colon and rectum—a newly recognized complication of CT colonography. Semin Ultrasound CT MR 2006; 27:161–5.

13. Belo-Oliveira P, Curvo-Semedo L, Rodrigues H, et al. Sigmoid colon perforation at CT colonography secondary to a possible obstructive mechanism: report of a case. Dis Colon Rectum 2007;50:1478–80.

14. Stevenson G. Normal anatomy and techniques of examination of the colon: barium, CT and MRI. In: Freeny PC, Stevenson GW, editors. Margulis and Burhenne's alimentary tract radiology. St Louis (MO): Mosby; 1994. p. 692–724.

15. Young BM, Fletcher JG, Earnest F, et al. Colonic perforation at CT colonography in a patient without known colonic disease. AJR Am J Roentgenol 2006; 186:119–21.

16. Bassett JT, Liotta RA, Barlow D, et al. Colonic perforation during screening CT colonography using automated CO2 insufflation in an asymptomatic adult. Abdom Imaging 2008;33:598–600.

17. Waye JD, Lewis BS, Yessayan S. Colonoscopy: a prospective report of complications. J Clin Gastroenterol 1992;15:347–51.

18. Anderson ML, Pasha TM, Leighton JA. Endoscopic perforation of the colon: lessons from a 10-year study. Am J Gastroenterol 2000;95:3418–22.

19. Sieg A, Hachmoeller-Eisenbach U, Eisenbach T. Prospective evaluation of complications in outpatient GI endoscopy: a survey among German gastroenterologists. Gastrointest Endosc 2001;53:620–7.

20. Tran DQ, Rosen L, Kim R, et al. Actual colonoscopy: what are the risks of perforation? Am J Surg 2001;67:845–7.
21. Korman LY, Overholt BF, Box T, et al. Perforation during colonoscopy in endoscopic ambulatory surgical centers. Gastrointest Endosc 2003;58:554–7.
22. Gatto NM, Frucht H, Sundarajan V, et al. Risk of perforation after colonoscopy and sigmoidoscopy: a population-based study. J Natl Cancer Inst 2003;95:230–6.
23. Bowles CJ, Leicester R, Romaya C, et al. A prospective study of colonoscopy practice in the UK today: are we adequately prepared for national colorectal cancer screening tomorrow? Gut 2004;53:277–83.
24. Han SY, Tishler JM. Perforation of the colon above the peritoneal reflection during the barium enema examination. Radiology 1982;144:253–5.
25. Blakeborough A, Sheridan MB, Chapman AH. Complications of barium enema examinations: a survey of consultant radiologists 1992–1994. Clin Radiol 1997;52:142–8.
26. Williams SM, Harned RK. Recognition and prevention of barium enema complications. Curr Probl Diagn Radiol 1992;20:123–51.
27. Blakeborough A, Sheridan MB, Chapman AH. Retention balloon catheters and barium enemas: attitudes, current practice, and relative safety in the UK. Clin Radiol 1997;52:62–4.
28. Berrington de Gonzalez A, Mahesh M, Kim KP, et al. Projected cancer risks from computed tomographic scans performed in the United States in 2007. Arch Int Med 2009;169(22):2071–7.
29. Sodickson A, Baeyens PF, Andriole KP, et al. Recurrent CT, cumulative radiation exposure, and associated radiation-induced cancer risks from CT of adults. Radiology 2009;251(1):175–84.
30. Committee to assess health risks from exposure to low levels of ionizing radiation, National Research Council. Health risks from exposure to low levels of ionizing radiation: BEIR VII. Washington, DC: National Academy of Sciences; 2005.
31. ICRP. The 2007 recommendations of the International Commission on Radiological Protection. New York: International Commission on Radiological Protection; 2007. ICRP Publication 103.
32. Nagel H. Radiation exposure in computed tomography. Hamburg: CTB Publications; 2002.
33. Brix G, Nagel HD, Stamm G, et al. Radiation exposure in multi-slice versus single-slice spiral CT: results of a nationwide survey. Eur Radiol 2003;13(8):1979–91.
34. Stamm G, Nagel HD. [CT-expo: a novel program for dose evaluation in CT]. Rofo 2002;174(12):1570–6 [in German].
35. Imaging Performance Assessment of Computed Tomography Group. ImPACT CT patient dosimetry calculator—version 0.99x. London: Imaging Performance Assessment of Computed Tomography Group; 2006.
36. Zankl M, Panser W, Drexler G. Part II: Organ doses from computed tomographic examinations in paediatric radiology. Tomographic anthropomorphic models. Munich (Germany): GSF-Bericht; 1993.
37. Zankl M, Panser W, Drexler G. Part VI: Organ doses from computed tomographic examinations. The calculation of dose from external photon exposures using reference human phantoms and Monte Carlo methods. Munich (Germany): GSF-Bericht; 1991.
38. Jones DG, Shrimpton PC. Survey of CT practice in the UK. Part 3: normalised organ doses calculated using Monte Carlo techniques (1991) NRPB R250. London: HMSO; 1991.
39. Shrimpton PC, Jones DG, Hillier MC, et al. Survey of CT practice in the UK. Part 2: dosimetric aspects (1991) NRPB R249. London: HMSO; 1991.

40. American College of Radiology. ACR practice guideline for the performance of computed tomography (CT) colonography in adults. Practice Guidelines and Technical Standards. Reston (VA): American College of Radiology; 2009.
41. Hara AK, Johnson CD, Reed JE, et al. Reducing data size and radiation dose for CT colonography. Am J Roentgenol 1997;168:1181–4.
42. van Gelder RE, Venema HW, Serlie IW, et al. CT colonography at different radiation dose levels: feasibility of dose reduction. Radiology 2002;224:25–33.
43. Macari M, Bini EJ, Xue X, et al. Colorectal neoplasms: prospective comparison of thin-section low-dose multi-detector row CT colonography and conventional colonoscopy for detection. Radiology 2002;224:383–92.
44. Graser A, Stieber P, Nagel D, et al. Comparison of CT colonography, colonoscopy, sigmoidoscopy and fecal occult blood tests for the detection of advanced adenoma in an average risk population. Gut 2009;58:241–8.
45. Iannaccone R, Laghi A, Catalano C, et al. Feasibility of ultra-low-dose multislice CT colonography for the detection of colorectal lesions: preliminary experience. Eur Radiol 2003;13:1297–302.
46. Iannaccone R, Laghi A, Catalano C, et al. Detection of colorectal lesions: lower-dose multi-detector row helical CT colonography compared with conventional colonoscopy. Radiology 2003;229:775–81.
47. Iannaccone R, Catalano C, Mangiapane F, et al. Colorectal polyps: detection with low-dose multi-detector row helical CT colonography versus two sequential colonoscopies. Radiology 2005;237:927–37.
48. Yee J, Kumar NN, Hung RK, et al. Comparison of supine, prone and both supine and prone scans in CT colonography. Radiology 2003;226:653–61.
49. Cohnen M, Vogt C, Beck A, et al. Feasibility of MDCT Colonography in ultra-low-dose technique in the detection of colorectal lesions: comparison with high-resolution video colonoscopy. Am J Roentgenol 2004;183:1355–9.
50. van Gelder RE, Venema HW, Florie J, et al. CT Colonography: feasibility of substantial dose reduction- comparison of medium to very low doses in identical patients. Radiology 2004;232:611–20.
51. Liedenbaum MH, Venema HW, Stoker J. Radiation dose in CT colonography–trends in time and differences between daily practice and screening protocols. Eur Radiol 2008;18(10):2222–8.
52. Mettler FA Jr, Huda W, Yoshizumi TT, et al. Effective doses in radiology and diagnostic nuclear medicine: a catalog. Radiology 2008;248(1):254–63.
53. Preston DL, Ron E, Tokuoka S, et al. Solid cancer incidence in atomic bomb survivors: 1958–1998. Radiat Res 2007;168(1):1–64.
54. Land CE. Estimating cancer risks from low doses of ionizing radiation. Science 1980;209(4462):1197–203.
55. Johnson CD, Chen MH, Toledano AY, et al. Accuracy of CT colonography for detection of large adenomas and cancers. N Engl J Med 2008;359(12):1207–17.
56. Brenner DJ, Georgsson MA. Mass screening with CT colonography: should the radiation exposure be of concern? Gastroenterology 2005;129(1):328–37.
57. Committee on the Biological Effects of Ionizing Radiation (BEIR V), National Research Council. Health effects of exposure to low levels of ionizing radiation: BEIR V. Washington, DC: National Academy of Sciences; 1990.
58. United Nations Scientific Committee on the Effects of Atomic Radiation. Sources and effects of ionizing radiation. New York: United Nations; 2006.
59. Pickhardt PJ, Hanson ME, Vanness DJ, et al. Unsuspected extracolonic findings at screening CT colonography: clinical and economic impact. Radiology 2008;249(1):151–9.

60. Yee J, Kumar NN, Godara S, et al. Extracolonic abnormalities discovered incidentally at CT colonography in a male population. Radiology 2005;236(2):519–26.
61. Gluecker TM, Johnson CD, Wilson LA, et al. Extracolonic findings at CT colonography: evaluation of prevalence and cost in a screening population. Gastroenterology 2003;124(4):911–6.
62. Kimberly JR, Phillips KC, Santago P, et al. Extracolonic findings at virtual colonoscopy: an important consideration in asymptomatic colorectal cancer screening. J Gen Intern Med 2009;24(1):69–73.

Finding Polyps at Colonoscopy Previously Noted on CT Colonography

Jerome D. Waye, MD[a,b,]*

KEYWORDS

- CT colonography • Colonoscopy
- Colon imaging • Colon polyps

From the standpoint of the colonoscopist, it is almost unbelievable that a polyp could be reported as a positive finding on CTC but not seen on a follow-up colonoscopy. Colonoscopy is the procedure that, because of its ability to visualize the mucosal surface of the colon and delineate stool from polyps, led to the barium enema losing its status as the primary imaging tool for the large bowel. Colonoscopy has the ability to suction pools of fluid from the large bowel, to see the surface in full color, to wash away debris such as fecal material or seeds, identify any protrusion as mucosal in origin, and, with a high degree of certainty, distinguish benign from malignant lesions. Because of the visual clarity of colonoscopy, it has been hailed as the standard for colon imaging since it was first introduced.

Vast strides in radiographic imaging have seen computed tomographic colonography (CTC) become a useful tool for screening of the large bowel. A lesion that is reported on CTC but not seen on colonoscopy is often counted as a false-positive radiographic reading. CTC lesions that are seen on colonoscopy are accepted as positive findings. In general, gastroenterologists, radiologists, and surgeons view optical colonoscopy as the "gold standard" for visualizing lesions in the large bowel. Because the colonoscope is an extension of the endoscopist's eye, having flexibility, tip deflection capability, wide-angle lenses, and the ability to detect colon pathology, it has widely replaced the barium enema (both single and double contrast) as the imaging modality for evaluation of the colon. It is not surprising that comparative studies have been performed that show the superiority of colonoscopy over the barium radiographic technique for large bowel screening. Two studies[1,2] have demonstrated extremely low sensitivity and specificity for the barium enema compared with

a Department of Medicine, Mount Sinai Medical Center, NY, USA
b 650 Park Avenue, NY 10065, USA
* 650 Park Avenue, NY 10065.
E-mail address: Jdwaye@aol.com

Gastrointest Endoscopy Clin N Am 20 (2010) 293–304
doi:10.1016/j.giec.2010.02.001
1052-5157/10/$ – see front matter © 2010 Elsevier Inc. All rights reserved.

giendo.theclinics.com

colonoscopy. The sensitivity of the barium radiographic colonography for polyp detection of any size was found to be poor, and even for polyps greater than 10 mm,[1] the ability to find polyps on barium enema is 50% that of colonoscopy. A study that retrospectively reviewed the reports of double contrast barium enema (DCBE) within 36 months prior to the diagnosis of colorectal cancer found that the overall rate of new or missed cancers was about 22%.[3] In this report, DCBE missed one-fifth of all subsequently surgically resected neoplasms. Several factors accounted for this apparent high rate of "missed lesions" in the colon. The 6 factors that were associated with missing the cancer were older age, female sex, previous abdominal pelvic surgery, diverticular disease, right-sided colorectal cancer, and having the radiographic examination performed in an office setting. The investigators' conclusion was that physicians who use DCBE to evaluate the colon must inform their patients that if a cancer is present, there is an approximately 1-in-5 chance that it will be missed.

Among the many benefits of computer technology has been the emergence of new, better, faster, and more specific radiographic imaging procedures such as the CTC. It was inevitable that the two radiographic imaging studies be compared. In a recent retrospective report[4] reviewing findings of patients with colon cancer who had either a DCBE or CTC, only 21 of 33 patients had their malignant neoplasm detected using DCBE whereas 32 of a similar cohort of 33 patients had the tumor detected on CTC.

A meta-analysis[5] reviewed the performance of DCBE versus CTC for the detection of colon polyps greater than or equal to 6 mm using colonoscopy as a gold standard. This comparison revealed that CTC markedly increased the ability to detect 6 mm polyps, and was also more sensitive than DCBE in detecting polyps of 6 to 9 mm. The conclusion was that DCBE has statistically lower sensitivity and specificity than CTC for detecting colorectal polyps greater than or equal to 6 mm.

In an editorial-type discussion, Stevenson[6] stated that, in comparison to DCBE radiographic examination of the colon, CTC is more accurate, is preferred by patients, has a shorter room time, fewer complications, and lower radiation exposure, and in addition reveals therapeutically significant extracolonic lesions in 5% to 10% of cases. He states that it is "rather irresponsible to continue to offer routine DCBE examinations."

A review of the recent medical literature on comparing CTC with colonoscopy has found many published studies that purportedly evaluate head-to-head comparisons of end results in screening average or high-risk populations for the presence of polyps or carcinoma. In several of these reports, a colonoscopic examination was performed after a full CTC examination with the colonoscopist "blinded" to the results of the CTC. Because the contrast used for CTC has been found not to interfere with the colonoscopy procedure, such a blind comparison would seem to be the ideal method to identify whether the CTC has missed any lesions and, conversely, should also reveal whether lesions seen on CTC could have been missed by the subsequent colonoscopic examination. Most of these reports have adopted colonoscopy as the gold standard for evaluation of CTC findings. Only a few articles have actually examined the possibility that colonoscopy may not find a true lesion reported on the CTC examination. A meta-analysis[7] reported on 47 articles in which CTC was compared with colonoscopy, with all using colonoscopy as a gold standard to affirm or rule out the presence of a lesion found on CTC. Several comparative reports have stated that they used the technique of "blind colonoscopy" performed after the CTC examination and that after each segment was examined by the colonoscopist, the finding on the CTC was revealed. It is unfortunate that most centers that used a "blind and revealed" protocol whereby CTC findings were given to the colonoscopist after viewing each segment have not reported on the actual number of lesions that were reported on

CTC but missed on the first blind colonoscopic examination, but then found on a second pass after the finding on CTC examination was revealed.

A study group of 15 clinical sites participated in the National CT Colonography Trial of the American College of Radiology Imaging Network,[8] designed to compare the finding of CTC with same-day colonoscopy for evaluation of large colorectal adenomas and cancers (equal to or greater than 10 mm in diameter). The colonoscopist was blinded to the CTC results but if the radiographic examination revealed a lesion equal to or greater than 10 mm in diameter and was not seen on the initial colonoscopy, the patient was advised to undergo an additional colonoscopic examination within 90 days. For the repeat colonoscopic examination, the CTC results were provided to the examiner before the examination. In a group of 2531 patients, 30 lesions measuring 10 mm or more were reported on the CTC in 27 participants, but not detected on the initial colonoscopic examination. Fifteen of these 27 patients, having 18 reported lesions, did have a second colonoscopic examination, and in this group, 5 of the 18 lesions were confirmed as true-positive CTC on the second colonoscopy examination. The diameters of these 5 lesions found on the second-look colonoscopy were 9 mm and 14 mm (inflammatory polyps), 10 mm and 11 mm (tubular adenomas), and a 35 mm tubulovillous adenoma. Overall, there were a total of 109 neoplasms (cancers or adenoma) equal to or greater than 10 mm found by CTC and eventually determined to be positive findings by colonoscopy. One of the problems of this study is that the original colonoscopic examiner was not provided with immediate feedback on the CTC location of polyps so that the area could be reexamined immediately during that procedure.

The most effective and accurate method to ensure that the CTC finding is a true positive has been addressed by Pickhardt and colleagues,[9] who enrolled 1253 asymptomatic adults to perform same-day CTC and colonoscopy. After interpretation of the CTC examination was available and reported, a colonoscopic examination was performed on the same day in all patients. After the colonoscopist examined each segment of the colon, the CTC results were revealed. If a reported polyp was not seen during the colonoscopy, the examiner reintubated that segment of the colon with the intention to verify or completely exclude the presence of a polyp. Because of CTC limitations, there was no attempt to include any polyp that measured 5 mm or less on either CTC or colonoscopy. In this study a total of 1310 polyps were found at CTC, with 511 of these polyps measuring 5 mm or greater in diameter. Of these 511 polyps, 55 (10.8%) were found only on the second-look colonoscopy after segmental unblinding of the written CTC report. Twenty-one of these polyps were adenomas (6 mm or larger) removed from 20 patients (mean diameter of 8.1 mm; range, 6–17 mm). The adenoma miss rate on the initial blinded prospective colonoscopy examination was 10.0% (21 of 210 adenomas), measuring at/or larger than 6 mm. These 20 patients who had missed adenomas (that measured 6 mm or larger) represented 11.9% of all patients with adenomas of that size that were found and removed during colonoscopy. The histology of these "missed" neoplasms found on the second-look colonoscopy after segmental unblinding showed that 17 were tubular adenomas, 3 were tubulovillous adenomas, and 1 was a small adenocarcinoma. Fifteen of these neoplasms were sessile, 4 pedunculated, and 2 flat. Ten of the 21 missed neoplasms were located in the proximal colon and 6 of the 11 distal lesions were in the rectum. During a repeat study of the CTC examinations, the majority of the nonrectal neoplasms (14 of 15) were located on a fold with 10 on the proximal aspect or the edge of folds. One adenoma (above the rectum) that was associated with a fold was located on the inner aspect of an acute bend in the colon. Five of the 6 missed adenomas in the rectum were within 10 cm of the anal verge on CTC.

This study involved 3 medical centers with 17 experienced colonoscopists (3 of the 21 findings of adenomas missed on the initial post-CTC colonoscopy were performed by colorectal surgeons and the rest by gastroenterologists). The lesson from this study is that colonoscopy can overlook polyps in the colon and that some reported lesions on CTC that are categorized as false positives by subsequent negative colonoscopy may actually exist but were overlooked on the colonoscopic examination. This report, by revealing that significant lesions may be overlooked on colonoscopy, is an important message for colonoscopists and indicates the need for continued improvements in colonoscopic technology. Areas that could be potentially "blind" to the colonoscopist are those that are on the proximal side of folds, the inner aspect of flexures, and in the rectum. In the Pickhardt series,[9] polyps located on the proximal side of a colonic fold accounted for two-thirds of missed adenomas (above the rectum).

The Pickhardt study should not come as a surprise, because missed lesions have been reported by colonoscopists for the last several years. The first report of back-to-back colonoscopies on the same day and immediately following each other was in 1991.[10] The next report of tandem colonoscopy appeared 6 years later,[11] and the most recent was in 2008.[12] The overall miss rates for adenomas in the earlier studies[10,11] were 15% to 24%. The large multicenter European study[12] found that the miss rate for all polyps was 28%, for hyperplastic polyps 31%, and for adenomas 21%. However, for those equal to or larger than 5 mm, the miss rate for all polyps was 12% and for adenomas 9%. Among the 14 polyps and 6 adenomas larger than 5 mm missed during the first examination, 5 polyps and 1 adenoma were sessile, 9 polyps and 5 adenomas were flat. Thirty-seven adenomas were overlooked in 286 patients with the median size being 3 mm; however, the range was from 1 to 18 mm. Three advanced adenomas were missed with a size from 15 to 18 mm. In this study, which reported a 27% rate of missed adenomas for lesions less than 5 mm in diameter, the miss rate for lesions greater than 5 mm in diameter was 9%. In a previous study of 183 patients having tandem colonoscopy, Rex and colleagues[11] reported a 27% miss rate for polyps smaller than 6 mm in diameter and only 6% for polyps larger than 9 mm. This rate represented 2 patients whose polyps were detected on a repeat colono-scopic examination. Benson and colleagues[13] evaluated the polyp miss rate on repeat colonoscopic examinations at 4 months, and then 1 year after the initial colonoscopic examination. Fifteen thousand colonoscopies were examined from multiple centers, for which the calculated miss rate for all polyps was 17% and the miss rate for neoplastic polyps 12%. However, the percentage of missed neoplastic polyps greater than 9 mm was only 2%. This report was a retrospective analysis of findings on a repeat colonoscopic examination between 3 and 7 years following the initial colono-scopic examination (assuming that large polyps had been overlooked in the initial colonoscopy), and stated that the overall miss rate for "advanced adenomas" (those larger than 10 mm) was 1.7%. However, this study was not a tandem colonoscopic examination and it was assumed that any lesion over 10 mm in diameter was missed on the original procedure.

A meta-analysis comparing CTC, air contrast barium enema, and colonoscopy[14] found 9 studies that reported segmental unblinding of the CTC findings for the colo-noscopist, but used the findings of a single colonoscopy as the factor that deter-mined whether a polyp was or was not present (colonoscopy was the gold standard). Another meta-analysis[7] comparing the accuracy of CTC with colono-scopy reviewed 47 studies in which the findings on CTC were corroborated or not by conventional colonoscopy or by surgery, and found the results were "highly heterogeneous." A report from Europe[15] compared CTC with segmental unblinding during colonoscopy, but there was no mention of any lesion missed by colonoscopy. In a more recent article,[16] same-day colonoscopy with segmental unblinding was performed, but this report did not reveal how many polyps found on CTC were actually missed by the colonoscopist after the CTC results were revealed. This report on 202 patients did mention that there was one polyp detected on CTC that was missed at initial colonoscopy but found on repeat colonoscopy. Another group[17] also performed segmental unblinding in a prospective same-day CTC and colonoscopy in 311 patients, but there was no mention of any lesion reported on CTC that was not discovered during the subsequent unblinded colonoscopic examination.

A study published in 2008[18] reported on the results of colonoscopy following a positive CTC examination whereby a polyp or mass was seen that was greater than 9 mm in diameter or at least 3 medium-sized polyps (6–9 mm) were reported. Most patients in this prospective report had colonoscopy within several hours of CTC. Although patients with large polyps typically were seen within several hours of CTC, the timing of colonoscopy had to be at most 30 days after CTC examination in order for the data to be included. In this study, the findings of colonoscopy examination were taken as the standard, and the colonoscopists were told exactly where the lesion was located. There was no attempt at performing a second colonoscopy if the first examination did not reveal an abnormality, and there was a false-positive CTC finding of 5% when the colonoscopy failed to locate a polyp.

In an early multicenter study[19] involving 600 participants, 9 clinical centers were recruited. Colonoscopies were performed with endoscopists blinded to the CTC results, with the CTC finding revealed after the colonoscopist examined each segment of the colon during scope withdrawal. In this study, conventional colonoscopy missed only one 7 mm lesion in the sigmoid colon and 19 lesions that ranged in size from 1 to 5 mm.

Colonoscopy was the reference standard in a 2009 article where CTC was evaluated for the detection of advanced neoplasia in persons at high risk for colon cancer.[20] The investigators noted that "colonoscopy itself may miss some lesions." In this study, where lesions less than 6 mm in size were reported as negative, a total of 93 cases had a positive CTC but lesions were not found on the subsequent "reference" colonoscopy performed about 3 hours after CTC. Each segment of the bowel was unblinded to the examiner once that area of the colon had been evaluated colonoscopically. In this study, a positive CTC result was recorded if the colonoscopic examination revealed at least one "advanced neoplasia 6 mm or larger" but if no polyp was seen on colonoscopy, the CTC was regarded as a false positive. Ninety-three cases were classified as CTC false positive when colonoscopy did not find a polyp. Blinded colonoscopy missed 2 advanced adenomas, a 13 mm pedunculated polyp in the cecum, and a 18 mm flat lesion in the ascending colon. This article did not state the number of colonoscopies when a lesion seen on CTC was missed on initial colonoscopy but was subsequently found on the second colonoscopic examination.

In a comparison of miss rates on colonoscopy with findings at surgical resection of an index lesion,[21] 16 more lesions were present on the surgical resection specimen in addition to all neoplasms detected at the presurgical colonoscopy. Most polyps were small and only one polyp greater than 1 cm was missed, and that tumor was in the ascending colon. It does seem that comparison of findings with either CT or colonoscopy would be best served by examining a surgical resected specimen to truly ascertain the miss rate of CTC or colonoscopy.

Despite the greater sensitivity for polyp discovery with CTC over DCBE, the US Preventive Services Task Force has not endorsed CTC as a diagnostic procedure for their guidelines on screening recommendations.[22,23] The recommendation of the US Preventive Services Task Force "concludes that for CT colonography there is insufficient evidence to permit a recommendation for colorectal cancer screening." This guideline was developed to assess and recommend preventive care services for any patient without signs or symptoms of the target condition.

The most recent guideline on screening for colorectal cancer from the American College of Gastroenterology (ACG)[24] stated that colonoscopy every 10 years, beginning at age 50, is the preferred colorectal cancer screening strategy, but in cases where colonoscopy may not be available or that persons are unwilling to undergo colonoscopy, then CTC every 5 years is an acceptable alternative. Another guideline has been issued by the American Cancer Society, the US Multisociety Task Force on Colorectal Cancer, and the American College of Radiology.[25] This study group does recommend CTC for screening purposes because of the "accumulation of evidence [...] the expert panel concludes that there are sufficient data to include CTC as an acceptable option for colorectal cancer screening."

It is not surprising that lesions may be missed on colonoscopy. There is not any endoscopist who performs colonoscopy who has not seen a polyp, lost sight of it while waiting for a snare or biopsy forceps, and then needed to search for it again. Similarly, polyps found during intubation and not removed may be very difficult to locate during removal of the instrument. Intubation of the colon is characteristically performed rather rapidly for several reasons, one of which is to minimize patient discomfort by shortening the examination. Another is to reduce spasm in the colon that will occur if the procedure is prolonged, and to avoid the necessity of overdistending the right colon with a slow intubation. Because of this, the colonoscopic examination is best performed during withdrawal of the instrument, which must be carefully controlled. This paradigm, performing a rapid insertion with little or no emphasis on inspection, followed by inspection during the withdrawal phase, has not been scientifically proven to be an optimal approach for achieving maximum detection of adenomas or cancer.[26] Because the extubation is the portion of the procedure during which time most adenomas are found, careful withdrawal is of utmost importance. In 2006, a combined task force of the ACG and the American Society for Gastrointestinal Endoscopy,[27] in a combined statement, recommended that the withdrawal phase of colonoscopy should be an average of 6 minutes in duration. A private practice group scrutinized their data and found that there was a strong correlation with withdrawal time and adenoma detection rate. In this study, Barclay and colleagues[28] reported that colonoscopists with an average withdrawal time of more than 6 minutes detected adenomas in 6.4% of screened patients compared with a 2.6% prevalence in colonoscopies performed by endoscopists whose withdrawal times averaged less than 6 minutes. The Mayo Clinic also validated the 6-minute withdrawal target as separating high from low adenoma detectors.[29] During the 6-minute withdrawal, the colonoscopist must make an assessment of each fold and try to visualize the area behind folds and on the inner aspect of angulations in the colon. The usual technique during withdrawal around a fold is rather complex, and requires skill and dexterity[26]: (A) withdraw air, which shortens the colon and moves the colonoscope tip proximal to the fold; (B) the tip is angulated toward the fold and withdrawn, with the colonoscope tip deflected in the direction of the fold; (C) this pulls on the fold and bends the fold toward the examiner, permitting visualization of the space behind the fold.

Whenever a fold or flexure is passed and a careful examination of its proximal aspect cannot be achieved, reinsertion, flexion of the tip, and repeat withdrawal is necessary. An attempt should be made to avoid a "red out" whereby nothing is seen when the tip is deflected behind a fold. The angle of deflection is controlled with the left thumb on the major up/down control knob as the instrument is withdrawn, moving the tip toward the fold, while permitting visualization of its hidden portion. A retroflexion should routinely be performed in the rectum.[30] It would seem that retroflexion of the instrument during the withdrawal phase at any location in the colon would be a worthwhile adjunct, but an article has stated that retroflexion in the right colon was not able to visualize any greater amount of any additional pathology than seen with straight end-on colonoscopy.[31] Various techniques have been attempted to increase the ability to see portions of mucosa hidden during the withdrawal phase. One of these techniques is to use a cap on the end of the instrument while another is to use a wide-angle instrument. Studies[32–34] have not identified improved overall adenoma detection using these devices. Pickhardt and colleagues,[9] in comparing colonoscopy with CTC, use a computer-simulated graphic representation of the area behind folds that cannot be seen with the straight end-on colonoscopic view during withdrawal of the instrument. Lieberman[35] commented in an editorial that "the data on colonoscopy accuracy [is] a humble reminder of the limitation of colonoscopy; nevertheless it remains the pre-eminent test for diagnosing and treating colonic neoplasia."

A more recent addition to the quest for a more thorough colonoscopic examination has been a mini-endoscope that permits both antegrade and retrograde visualization simultaneously during colonoscopic withdrawal. This device is called the Third Eye Retroscope (TER). When placed through the instrument channel of a standard colonoscope it flexes 180° as it emerges from the tip and extends into the lumen (**Fig. 1**). The device carries a light source and a viewing chip. The light from the retroverted instrument illuminates the areas distal to the colonoscope tip, permitting the device to visualize the proximal portions of folds and the valleys in between these folds as the colonoscope simultaneously is looking forward (**Fig. 2**). The TER has shown an increased detection rate for polyps and adenomas. It has been suggested that this instrument is "one of the most promising devices for improvement of mucosal exposure during colonoscopy"[36] (**Fig. 3**). Preliminary reports of the TER have been published.[37,38] A prospective multicenter study by 14 endoscopists at 8 sites studied 249 patients who presented for screening or surveillance colonoscopy.[39] Following cecal intubation, the disposable TER was inserted through the instrument channel of the colonoscope. During withdrawal, the forward and retrograde video images were observed side by side simultaneously on a wide-screen monitor. The number and sizes of lesions detected with the standard colonoscope were recorded, as were the number and sizes of lesions found that were first detected with the TER, but not with the forward viewing colonoscope. (**Fig. 4**) In these subjects, 257 polyps

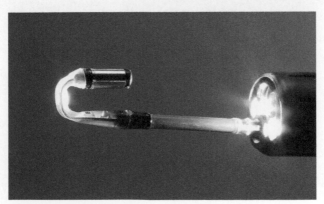

Fig. 1. The retroscope flexes 180° as it emerges from the tip of the colonoscope. The light source is at the bend of the device, and the video chip at the tip of the Third Eye Retroscope (TER) looks backward toward the shaft of the colonoscope.

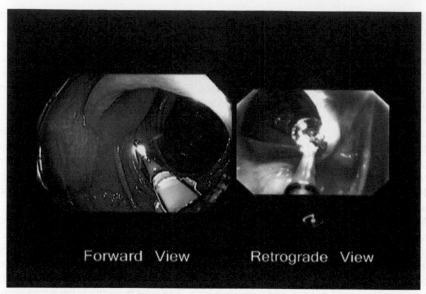

Forward View   Retrograde View

Fig. 2. Standard monitor view showing simultaneously the standard colonoscope image on the left (forward view), and the retrograde view from the Third Eye device on the right. In the forward view, the light of the TER is seen at the bend of the device. The TER visualizes the area behind the colonoscope as well as being able to see behind the fold on which the colonoscope is resting.

including 136 adenomas were identified with the colonoscope. The TER detected 34 additional polyps with (a 13.2% increase over standard forward viewing colonoscopy). These 34 polyps included 15 adenomas (an 11% increase over those seen with the standard forward viewing colonoscope). The additional detection rate with the TER

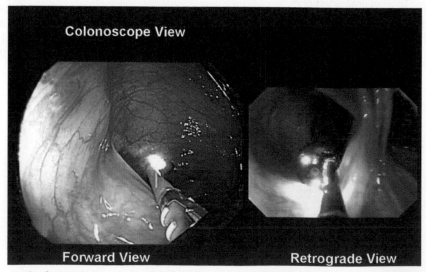

Colonoscope View

Forward View   Retrograde View

Fig. 3. The forward view shows the Third Eye extended beyond the tip of the colonoscope. The simultaneous view at the splenic flexure demonstrates both the transverse colon on the right and a view down the descending colon to the left of the flexure.

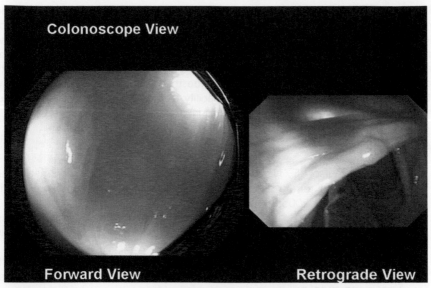

Fig. 4. The forward view from the colonoscope demonstrates a fold, and the retrograde view shows a small polyp that was on the opposite side of the fold. This polyp could not be seen with the colonoscope, which is transilluminating the same fold.

compared with standard colonoscopy for any lesion greater than or equal to 10 mm was 30.8% for all polyps and 33.3% for adenomas. Every polyp detected with the TER was subsequently located with the colonoscope and removed. Another prospective multicenter study[40] involving 17 investigators and 298 patients at 9 sites had a study design that was similar except that the endoscopists were initially naïve to the Third Eye device and were followed through the "learning curve" over 20 procedures. Their overall additional detection rates for the Third Eye compared to the colonoscope alone were 14.8% for all polyps and 16.0% for adenomas. For procedures performed after each endoscopist had completed 15 cases using the device, mean additional detection rates with the Third Eye were 17.0% for all polyps and 25.0% for adenomas. As in the prior multicenter study[39], additional adenoma detection rates with the Third Eye were greater for larger lesions compared to smaller lesions, suggesting that at least some of the lesions that were hidden from the view of the colonoscope might have been missed during previous exams.

SUMMARY

The search for the perfect imaging tool for the colon is an ongoing quest. For many years, the barium enema and rigid sigmoidoscope were the only methods to evaluate the large bowel, and they were imperfect instruments. When colonoscopy was introduced, it far surpassed the capability of both the barium enema and the sigmoidoscope, and became the procedure of choice for visualization of the large bowel. The explosion of computer technology led to high-level radiographic processors that permit CTC to be a more rapid examination than colonoscopy, to require no sedation, and to have fewer complications. Several studies have demonstrated the capability of CTC and colonoscopy. Both techniques have been shown to miss lesions in the colon, and reports of tandem colonoscopy studies reveal significant miss rates.

The goal of all these procedures is better patient care, seeking to prevent colon cancer by finding precursor lesions at a stage before they become malignant. Technology is changing rapidly on all fronts, and whether adenomas are found by newer multislice CTC or on a retroversion view colonoscopy device, the lesions discovered need to be carefully evaluated by the colonoscopist because the colonoscope, frequently the reference standard, may not be the gold standard. Slow withdrawal of the colonoscope coupled with the capability to fully visualize the entire mucosal surface will lead to a further decrease in the incidence of colon and rectal cancer.

REFERENCES

1. Rockey DC, Paulson E, Niedzwiecki D, et al. Analysis of air contrast barium enema, computed tomographic colonography, and colonoscopy: prospective comparison. Lancet 2005;365:305–11.
2. Winawer SJ, Stewart ET, Zauber AG, et al. A comparison of colonoscopy and double-contrast barium enema for surveillance after polypectomy. National Polyp Study Work Group. N Engl J Med 2000;342:1766–72.
3. Toma J, Paszat LF, Gunraj N, et al. Rates of new or missed colorectal cancer after barium enema and their risk factors: a population-based study. Am J Gastroenterol 2008;103:3142–8.
4. Thomas S, Atchley J, Higginson A. Audit of the introduction of CT colonography for detection of colorectal carcinoma in a non-academic environment and its implications for the national bowel cancer screening programme. Clin Radiol 2009;64:142–7.
5. Sosna J, Sella T, Sy O, et al. Critical analysis of the performance of double-contrast barium enema for detecting colorectal polyps > or = 6 mm in the era of CT colonography. AJR Am J Roentgenol 2008;190:374–85.
6. Stevenson G. Colon imaging in radiology departments in 2008: goodbye to the routine double contrast barium enema. Can Assoc Radiol J 2008;59: 174–82.
7. Chaparro M, Gisbert JP, Del Campo L, et al. Accuracy of computed tomographic colonography for the detection of polyps and colorectal tumors: a systematic review and meta-analysis. Digestion 2009;80:1–17.
8. Johnson CD, Chen MH, Toledano AY. Colorectal cancer screening with computed tomographic colonography. N Engl J Med 2008;359:1207–17.
9. Pickhardt PJ, Nugent PA, Mysliwiec PA, et al. Location of adenomas missed by optical colonoscopy. Ann Intern Med 2004;141:352–9.
10. Hixson LJ, Fennerty MB, Sampliner RE, et al. Prospective blinded trial of the colonoscopic miss-rate of large colorectal polyps. Gastrointest Endosc 1991;37: 125–7.
11. Rex DK, Cutler CS, Lemmel GT, et al. Colonoscopic miss rates of adenomas determined by back-to-back colonoscopies. Gastroenterology 1997;112: 24–8.
12. Heresbach D, Barrioz T, Ponchon T. Miss rate for colorectal neoplastic polyps: a prospective multicenter study of back-to-back video colonoscopies. Endoscopy 2008;40:284–90.
13. Bensen S, Mott LA, Dain B, et al. The colonoscopic miss rate and true one-year recurrence of colorectal neoplastic polyps. Polyp Prevention Study Group. Am J Gastroenterol 1999;94:194–9.
14. Rosman AS, Korsten MA. Meta-analysis comparing CT colonography, air contrast barium enema, and colonoscopy. Am J Med 2007;120:203–10.

15. Chaparro Sánchez M, del Campo Val L, Maté Jiménez J, et al. Computed tomography colonography compared with conventional colonoscopy for the detection of colorectal polyps. Gastroenterol Hepatol 2007;30:375–80.
16. Roberts-Thomson IC, Tucker GR, Hewett PJ, et al. Single-center study comparing computed tomography colonography with conventional colonoscopy. World J Gastroenterol 2008;14:469–73.
17. Graser A, Stieber P, Nagel D, et al. Comparison of CT colonography, colonoscopy, sigmoidoscopy and faecal occult blood tests for the detection of advanced adenoma in an average risk population. Gut 2009;58:241–8.
18. Cornett D, Barancin C, Roeder B, et al. Findings on optical colonoscopy after positive CT colonography exam. Am J Gastroenterol 2008;103:2068–74.
19. Cotton PB, Durkalski VL, Pineau BC, et al. Computed tomographic colonography (virtual colonoscopy): a multicenter comparison with standard colonoscopy for detection of colorectal neoplasia. JAMA 2004;291:1713–9.
20. Regge D, Laudi C, Galatola G, et al. Diagnostic accuracy of computed tomographic colonography for the detection of advanced neoplasia in individuals at increased risk of colorectal cancer. JAMA 2009;301:2453–61.
21. Postic G, Lewin D, Bickerstaff C, et al. Colonoscopic miss rates determined by direct comparison of colonoscopy with colon resection specimens. Am J Gastroenterol 2002;97:3182–5.
22. Whitlock EP, Lin JS, Liles E, et al. Screening for colorectal cancer: a targeted, updated systematic review for the U.S. Preventive Services Task Force. Ann Intern Med 2008;149:638–58.
23. U.S. Preventive Services Task Force. Screening and surveillance for the early detection of colorectal cancer and adenomatous polyps, 2008: a joint guideline from the American Cancer Society, the US Multi-Society Task Force on Colorectal Cancer, and the American College of Radiology. Ann Intern Med 2008;149:627–37.
24. Rex DK, Johnson DA, Anderson JC, et al. American College of Gastroenterology guidelines for colorectal cancer screening 2009. Am J Gastroenterol 2009;104:739–50 [corrected].
25. Levin B, Lieberman DA, McFarland B, et al. Screening and surveillance for the early detection of colorectal cancer and adenomatous polyps, 2008: a joint guideline from the American Cancer Society, the US Multi-Society Task Force on Colorectal Cancer, and the American College of Radiology. Gastroenterology 2008;134:1570–95.
26. Huh KC, Rex DK. Missed neoplasms and optimal colonoscopic withdrawal technique. In: Waye JD, Rex DK, Williams CB, editors. Colonoscopy principles and practice. Second Edition. London: Blackwell Publishing; 2009. Chapter 41.
27. Rex DK, Petrini JL, Baron TH, et al. Quality indicators for colonoscopy. Am J Gastroenterol 2006;101:873–85.
28. Barclay RL, Vicari JJ, Doughty AS, et al. Colonoscopic withdrawal times and adenoma detection during screening colonoscopy. N Engl J Med 2006;355:2533–41.
29. Simmons DT, Harewood GC, Baron TH, et al. Impact of endoscopist withdrawal speed on polyp yield: implications for optimal colonoscopy withdrawal time. Aliment Pharmacol Ther 2006;24:965–71.
30. Waye JD. What constitutes a total colonoscopy? Am J Gastroenterol 1999;94:1429–30.
31. Rex DK, Chen SC, Overhiser AJ. Colonoscopy technique in consecutive patients referred for prior incomplete colonoscopy. Clin Gastroenterol Hepatol 2007;5:879–83.

32. Fatima H, Rex DK, Rothstein R, et al. Cecal insertion and withdrawal times with wide-angle versus standard colonoscopes: a randomized controlled trial. Clin Gastroenterol Hepatol 2008;6:109–14.

33. Rex DK, Chadalawada V, Helper DJ. Wide angle colonoscopy with a prototype instrument: impact on miss rates and efficiency as determined by back-to-back colonoscopies. Am J Gastroenterol 2003;98:2000–5.

34. Deenadayalu VP, Chadalawada V, Rex DK. 170 degrees wide-angle colonoscope: effect on efficiency and miss rates. Am J Gastroenterol 2004;99:2138–42.

35. Lieberman D. Colonoscopy: as good as gold? Ann Intern Med 2004;141:401–3.

36. Rex DK. Third Eye Retroscope: rationale, efficacy, challenges. Rev Gastroenterol Disord 2009;9:1–6.

37. Triadafilopoulos G, Watts HD, Van Dam J. A novel retrograde-viewing auxiliary imaging device (Third Eye Retroscope) improves the detection of simulated polyps in anatomic models of the colon. Gastrointest Endosc 2007;65:139–44.

38. Triadafilopoulos G, Li J. A pilot study to assess the safety and efficacy of the Third Eye Retrograde auxiliary imaging system during colonoscopy. Endoscopy 2008; 40:478–82.

39. Waye JD, Heigh RI, Rex DK, et al. A retrograde-viewing device improves detection of adenomas in the colon: a prospective efficacy evaluation. Gastrointest Endosc 2010;71:551–6.

40. DeMarco DC, Odstrcil E, Lara LF, et al. Impact of experience with a retrograde-viewing device on adenoma detection rates and withdrawal times during colonoscopy: the third eye retroscope study group. Gastrointest Endosc 2010;71: 542–50.

Extracolonic Findings at CT Colonography

Judy Yee, MD[a,*], Srikant Sadda, MD[b], Rizwan Aslam, MD[a], Benjamin Yeh, MD[a]

KEYWORDS

• CTC • Extracolonic findings • AAA • Colorectal cancer

Computed tomographic colonography (CTC) is a validated tool for the evaluation of the colon for polyps and cancer. The technique employed for CTC includes a low-dose CT scan of the abdomen and pelvis that is typically performed without the administration of intravenous contrast. Using this technique it is possible to discover findings outside of the colon. By far, most extracolonic findings are determined to be clinically inconsequential on CTC and most patients are not recommended for further testing. However, some findings may result in additional diagnostic evaluation or intervention, which can lead to patient anxiety and increased morbidity and health care costs. Alternatively, some findings can lead to the earlier diagnosis of a clinically significant lesion, which could result in decreased patient morbidity and mortality as well as overall savings in downstream health care costs. The controversies of detecting and evaluating these incidental extracolonic findings on CTC are discussed.

BENEFITS

CTC is the only colorectal cancer–screening tool that can directly image both the colon and extracolonic structures and organs. The findings outside of the colon may be completely incidental or they may be the actual cause of the patient's presenting symptom, such as abdominal pain. This unique ability can be viewed as a benefit by patients who are becoming more interested in being advocates for their own health care and by patients who would like to be able to pursue preventive care. Some of the more commonly identified extracolonic findings on CTC include benign lesions or lesions that do not affect the management of the asymptomatic patient, such as simple renal and hepatic cysts, gallstones, and renal stones. Other findings such as

[a] San Francisco Veterans Affairs Medical Center, University of California, San Francisco, 4150 Clement Street, San Francisco, CA 94121, USA
[b] Department of Radiology and Biomedical Imaging, Mount Sinai Medical Center, 4300 Alton Road, Miami Beach, FL 33140, USA
* Corresponding author. San Francisco Veterans Affairs Medical Center, University of California, 4150 Clement Street, San Francisco, CA 94121.
E-mail address: Judy.yee@radiology.ucsf.edu

Gastrointest Endoscopy Clin N Am 20 (2010) 305–322
doi:10.1016/j.giec.2010.02.013
1052-5157/10/$ – see front matter. Published by Elsevier Inc.

abdominal aortic aneurysm (AAA) and extracolonic malignancies can benefit patients in early detection and treatment.

CTC has the ability to simultaneously screen for AAA and colorectal carcinoma. The diagnosis and sizing of AAA by CT scan does not require the administration of intravenous contrast, and thus unenhanced-screening CTC is well suited for evaluation of AAA. Patients with AAA benefit from early diagnosis because the natural history of these aneurysms is to continually enlarge over a period of years, which can potentially lead to rupture. The strongest risk factor for rupture of an AAA is its large size, particularly when it is 5.5 cm or larger in diameter. Each year there are about 15,000 deaths caused by AAA in the United States.[1] An AAA is defined as having an infrarenal aortic diameter larger than 3.0 cm. Small AAAs measure between 3.0 and 3.9 cm, intermediate-sized AAAs measure from 4.0 to 5.4 cm, and those that are 5.5 cm or larger in diameter are considered large. The major risk factors for the development of AAAs include male gender, smoking history, and an age of 65 years or older.[2] Thus AAA and colorectal carcinoma tend to occur with increasing frequency in similar-aged patient cohorts. In 2005, the US Preventive Services Task Force recommended the performance of one-time screening for AAA by ultrasonography in men between 65 and 75 years who have ever smoked.[2] In 2007, the Screening Abdominal Aortic Aneurysms Very Efficiently (SAAAVE) act became law, enabling Medicare to cover the costs of AAA screening by ultrasonography.[3] The prevalence of asymptomatic AAAs in screening programs using ultrasonography has been found to be about 5% in men aged 65 years and older.[3,4]

AAAs do not typically cause symptoms, and they are often identified as incidental findings on imaging studies such as CTC. In a study of 243 patients undergoing elective repair of AAA, 62% of cases were identified incidentally on radiologic examinations.[5] The diagnosis of AAA was often missed on physical examination alone. In this study, 43% of patients with AAAs detected by imaging had palpable aneurysms that should have been detected on physical examination but were missed.

The early detection of AAA allows appropriate follow-up for its increasing size, and those that are 5.5 cm or larger require surgical or endovascular repair. The mortality rate associated with elective AAA repair is 5% or less, whereas the mortality rate for surgery after aneurysm rupture is significantly higher ranging between 80% and 95%.[6,7] It has been found that open surgical repair of AAAs measuring at least 5.5 cm in diameter leads to about 43% decrease in mortality in older men undergoing screening.[2] Screening for asymptomatic AAAs can reduce the incidence rate of ruptured AAAs by 49%.[8]

Malignant tumors outside of the colon may also be identified by CTC. These typically appear as complex cystic or solid masses of the abdominal or pelvic organs. In unenhanced low-dose CTC, extracolonic malignancies are more easily visualized when they protrude from or deform the contour of an organ. Adenopathy located in the retroperitoneum or mesenteric fat may also be identified. Intravenous contrast may be administered for diagnostic CTC when the patient has symptoms or prior studies suspicious for colorectal cancer. Contrast-enhanced diagnostic CTC allows improved visualization of extracolonic carcinomas, although higher dose CT technique using increased tube current is necessary.

It is recognized that patients with renal cell carcinoma often have no symptoms and that most of these tumors are diagnosed as an incidental finding. Renal cell carcinomas that are identified incidentally on CTC may be found at an earlier stage when they are more likely to be curable. Tsui and colleagues[9] retrospectively evaluated 633 consecutive patients with renal cell carcinoma who underwent radical or partial nephrectomy. The investigators found that 15% of patients had incidentally detected renal cell carcinoma and that these patients had significantly lower stage and lower grade tumors compared with patients who had symptoms leading to their diagnosis. Stage 1 lesions were found in 62% of patients with incidental renal cell carcinoma when compared with 23% of the patients with symptomatic renal cell carcinoma. The 5-year survival rate was significantly higher at 85% for incidentally discovered renal cell carcinoma compared with 63% for symptomatic tumors. Similarly, the local and distal recurrence rates were higher for symptomatic lesions. Other studies have also found that there is improved prognosis and patient outcome for incidentally discovered renal cell carcinomas that are more often found at an earlier pathologic stage than symptomatic tumors.[10,11]

In recognition of the increasing number of incidental renal masses identified by imaging, management recommendations for cystic and solid masses have been developed. Management of cystic renal masses is typically based on the Bosniak classification scheme.[12] Most incidentally identified renal cystic lesions are small and if simple appearing these are to be considered benign. Bosniak suggests that cystic lesions smaller than 1 cm that measure between 0 and 20 Hounsfield units and without evidence of calcifications, septations, nodularity, or enhancement can be presumed to be benign and do not need any additional workup.[13] Surgery is suggested for solid renal masses larger than 1 cm. Very small solid masses less than 1 cm may be observed by follow-up imaging because these have a reasonable chance of being benign and they are often not well characterized and difficult to biopsy because of their small size.[12] Specific recommendations for the management of incidental renal lesions identified on low-dose CTC need to be defined. A standardized framework for defining, managing, and reporting incidental findings is being developed by the Incidental Findings Committee under the Commission on Body Imaging of the American College of Radiology.[14]

The identification of disease at an earlier stage allows for more timely intervention, which can avoid the high costs of health care required for more extensive diagnostic tests, treatments such as chemotherapy, extended hospitalizations, and surgery from later presentation of disease. Although some extracolonic carcinomas that are discovered may be too advanced for surgical management, they may be found when the patient is relatively symptom free offering a wider window of time for the patient and family to plan for the future, before the onset of significant symptoms. Similarly, if metastases are identified at the time of diagnosis of colon carcinoma on CTC, this can help direct patient management without additional diagnostic evaluation or intervention.

LIMITATIONS

In the debate about the effect of the discovery of incidental findings, it is important to consider the potential for the evaluation and treatment of these lesions to have negative economic, societal, and medical effects. Although these issues are actually relevant for most cross-sectional imaging studies, the proposed widespread use of CTC for colorectal screening in asymptomatic patients has made it significant. The workup and management of extracolonic findings on CTC may lead to increased health care costs, cause patient morbidity or mortality, and expose patients to unnecessary radiation. Patients can experience undue distress and inconvenience associated with the discovery and workup of incidental findings that are eventually determined to be benign. These disadvantages must be considered along with the potential benefits associated with the early detection of clinically important or malignant incidental lesions on CTC. Cost effectiveness as estimated by the number of life years saved due to incidental lesions is not known. Including incidental lesions into cost-benefit analysis is difficult because the outcome of patients is often uncertain.[15] In addition, substantial numbers of patients who receive recommendations to have follow-up of incidental lesions do not return for workup. Another confounding issue occurs when patients with incidental findings proceed to workup and management that are not indicated or recommended based on imaging.

In an analogous evaluation, the psychological side effects of breast cancer screening were studied.[16] Increased anxiety that affected mood (26%) and daily functioning (17%) was experienced by women who underwent additional evaluation of suspicious mammographic findings for breast lesions that were later found to be benign. Overall, women with abnormal mammograms reported significantly stronger intentions to obtain mammograms in the next year compared with women with normal mammograms. Today, the discovery of incidental findings is a growing part of medicine, with a concurrent increase in the use of imaging techniques in health care. Clinical decision analysis and cost-effective analysis must take into account both the risks and benefits of the management of incidental lesions.

CTC PROTOCOL

The development of multidetector CT scanner technology has allowed scanning of the entire abdomen and pelvis by CTC using thinner slices while lowering radiation dose. The slice thickness ranges between 1 and 2.5 mm for 4- and 8-detector CT scanners and between 0.625 and 1.25 mm for 16- and 64-detector CT scanners. The American College of Radiology Practice Guidelines for the Performance of CT Colonography in Adults were recently revised and recommend an optimal slice thickness of 3 mm or less with a reconstruction interval of 2.0 mm or less.[17] A breathhold of 25 seconds or less is suggested. Standard CTC protocol requires scanning in 2 opposing positions, typically supine and prone, which has been shown to improve segmental colonic distention and cleansing leading to increase in polyp detection ability.[18] Current multidetector CTC protocol performed for screening of colorectal cancer uses low tube current (50–80 effective mAs) for a tube potential of 120 kVp, which helps to maintain a low radiation dose to the patient. Generally, this is equivalent to a CT dose index volume of 6.26 mGy per position or a total of 12.5 mGy for dual-position CTC.[17]

The detection of extracolonic findings is performed on the axial images, and evaluation is best performed at the time of review of the colon. Multiplanar reformats may be used to correlate with the axial images for further evaluation of questionable lesions. CTC scans allow visualization of the lung bases in addition to structures in the abdomen and pelvis. Similar to the interpretation of a CT scan of the abdomen and pelvis, CTC requires review of the data set using various window widths and levels when evaluating for extracolonic lesions. A soft tissue window (width 400, level 40) is best for evaluation of the solid organs and most structures in the abdomen and pelvis. Lung windows (width 1500, level −700) are used to review the lung bases. Bone windows (width 2000, level 300) are useful to evaluate the skeleton.

The use of low tube current for CTC decreases the number of photons that reach the detectors and consequently increases image noise. Studies have shown that low-dose CTC protocols allow for similar excellent sensitivity and specificity in polyp detection when compared with higher-dose CT protocols.[19–22] However, even with these lower-dose protocols, detection of extracolonic pathology is feasible. Ultra-low-dose CTC using 10 mAs has been found to successfully detect colorectal polyps and cancers, resulting in a 40% to 70% decrease in radiation dose compared with prior studies.[23] The use of low-dose CT technique still allows the detection of colorectal polyps and cancers because of the high contrast between the low density of the gas-distended lumen and the soft tissue density of the colonic wall. However, increased image noise may compromise the evaluation of extracolonic lesions. Newer iterative reconstruction or denoising CT image reconstruction techniques promise to improve the image quality of low-dose scans in the near future. Additional studies are needed to define the ability of CTC to detect and characterize extracolonic findings using low-dose unenhanced CT technique.

HOW TO CLASSIFY EXTRACOLONIC FINDINGS

Various classification schemes have been used to categorize extracolonic findings. Extracolonic findings are often classified as having high, moderate, or low clinical importance. Extracolonic findings may also be categorized as simply clinically significant or clinically insignificant based on whether or not the lesion requires additional workup as determined at the time of the CTC. Specific parameters such as lesion size or location can also affect the clinical significance of an extracolonic finding.

Extracolonic findings of high clinical importance are typically those that require timely or immediate additional evaluation or medical attention. A change in clinical management results from this type of finding and can include further imaging, testing, or surgery. Extracolonic findings of high clinical importance include AAAs larger than 3 cm, (**Fig. 1**)[24] masses of the abdominal organs suspicious for malignancy (**Fig. 2**), indeterminate pulmonary nodules (**Fig. 3**), and adenopathy. Findings requiring immediate communication with the referring clinician include previously unknown pneumothorax and pneumoperitoneum. Findings of active infection or inflammation in which the patient requires immediate medical attention include pneumonia, pancreatitis, diverticulitis, and appendicitis.

Extracolonic findings of moderate importance are those that are likely benign but may need further workup or treatment at a later time if the patient becomes symptomatic (**Fig. 4**). Nonobstructing cholelithiasis and nephrolithiasis (**Fig. 5**), splenomegaly, cardiomegaly, and pleural effusion are examples of findings considered to be of moderate importance. Asymptomatic ventral, inguinal, or other hernias are also considered to be of moderate importance.

Extracolonic findings of minor importance are benign and do not require any additional workup. These findings include simple renal and hepatic cysts, fatty liver, calcified granuloma, lipoma, vertebral hemangioma, and arterial calcifications. Asymptomatic small hiatal hernias are also of minor importance.

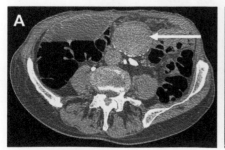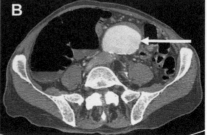

Fig. 1. (*A*) Large, incidentally discovered infrarenal AAA (*arrow*) seen on screening CTC. (*B*) Contrast-enhanced CT performed for follow-up again shows the aneurysm (*arrow*).

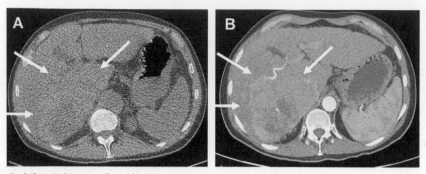

Fig. 2. (*A*) Axial image from low-dose unenhanced screening CTC demonstrates heterogeneous mass (*arrows*) in the right hepatic lobe. (*B*) The lesion (*arrows*) is better seen on post-contrast CT during arterial phase. The biopsy confirmed hepatocellular carcinoma.

In 2005, the Working Group on Virtual Colonoscopy developed a consensus proposal for the CTC reporting and data system (C-RADS) in 2005. A classification system for extracolonic findings is also included that consists of 5 categories.[25] This system is increasingly used for practical documentation and reporting of extracolonic findings. Category E0 represents a nondiagnostic study due to significant compromise of image quality related to technical factors or artifact. Category E1 represents a normal study with no extracolonic abnormalities visible or if there are anatomic variants only. Category E2 represents clinically unimportant findings that do not require further workup. Category E3 represents findings that are likely unimportant but are not well characterized and may require additional workup according to specific local practice guidelines. Category E4 findings are of major importance that require prompt or immediate evaluation. More widespread use of this classification scheme helps to standardize documentation and reporting of extracolonic findings.

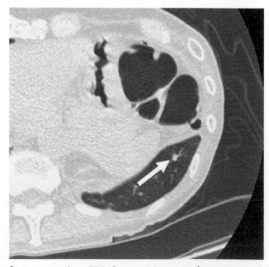

Fig. 3. Axial image from screening CTC shows a 5-mm pulmonary nodule at the left lower lobe (*arrow*).

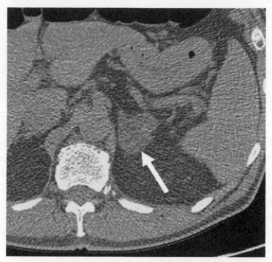

Fig. 4. Three-centimeter low-density lesion of the left adrenal gland (*arrow*) consistent with a benign adenoma, which does not typically require additional imaging.

LITERATURE REVIEW OF EXTRACOLONIC FINDINGS

There are multiple variables to consider when comparing studies evaluating extracolonic findings on CTC. These include the classification systems and definitions of extracolonic findings used as well as the type of patient population being evaluated. The tube current used and cost-assessment methodology are also important criteria. Screening CTC typically uses low tube current of 50 to 80 effective mAs, which may not be optimal for the evaluation of extracolonic findings. The use of intravenous contrast can alter sensitivity of extracolonic findings and affect potential further

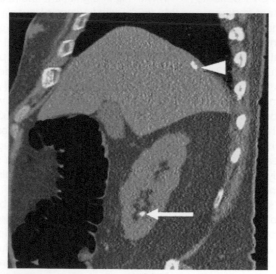

Fig. 5. Nonobstructing 3-mm right renal calculus (*arrow*) and 8-mm calcified liver granuloma (*arrowhead*) demonstrated on sagittal reformat.

workup. It is also important to exclude previously known extracolonic findings, because these are typically not used in data analysis. A comparison of original studies evaluating extracolonic findings on CTC is provided in **Table 1**.

In 2000, a study by Hara and colleagues[26] produced the first report in the literature evaluating extracolonic findings on CTC. CTC was performed in 264 patients who were at high risk for colorectal carcinoma, using 5-mm collimation and a tube current of 70 mA. Extracolonic findings were categorized as having high, moderate, or low importance. The range of follow-up after CTC was 7 to 22 months. Extracolonic findings were seen in 109 (41%) patients, with highly important findings seen in 30 (11%) patients. A total of 151 lesions were identified. Of these, 34 (23%) were highly important, 49 (32%) were of moderate importance, and 68 (45%) were of low importance. Of the 30 patients with highly important lesions, 12 had findings that were previously known. The remaining 18 (7% of all patients) had further diagnostic evaluation, with 6 going on to surgery. Two of the postsurgical cases proved to be malignant lesions. Total additional workup cost resulting from extracolonic findings was $7234 ($28 per CTC examination). Of the total additional cost, 23% was spent on evaluation of what ultimately proved to be malignant or surgical pathology, 44% on indeterminate lesions, and 33% on benign etiologies.

A trial evaluating 100 patients (mean age, 65 years) was performed by Edwards and colleagues.[27] The CTC protocol consisted of 5-mm collimation and an effective dose of 70 mAs. A total of 15 patients (15%) were identified with extracolonic lesions, significantly lower than in other studies. Notable findings included a probable renal cell cancer (not further assessed due to patient death from unrelated causes) and an AAA. Also 2 liver lesions and 3 ovarian cysts were seen. Of these 15 patients, 11 had further workup, including 2 patients who had surgery for large ovarian cysts (benign on pathology).

A large study of extracolonic findings in 681 asymptomatic, screening patients (median age, 64 years) who underwent CTC was performed by Gluecker and colleagues.[28] CTC was performed using 5-mm collimation and a tube current of either 40 mA or 70 mA. Extracolonic findings were categorized as high, medium, or low clinical importance. A total of 858 extracolonic findings were identified in 469 of 681 (69%) patients. There were 71 patients (10%) with highly significant findings, 183 (27%) with moderately important findings, and 341 (50%) with findings of low clinical importance. Follow-up investigation (mean interval, 31 months) revealed a total of 94 procedures for highly important lesions, with 1.3% of patients requiring medical or surgical intervention. Additional cost amounted to $34.33 per CTC examination performed.

Another large study of 1233 asymptomatic screening patients undergoing CTC was performed by Pickhardt and colleagues.[29] CTC protocol consisted of multidetector CT with 1.25- to 2.5-mm collimation and 100 mA tube current. Findings were categorized as having high, moderate, or low clinical significance. Only 56 of 1233 (4.5%) patients demonstrated highly significant findings, a lower percentage than found by Gluecker and colleagues, which may be partially related to the younger mean age of the patients (58 years vs 64 years). Extracolonic malignancies were identified in 5 of 1233 (0.4%) patients. This study suggested a lower incidence of extracolonic findings in an asymptomatic population.

Ginnerup Pedersen and colleagues[30] evaluated an asymptomatic but high-risk population (history of previous adenomatous polyps or cancer) of 75 patients (median age, 61 years). CTC protocol consisted of 2.5-mm collimation and an effective dose of 70 mAs. Chart review was performed 6 months after CTC. After excluding preexisting lesions, 68 new extracolonic lesions were identified in 49 (65%) patients, with recommendations for additional workup in 9 (12%) patients. Two patients (3%) had surgery related directly to the extracolonic finding or from a complication of the workup.

Table 1
Extracolonic findings on unenhanced CTC

Study	Cohort Size	Cohort Type	Tube Current (or Effective Dose)	Length of Follow-up (mo)	Overall Percentage of Subjects with ECFs	Subjects with Major ECFs (%)	Subjects Receiving Further Workup for ECFs (%)	Subjects Having Surgery Related to ECF (%)	Cost/CTC Performed
Hara et al[26] (2000)	264	High risk/symptomatic	70 mA	7–22	41	11	7	2.3	$28
Edwards et al[27] (2001)	100	High risk/symptomatic	70 mAs	—	15	—	11	2	—
Gluecker et al[28] (2003)	681	Asymptomatic	40–70 mA	31 (mean)	69	10	10	1.3	$34.33
Pickhardt et al[29] (2003)	1,233	Asymptomatic	100 mA	—	—	4.5	4.5	—	—
Ginnerup Pedersen et al[30] (2003)	75	High risk/symptomatic	70 mAs	6	65	12	—	3	$12
Hellstrom et al[31] (2004)	111	High risk/symptomatic	125 mAs	36 (maximum)	85	23	13	—	—
Rajapaksa et al[32] (2004)	250	High risk/symptomatic	50 mAs	17 (median)	33	12.5	4.4	<1	—
Chin et al[33] (2005)	432	Asymptomatic	79–96 mA	24 (maximum)	27	7.4	7.4	—	$24.37[a]
Yee et al[34] (2005)	500	Mixed	150 mA	42 (mean)	63	9	5	1	$28.12
Pickhardt et al[35] (2008)	2195	Asymptomatic	Low dose	18 (mean)	—	9.3	6.1	—	$98.58[a]
Flicker et al[36] (2008)	366	Mixed	80–100 mAs	18 for E3 lesions; 1.5 for E4 lesions	72	18	—	—	$13.07
Kimberly et al[37] (2009)	136	Mixed	180 mA/80 mA	38 mo (median)	98	18.4	32.5	—	$248[a]
Stitt et al[38] (2009)	749	Asymptomatic	Low dose	—	—	—	—	1.2	—

Abbreviation: ECFs, extracolonic findings.

[a] Included costs of surgical and/or clinical evaluation.

Extracolonic findings were evaluated in a cohort of 111 symptomatic patients (median age, 66 years) on CTC in a study by Hellstrom and colleagues.[31] CTC protocol consisted of 5-mm collimation and an effective dose of 125 mAs. Extracolonic lesions were categorized as having major, moderate, or minor clinical importance, and patients were followed up to 3 years after CTC. Prevalence of extracolonic findings was high, with lesions detected in 94 (85%) patients. There were 26 (23%) patients with highly important findings, 58 (52%) with moderately important findings, and 46 (41%) with either no findings or findings of low importance. The investigators suggested the high prevalence of extracolonic findings may be related to the high-risk, symptomatic patient cohort. Of the 26 patients with highly important findings, 13 had findings which were previously unknown.

Extracolonic findings on CTC were studied in a cohort of 250 patients by Rajapaksa and colleagues.[32] The patient population included mostly men and symptomatic patients, with a mean age of 62.5 years. Low-dose CTC protocol consisted of 1-mm collimation and an effective dose of 50 mAs. Extracolonic findings were reported as having high, moderate, or low clinical significance, with a median follow-up time of approximately 17 months. A total of 136 extracolonic findings were reported in 83 (33%) patients, notably less than in the Hellstrom and colleagues study, despite a similar high-risk patient population. Of the 136 extracolonic findings, 17 (12.5%) extracolonic findings were reported as highly significant, 53 (39%) as moderately significant, and 66 (49%) as having low significance. Of the 17 major findings, 14 (82%) were newly identified at the time of CTC, with additional testing performed in 11 of 250 (4.4%) patients.

In a study of 432 asymptomatic patients from a screening population (mean age 58.6 years), Chin and colleagues[33] investigated the incidence and cost of follow-up of extracolonic findings on CTC. Collimation of either 3 or 5 mm and a tube current of 70 mA or 96 mA was used. Extracolonic findings were labeled as clinically relevant if further medical or surgical attention or follow-up imaging was needed for the finding. Only lesions that were newly discovered or showed significant interval change were included. A total of 146 extracolonic findings were detected in 118 patients (27%), and 32 clinically relevant lesions (32 out of 146, 21.9%) were identified in 32 patients (32 out of 432, 7.4%). The most common finding was AAA, which was seen in 6 patients. Patients' records were reviewed up to 2 years after CTC. The total cost of follow-up was $10,527.99 ($24.37 per CTC); $6469 of this total cost was for additional imaging studies, with $792 for pathologic evaluation and $3265 for clinical evaluation. The cost of extracolonic finding workup was similar to previous studies.

Yee and colleagues[34] evaluated extracolonic findings in a large cohort of male patients, with a mean age of 62.5 years. Of the 500 patients, there was a mixture of screening, asymptomatic patients (39%) and high-risk or symptomatic patients (61%). CTC technique for this study consisted of 2.5- to 3-mm collimation and a tube current of 120 to 150 mA. Extracolonic findings requiring further diagnostic testing or follow-up imaging were labeled as clinically significant. A total of 596 extracolonic findings were present in 315 patients (315 out of 500, 63%). Fifty clinically significant lesions were seen in 45 patients (9% of all patients), with 36 new findings occurring in 35 patients. The frequency of significant lesions was similar in both high-risk and screening patients. The mean follow-up time was longer than other studies at 3.6 years. Out of the 35 patients with new findings, 12 (34%) had benign lesions, 13 (37%) had clinically significant lesions, and 10 (29%) did not receive their recommended additional imaging. In summary, 25 patients (25 out of 500, 5%) had their management changed, with 13 having proven clinically important findings on follow-up imaging or surgery. The additional imaging costs totaled $14,058 ($28.12

per CTC examination). Of this amount, 35% ($4872) was used in evaluating lesions that were confirmed as clinically significant.

In a trial by Pickhardt and colleagues,[35] extracolonic findings were tabulated in 2195 asymptomatic, screening patients (mean age, 58 years) who underwent CTC. Low-dose CTC protocol consisted of slices of 5 mm thickness. Extracolonic findings of moderate or greater clinical importance were used for further analysis. A total of 204 of 2195 (9.3%) patients had findings of at least moderate clinical importance. Of these 204 patients, 189 (86%) were newly identified. The mean total follow-up time was 544 days. A total of 133 patients (133 out of 2195, 6.1%) underwent further evaluation, including 18 patients who were not recommended for follow-up imaging by the radiologist. In 55 of these 133 (or 55 out of 2195 2.5% of total) patients, findings of at least moderate or greater importance were observed after further workup, with the remainder proving to be of minor clinical importance. The total cost for further evaluation was $216,347 ($98.58 per CTC examination); of which, $146,247 ($67.54 per CTC examination) was for follow-up surgical costs and $68,093 ($31.02 per CTC examination) was for nonsurgical follow-up procedures, including imaging. Unlike other trials, this study included the cost of surgery required for management of clinically significant extracolonic findings.

In another study, Flicker and colleagues[36] evaluated extracolonic findings in 376 patients (mean age, 61 years) on CTC. The patient cohort consisted of 210 screening patients and 166 high-risk patients. Variable CTC technique was used with an effective dose ranging between 50 and 100 mAs. Extracolonic findings were reported based on the C-RADS criteria (E0–E4). A total of 520 extracolonic lesions were described in 272 of 376 (72%) patients. A total of 447 out of 520 lesions (86%) were rated E2, 56 out of 520 (11%) were identified as E3 lesions in 51 (51 out of 376, 13.6%) patients, and 17 out of 520 (3%) E4 lesions were reported in 16 (16 out of 376, 4.3%) patients. There were 6 (2.8%) screening patients and 10 (6%) high-risk patients with E4 lesions. The mean follow-up time was 18 months for E3 lesions and 1.5 months for E4 lesions. A total of 14 additional imaging studies were performed at a cost of $4914 ($13.07 per CTC). The frequency of E4 lesions was significantly greater in the high-risk group (2.8% vs 6%).

In a study by Kimberly and colleagues,[37] 136 patients (median age, 57 years) underwent CTC with 5-mm collimation and a tube current of 180 mA supine and 80 mA prone. Extracolonic findings were classified as having high, moderate, or low importance. A total of 423 extracolonic findings were detected in 134 (98%) patients, with 25 extracolonic findings of high importance detected in 25 (18.4%) patients. The most common highly important finding was a pulmonary nodule, which was seen in 23 patients. A total of 53 findings of moderate importance were present in 35 patients, and 345 findings of low importance were identified in 74 patients. The median follow-up time was 38 months. Further workup was performed in 32 (32 out of 136, 23.5%) patients. There were 73 imaging studies performed at a cost of $25,227 ($185 per CTC). Laboratory studies totaled $1080 ($8 per CTC). Five patients underwent procedures, costing $5163 ($38 per CTC). Follow-up clinic visits that were attributed to extracolonic findings from CTC amounted to $2279 ($17 per CTC). The combined cost for follow-up workup was $33,690 ($248 per patient). This is greater than in the previous studies, likely related to incorporation of clinic and laboratory test costs into the analysis. The large number of pulmonary nodules also added to the higher costs.

In a study of 749 women (mean age, 61.2 years) undergoing low-dose CTC, Stitt and colleagues[38] evaluated extracolonic findings of gynecologic origin. All patients were asymptomatic for gynecologic disease. Only extracolonic findings of gynecologic nature were included in this study. Gynecologic findings were identified in 71 of 749 (9.5%) patients, of whom 57 (57 out of 71, 80%) had findings that were considered benign at the time of CTC. Additional evaluation was performed in 14 (20%) patients. Recommended imaging was performed in 13 patients, and 9 patients underwent surgery. All lesions were benign on pathology. This study showed that although gynecologic findings occur in almost 10% of female patients undergoing CTC, these lesions are typically proven to be benign.

The American College of Radiology Imaging Network's (ACRIN's) National CTC Trial reported a 66% incidence of extracolonic findings, with 16% of findings requiring additional workup or clinical correlation.[39] There were a total of 2531 participants, with a mean age of 58 years. However, these results are preliminary as the data included extracolonic findings that were previously known to the subjects and their health care provider. Therefore, the number of new findings requiring additional workup or urgent care will be lower.

Xiong and colleagues[40] performed a meta-analysis of primary studies of extracolonic findings on CTC published between 1993 and 2004. In total, 3488 patients were identified from 17 studies, including 13 full-length articles and 4 abstracts. A total of 2015 extracolonic lesions were seen in 1362 (39%) patients, with 188 of them undergoing further workup and 17 of 2237 patients (0.8%) requiring immediate treatment. Extracolonic malignancies were identified in 81 of 3005 patients (2.7%), with almost half (42%) detected at an early stage. This study confirmed that there is a low overall prevalence of extracolonic lesions found on CTC that are of clinical importance.

Intravenous Contrast

Screening CTC consists of a low-dose unenhanced scan that still allows the detection of findings outside the colon (**Table 2**). Diagnostic CTC often requires the use of intravenous contrast and higher tube current. Intravenous contrast is also often required to problem solve indeterminate lesions found on unenhanced CTC. Contrast-enhanced CT allows improved characterization of indeterminate low-density lesions in the kidney and liver and allows identification of intraluminal vascular disease.

Hara[41] evaluated extracolonic findings in 163 patients who underwent CTC with and without intravenous contrast, with an effective dose of 180 mAs. Extracolonic lesions of high significance were identified in 24% of precontrast studies and 17% of postcontrast studies. The lower rate of findings on postcontrast scans may be attributed to improved characterization of lesions as benign with the use of intravenous contrast. Follow-up imaging was requested more often with noncontrast CTC than with postcontrast CTC.

Extracolonic findings were evaluated by Spreng and colleagues[42] in a cohort of 102 symptomatic patients who underwent CTC. Comparison was made between 72 patients who had contrast-enhanced CTC and 30 patients who underwent noncontrast studies. CTC protocol consisted of 2-mm collimation and an effective dose of 200 mAs. Extracolonic findings were categorized as either needing further evaluation or no evaluation. There were 91 (89%) patients with a total of 303 extracolonic findings. Further evaluation or change in management was recommended in 26 of 102 (25%) patients, and 22 of these 26 patients had undergone contrast-enhanced CTC. The investigators concluded that contrast-enhanced CTC resulted in a higher percentage of extracolonic findings that needed additional evaluation compared with unenhanced CTC, which is in contrast to Hara and colleagues' (2005) results.

Khan and colleagues[43] evaluated 225 older patients at high risk for colon carcinoma who underwent CTC. The median age of the patients was 74 years, which is much

Table 2
Extracolonic findings on contrast-enhanced CTC

Study	Cohort Size	Cohort Type	Tube Current (or Effective dose)	Length of Follow-up (mo)	Overall Percentage of Subjects with ECFs	Subjects with Major ECFs (%)	ECFs on Precontrast CTC (%)	ECFs on Postcontrast CTC (%)
Hara[41] (2005)	163	—	180 mAs		—	—	24 (significant lesions only)	17 (significant lesions only)
Spreng et al[42] (2005)	102	Symptomatic	200 mAs		89	25	29	71
Khan et al[43] (2007)	225	High risk	220 mAs supine/ 50 mAs prone	12 (maximum)	52	23	24	62.3
Kim et al[44] (2007)	2,230	Asymptomatic	120 mAs supine/ 50 mAs prone	19 (mean)	66.5	5.1	—	66.5
Park et al[45] (2009)	920	Mixed	30–200 mAs	6	58	58	—	58

Abbreviation: ECFs, extracolonic findings.

older than in other studies. CTC was performed with 2.5-mm collimation and an effective dose of 220 mAs supine and 50 mAs prone. Intravenous contrast was given in 162 (72%) patients. A total of 211 extracolonic findings were identified in 116 (52%) patients. A higher number of extracolonic findings were identified in patients who underwent contrast-enhanced CTC than in patients who underwent unenhanced CTC (62% vs 24%). Medical records were reviewed up to 12 months after CTC. Patients with previously known findings or colon cancer metastases were excluded from evaluation. Of 104 patients with newly discovered extracolonic findings, 24 (23%) had additional testing, with 12 patients undergoing 14 surgical procedures.

In a large trial, Kim and colleagues[44] evaluated 2230 asymptomatic screening patients (mean age, 57.5 years) undergoing contrast-enhanced CTC. The study protocol consisted of 2 mm and an effective dose of 120 mAs supine and 50 mAs prone. Findings were divided into potentially important, likely unimportant, and clinically unimportant categories. In total, 2186 extracolonic findings were found in 1484 patients (66.5%). Of these, 121 findings were potentially important (5.5%), with 6 lesions that were previously known, leaving 115 new lesions in 115 patients. The mean follow-up time was 1.6 years. Of the 115 patients with new, potentially important findings, 100 (87%) had additional imaging. Of these 100 patients, 51 (51%) ultimately had findings requiring treatment or were deemed clinically important after follow-up evaluation (51 out of 2230, 2.3% of total population). The low rate of potentially important findings was attributed to the young, screening population cohort. It was concluded that the improved lesion characterization from contrast-enhanced CTC leads to decreased cost of follow-up.

Park and colleagues[45] evaluated 920 patients (mean age, 57 years) undergoing CTC. Contrast-enhanced CTC was performed in 764 patients, and noncontrast CTC was performed in 156 patients. CTC protocol consisted of 1.25- to 5-mm collimation and an effective dose of 30 to 200 mAs. Lesions were classified as having high, intermediate, or low significance. A total of 692 extracolonic findings were identified in 532 out of 920 (58%) patients. Of the 692 lesions 60 (8.7%) were reported as highly significant, 250 (36.1%) as moderately significant, and 382 (55.2%) were reported as having low significance. A total of 459 of 764 (60%) patients had extracolonic findings on contrast-enhanced CTC, whereas 73 of 156 patients (47%) had lesions identified on noncontrast CTC. Treatment was performed for highly significant lesions in 49 of 60 (81.7%) patients and for moderately significant lesions in 52 of 250 patients (20.8%). Only 11 of 382 (2.9%) patients received treatment for lesions of low significance. There was a greater incidence of extracolonic findings on contrast-enhanced CTC than on noncontrast CTC in this study, similar to the results from Khan and colleagues and Spreng and colleagues.

ECONOMIC CONSIDERATIONS

There have been several studies that have evaluated the cost of follow-up care for incidental findings detected on CTC. Multiple studies have found that there is an additional cost ranging from $12 to $34 per CTC study.[26,28,33,34,36] These studies were consistent in showing that the cost of workup of clinically relevant extracolonic lesions is low when balanced with the potential ability to detect serious findings that positively affect health care. An exception to these findings were the results of a study by Kimberly and colleagues[37] that showed an additional cost of $248 per CTC study, of which $185 per CTC was from additional imaging. This was likely related to the high frequency of incidental pulmonary nodules detected. Size criteria for nodules were not given in the study.

The costs presented in these studies consisted of additional diagnostic workup, and in some cases included clinical workup,[33,37] but did not include the cost of interventional procedures such as surgery, which would lead to higher total costs. In an assessment of the clinical resources and costs associated with the evaluation and treatment of extracolonic lesions in the United Kingdom, 225 symptomatic patients were evaluated.[46] Extracolonic findings were detected in 116 (52%) patients with 24 (11%) patients requiring further workup or treatment. It was found that surgical procedures accounted for the majority (87%) of the total costs. The resources that were used due to the workup of extracolonic lesions almost doubled the cost of diagnostic CTC. It was noted that the higher costs in this study may have partially been related to the higher mean age of 74 years in the symptomatic cohort. In a trial by Pickhardt and colleagues,[35] surgery was the costliest element of extracolonic lesion evaluation, accounting for $67.54, or 68% of the total additional cost per CTC examination, when compared with follow-up imaging, which added only an additional $28 per examination. These studies demonstrate that costs increase significantly when including surgical evaluation. However, this needs to be weighed against the potentially higher costs incurred if clinically significant lesions are detected at an advanced stage.

Hassan and colleagues[47] modeled the effect of incorporating the detection of extracolonic cancers and AAAs into CTC screening. Using a computerized Markov model to simulate the occurrence of colorectal neoplasia, extracolonic neoplasm, and AAA in a cohort of 100,000 subjects who were 50 years of age, substantial gains in life years by CTC screening over colonoscopy-based screening were found. This work was then applied to an older age group of 65 years and more.[48] Results demonstrated that CTC resulted in 7786 and 7027 life years gained at 5- and 10-year intervals (using a 6-mm polyp size threshold to recommend optical colonoscopy), respectively, compared with 6032 life years gained with 10-year optical colonoscopy. The improved efficacy of CTC was attributed to the prevention of AAA rupture, because CTC and optical colonoscopy were similar in colorectal cancer detection rates and prevention. All 3 strategies were highly cost effective compared with no screening, with an incremental cost-effectiveness ratio (ICER) of $6088, $1251, and $1104 per life year gained for 5-year CTC, 10-year CTC, and 10-year optical colonoscopy, respectively. Both CTC strategies remained cost effective against colonoscopy with ICER values of $23,234 and $2,144 for 5-year and 10-year CTC, respectively. Both studies demonstrated that CTC is a highly cost effective and clinically effective strategy given its ability to simultaneously screen for both colorectal cancers and AAAs.

SUMMARY

The ability to identify extracolonic findings on CTC has the potential benefit of allowing earlier detection of clinically significant disease leading to earlier intervention. This can prolong or save lives. However, potential limitations include increased health care costs because of the workup of extracolonic findings that are ultimately determined to be benign. There are also detrimental effects on the psychological well being of patients and the possibility of increased patient morbidity.

CTC is typically performed in older patients starting at 50 years, and therefore, as demonstrated in multiple published studies, most patients will have extracolonic findings. However, most of these extracolonic lesions are not clinically relevant. The incidence of findings of high clinical importance is likely dependent on the specific type and age of the patient cohort being evaluated. Patients at high risk for colon cancer or who are symptomatic have been found to have 11% to 23% incidence of highly important findings, whereas asymptomatic screening patients have a lower incidence (4.5%–16%). Although most patients suspected of having an extracolonic finding of major importance will end up having a benign lesion, about 1% to 3% of patients will have surgery for the previously unsuspected extracolonic finding.

Several studies have shown that the additional cost per study for the evaluation and follow-up of extracolonic findings is low. This can be confirmed by performing additional larger studies on asymptomatic versus symptomatic patients. Screening CTC is a low-dose unenhanced scan. Low-dose CT technique results in images with increased noise, which can limit the ability to detect and characterize extracolonic findings on CTC. Specific criteria for the workup of these extracolonic findings identified on low-dose unenhanced CTC should be developed.

REFERENCES

1. Lesperance K, Andersen C, Singh N, et al. Expanding use of emergency endovascular repair for ruptured abdominal aortic aneurysm: disparities in outcomes from a nationwide perspective. J Vasc Surg 2008;47:1165–70.
2. United States Preventive Services Task Force. Screening for abdominal aortic aneurysm: recommendation statement. Ann Intern Med 2005;142:198–202.
3. Lee E, Pickett E, Hedayati N, et al. Implementation of an aortic screening program in clinical practice: implications for the Screen for Abdominal Aortic Aneurysm Very Efficiently (SAAAVE) act. J Vasc Surg 2009;49:1107–11.
4. Kyriakides C, Byrne J, Green S, et al. Screening of abdominal aortic aneurysm: a pragmatic approach. Ann R Coll Surg Engl 2000;82:59–63.
5. Chervu A, Clagett GP, Valentine RJ, et al. Role of physical examination in the detection of abdominal aortic aneurysms. Surgery 1995;117:454–7.
6. Nevitt MP, Ballard DJ, Hallett JW. Prognosis of abdominal aortic aneurysms: a population-based study. N Engl J Med 1989;321:1009–14.
7. Johansson G, Swedenborg J. Ruptured abdominal aortic aneurysms: a study of incidence and mortality. Br J Surg 1986;73:101–3.
8. Wilmink T, Quick C, Hubbard C, et al. The influence of screening on the incidence of ruptured abdominal aortic aneurysms. J Vasc Surg 1999;30:203–8.
9. Tsui K, Shvarts O, Smith R, et al. Renal cell carcinoma: prognostic significance of incidentally detected tumors. J Urol 2000;163:426–30.
10. Homma Y, Kawabe K, Kitamura T, et al. Increased incidental detection and reduced mortality in renal cancer: recent retrospective analysis at eight institutions. Int J Urol 1995;2:77–80.
11. Sweeney JP, Thornhill JA, Graiger R, et al. Incidentally discovered renal cell carcinoma: pathologic features, survival trends and implications for treatment. Br J Urol 1996;78:351–3.
12. Silverman SG, Israel GM, Herts B, et al. Management of the incidental renal mass. Radiology 2008;249:16–31.
13. Bosniak MA, Rofsky NM. Problems in the detection and characterization of small renal masses. Radiology 1996;198:638–41.
14. Berland L. Incidental extracolonic findings on CT colonography: the impending deluge and its implications. J Am Coll Radiol 2009;6:14–20.
15. Westbrook JI, Braithwaite J, McIntosh JH. The outcomes for patients with incidental lesions: serendipitous or iatrogenic? AJR Am J Roentgenol 1998;171:1193–6.
16. Lerman C, Trock B, Rimer BK, et al. Psychological side effects of breast cancer screening. Health Psychol 1991;10:259–67.

17. ACR practice guideline for the performance of computed tomography (CT) colonography in adults. In: Practice guidelines and technical standards 2009. Reston (VA): American College of Radiology; 2009. p. 295–9.

18. Yee J, Kumar NN, Hung RK, et al. Comparison of supine, prone and both supine and prone scans in CT colonography. Radiology 2003;226:653–61.

19. van Gelder RE, Venema HW, Serlie IW, et al. CT colonography at different radiation dose levels: feasibility of dose reduction. Radiology 2002;224:25–33.

20. Macari M, Bini EJ, Xue X, et al. Colorectal neoplasms: prospective comparison of thin-section low-dose multi-detector row CT colonography and conventional colonoscopy for detection. Radiology 2002;224:383–92.

21. Iannaccone R, Laghi A, Catalano C, et al. Detection of colorectal lesions: lower-dose multi-detector row helical CT colonography compared with conventional colonoscopy. Radiology 2003;229:775–81.

22. Iannaccone R, Catalano C, Mangiapane F, et al. Colorectal polyps: detection with low-dose multi-detector row helical CT colonography versus two sequential colonoscopies. Radiology 2005;237:927–37.

23. Iannaccone R, Laghi A, Catalano C, et al. Feasibility of ultra-low-dose multislice CT colonography for the detection of colorectal lesions: preliminary experience. Eur Radiol 2003;13:1297–302.

24. Johnston KW, Rutherford RB, Tilson MD, et al. Suggested standards for reporting on arterial aneurysms. Subcommittee on Reporting Standards for Arterial Aneurysms, Ad Hoc Committee on Reporting Standards, Society for Vascular Surgery and North American Chapter, International Society for Cardiovascular Surgery. J Vasc Surg 2001;13:452–8.

25. Zalis M, Barish M, Choi R, et al. CT colonography reporting and data system (C-RADS): a consensus statement. Radiology 2005;236:3–9.

26. Hara AK, Johnson CD, MacCarty RL, et al. Incidental extracolonic findings at CT colonography. Radiology 2000;215:353–7.

27. Edwards JT, Wood CJ, Mendelson RM, et al. Extracolonic findings at virtual colonoscopy: implications for screening programs. Am J Gastroenterol 2001;96:3009–12.

28. Gluecker TM, Johnson CD, Wilson LA, et al. Extracolonic findings at CT colonography: evaluation of prevalence ad cost in a screening population. Gastroenterology 2003;124:911–6.

29. Pickhardt PJ, Choi R, Hwang I, et al. Computed tomographic virtual colonoscopy to screen for colorectal neoplasia in asymptomatic adults. N Engl J Med 2003;349:2191–200.

30. Ginnerup Pedersen B, Rosenkilde M, Christiansen TE, et al. Extracolonic findings at computed tomography colonography are a challenge. Gut 2003;52:1744–7.

31. Hellstrom M, Svensson MH, Lasson A. Extracolonic and incidental findings on CT colonography (virtual colonoscopy). AJR Am J Roentgenol 2004;182:631–8.

32. Rajapaksa RC, Macari M, Bini E. Prevalence and impact of extracolonic findings in patients undergoing CT colonography. J Clin Gastroenterol 2004;38:767–71.

33. Chin M, Mendelson R, Edwards J, et al. Computed tomographic colonography: prevalence, nature, and clinical significance of extracolonic findings in a community screening program. Am J Gastroenterol 2005;100:2771–6.

34. Yee J, Kumar N, Godara S, et al. Extracolonic abnormalities discovered incidentally at CT colonography in a male population. Radiology 2005;236:519–26.

35. Pickhardt PJ, Hanson ME, Vanness DJ, et al. Unsuspected extracolonic findings at screening CT colonography: clinical and economic impact. Radiology 2008;249:151–9.

36. Flicker M, Tsoukas AT, Hazra A, et al. Economic impact of extracolonic findings at computed tomographic colonography. J Comput Assist Tomogr 2008;32: 497–503.
37. Kimberly J, Phillips C, Santago P, et al. Extracolonic findings at virtual colonoscopy: an important consideration in asymptomatic colorectal cancer screening. J Gen Intern Med 2009;24(1):69–73.
38. Stitt IA, Stany MP, Moser RP, et al. Incidental gynecological findings on computed tomographic colonography: prevalence and outcomes. Gynecol Oncol 2009;115: 138–41.
39. Johnson CD, Chen MH, Toledano AY, et al. The National CT colonography trial: multicenter assessment of accuracy for detection of large adenomas and cancers. N Engl J Med 2008;359:1207–17.
40. Xiong T, Richardson M, Woodroffe R, et al. Incidental lesions found on CT colonography: their nature and frequency. Br J Radiol 2005;78:22–9.
41. Hara AK. Extracolonic findings at CT Colonography. Semin Ultrasound CT MR 2005;26:24–7.
42. Spreng A, Netzer P, Mattich J, et al. Importance of extracolonic findings at IV contrast medium-enhanced CT colonography versus those at non-enhanced CT colonography. Eur Radiol 2005;15:2088–95.
43. Khan KY, Xiong T, McCafferty I, et al. Frequency and impact of extracolonic findings detected at computed tomographic colonography in a symptomatic population. Br J Surg 2007;94:355–61.
44. Kim YS, Kim N, Kim SY, et al. Extracolonic findings in an asymptomatic screening population undergoing intravenous contrast-enhanced computed tomography colonography. J Gastroenterol Hepatol 2008;23:49–57.
45. Park SK, Park DI, Lee SY, et al. Extracolonic findings of computed tomographic colonography in Koreans. World J Gastroenterol 2009;15:1487–92.
46. Xiong T, McEvoy K, Morton DG, et al. Resources and costs associated with incidental extracolonic findings from CT colonography: a study in a symptomatic population. Br J Radiol 2006;79:948–61.
47. Hassan C, Pickhardt PJ, Laghi A, et al. Computed tomographic colonography to screen for colorectal cancer, extracolonic cancer, and aortic aneurysm. Arch Intern Med 2008;168:696–705.
48. Pickhardt PJ, Hassan C, Laghi A, et al. Colonography to screen for colorectal cancer and aortic aneurysm in the Medicare population: cost-effectiveness analysis. AJR Am J Roentgenol 2009;192:1332–40.

MR Colonography and MR Enterography

Lewis K. Shin, MD[a,b,*], Peter Poullos, MD[a],
R. Brooke Jeffrey, MD[a,c]

KEYWORDS

- Magnetic resonance colonography
- Magnetic resonance enterography • Virtual colonoscopy
- Polyp • Inflammatory bowel disease • Enteroclysis

The bowel is a common site for pathologic processes, including malignancies and inflammatory disease. The American Cancer Society estimated 146,970 new cases of colorectal cancer with 49,920 deaths in 2009.[1] Colorectal cancer accounts for 10% of all new cancers and 9% of cancer deaths.[1] From the early 1990s to 2005, there was a significant decrease in the incidence of colorectal cancer and cancer death rates, which has been attributed to screening measures, earlier detection, and improved therapies.

Virtual colonoscopy (VC), also known as computed tomography colonography (CTC), is an effective method for detecting small (6–9 mm) and larger (≥10 mm) polyps.[2–4] However, in light of increasing concerns about ionizing radiation exposure from medical imaging and potential increased risk of future radiation-induced malignancies,[5–8] magnetic resonance imaging (MRI) is seen as an increasingly attractive alternative. Improvements in MRI technology, which include multicoil designs with parallel imaging[9,10] and higher field strength magnets,[10–12] now permit three-dimensional (3D) volumetric imaging of the entire colon in a single breath hold at high spatial resolution, making VC with MRI possible.

MR COLONOGRAPHY TECHNIQUES

Early research in the late 1990s on MR colonography (MRC) showed the feasibility of this technique.[13] Two major imaging strategies have evolved: dark-lumen MRC

[a] Department of Radiology, Stanford University School of Medicine, 300 Pasteur Drive, Room H-1307, Stanford, CA 94305-5105, USA
[b] Department of Radiology, The Lucas Center for MR Spectroscopy and Imaging, Stanford University, MC#5488, Route 8, Stanford, CA 94305-5488, USA
[c] Abdominal Imaging, Department of Radiology at Stanford University Medical Center, 300 Pasteur Drive, Room H-1307, Stanford, CA, USA
* Corresponding author. Department of Radiology, The Lucas Center for MR Spectroscopy and Imaging, Stanford University, MC#5488, Route 8, Stanford, CA 94305-5488.
E-mail address: lshin@stanford.edu

Gastrointest Endoscopy Clin N Am 20 (2010) 323–346
doi:10.1016/j.giec.2010.02.010
1052-5157/10/$ – see front matter. Published by Elsevier Inc.

giendo.theclinics.com

(**Fig. 1**)[10,14–16] and bright-lumen MRC.[15,17–20] As the respective names suggest, there terms refer to the intraluminal signal intensity. Regardless of which technique is chosen, adequate colonic distension is mandatory for accurate evaluation.

Dark-lumen MRC typically requires 2 L of a warm, tap-water enema.[12,14,21,22] Alternative agents include room air[16,23,24] and CO_2.[25] However, gas can cause imaging artifacts and it is uncertain whether gas-distension techniques are feasible at 1.5-T MRI field strengths. Some studies have shown that air does not produce significant degradation of image quality,[26] whereas others have shown severe artifacts (15% of colonic segments) compared with water-distension techniques (0.3%).[23] Specifically, the majority (54.4%) of the artifacts in the former group were attributed to air-related artifacts.[23] These air-related artifacts are exacerbated with increasing field strength; thus MRC with gaseous distension at 3 T would be even more challenging. Dark-lumen MRC typically involves injection of intravenous (IV) gadolinium (Gd) contrast agents that can aid in differentiating polyps and carcinoma from stool, as the latter does not enhance.[27]

Bright-lumen techniques typically involved colonic distension with water enemas spiked with MRI contrast (eg, Gd agents).[15,17,20,28] Another novel bright-lumen technique is achieved after the bile (and thus stool) is tagged after gadobenate dimeglumine (MultiHance, Bracco Diagnostics Inc, Princeton, NJ, USA; an agent with partial biliary excretion) is administered intravenously.[29] Alternatively, water enemas using T2-weighted imaging can also achieve a bright-lumen contrast (**Fig. 2**).

Although dark- and bright-lumen techniques are currently in use, Lauenstein and colleagues[30] illustrate many advantages of dark-lumen MRC. If intraluminal Gd is used, bright-lumen MRC is more expensive because the amount of contrast required for the enema solution exceeds that required for IV administration for dark-lumen MRC. With bright-lumen techniques, air can cause confusion by appearing as an intraluminal filling defect.[30] Dark-lumen MRC can theoretically better characterize suspected colonic conditions by directly evaluating for enhancement rather than relying only on the presence of filling defects or wall thickening.[30] Post-IV contrast-enhanced

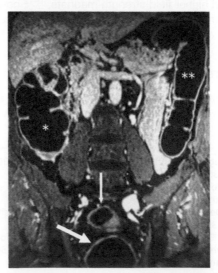

Fig. 1. Dark-lumen MRC after IV contrast administration shows enhancing colonic wall and dark signal of distended right colon (*asterisk*), left colon (*double asterisks*), sigmoid (*small arrow*), and rectum (*large arrow*).

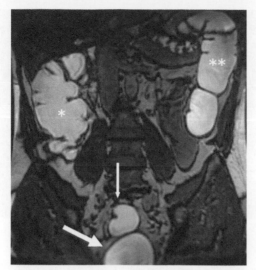

Fig. 2. Bright-lumen MRC without contrast administration shows dark colonic wall and bright signal of distended right colon (*asterisk*), left colon (*double asterisks*), sigmoid (*small arrow*), and rectum (*large arrow*).

imaging can better characterize extraluminal disease (eg, enhancing liver/renal lesions) than noncontrast imaging alone.[30]

PATIENT SELECTION

Several considerations need to be addressed to perform MRC successfully. As with all MR examinations, proper screening is necessary to exclude patients with contraindications such as pacemakers and metallic implants (ie, aneurysm clips) as well as to identify those with claustrophobia. Hip prostheses are typically not a contraindication to MR, but can cause severe artifacts in the rectum, producing nondiagnostic images.[31] Screening patients for impaired renal function is necessary if IV contrast is administered to reduce the risk of nephrogenic systemic fibrosis, which seems to be related to the IV administration of Gd-containing contrast agents.[32]

PREPARATION

A cathartic preparation is generally mandatory to eliminate residual stool, which can potentially be misinterpreted as a pathologic, intraluminal filling defect (polyp, malignancy) (**Fig. 3**). In addition, large amounts of residual stool can obscure underlying disease. Similar to conventional colonoscopy (CC), a typical bowel-cleansing regimen requires ingestion of 3 to 4 L of polyethylene glycol (PEG) solution the previous day of examination.

STOOL TAGGING

Several techniques have been developed to deliberately alter the signal of stool to render it invisible. This goal is accomplished by ingesting an oral contrast agent that causes the stool to match the signal of the enema (eg, bright stool for bright-lumen MRC and dark stool for dark-lumen MRC). This process is analogous to fecal tagging with electronic subtraction in CTC. As with CTC, the use of stool tagging has the potential to reduce or even eliminate the arduous cathartic preparation.[23] Robust

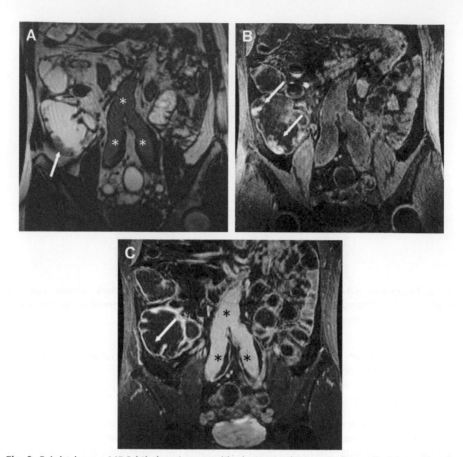

Fig. 3. Bright-lumen MRC (*A*) showing masslike lesion in the cecum (*arrow*) with previously unknown aortoiliac aneurysm (*asterisks*) with mural thrombus. Dark-lumen MRC (*B*) shows 2 masses (*arrows*), both bright before IV contrast administration. Dark-lumen MRC after IV contrast administration (*C*) shows cecal masses are artifacts caused by residual stool. Pseudo-masses do not enhance and have migrated (*arrow*) with patent lumen of aortoiliac aneurysm (*asterisks*) shown.

tagging decreases false-positive examinations by preventing misinterpretation of filling defects as colonic pathology; false-negative examinations also decrease as potential lesions are obscured by residual stool. Conversely, inadequate tagging has been shown to lead to nondiagnostic evaluation of approximately 5% of colonic segments.[33–35]

Tagging was first described in bright-lumen MRC (Gd-water enema) by Weishaupt in 1999.[36] Since then, many tagging agents and combinations of regimens have been tested, and it is an area of active research. The ideal tagging agent is inexpensive, well tolerated and provides robust, uniform stool tagging without generating image-comprising artifacts. Generally, MRC protocols involve ingestion of the tagging agents with meals consisting of a low-fiber and low-manganese diet for up to 2 days before MRC.[27,37] Manganese-rich foods like fruits and chocolate can result in bright signal stool artifacts on dark-lumen examinations and should be avoided. Gd tagging can be expensive because additional Gd is administered via enema at the time of the examination.[38] Barium oral contrast has been used as a less expensive alternative.[23,30,33] Because barium renders the stool dark on MR imaging, this method is reserved for dark-lumen MRC. Ferumoxsil (Lumirem, Guerbet Group, Paris, France) is another dark-lumen agent composed of small iron particles that also causes low signal on dark-lumen MRC.[30]

Patient acceptance of MRC stool-tagging regimens is variable. Florie and colleagues[20] found favorable results in a screening population undergoing MRC with Gd-based stool tagging for bright-lumen MRC, with most (69%) patients preferring MRC to a cathartic preparation (PEG) with CC (22%). However, Goehde and colleagues[39] reported low acceptance when tagging regimens involved only high concentration of oral barium contrast. Forty-two patients surveyed in a barium-only tagging MRC trial rated the barium slightly worse than the CC cathartic preparation. One hundred and fifty milliliters of 100% barium were given 6 times in the 36 hours before MRC. These investigators point out that in addition to the ingestion of barium, related feelings of constipation and abdominal pain were problematic. Conversely, Rodriguez Gomez and colleagues[23] found favorable results in their barium-only tagging protocol of 200 mL with each main meal for 48 hours before MRC, with 78.3% of 83 patients studied preferring MRC compared with 21.7% for CC for future examinations.

Barium contrast can be thick and heavy when ingested alone, and nausea has been reported in up to 50% of patients.[37] Thinner barium solutions mixed with other agents have subsequently been explored. Barium with 5% diatrizoate meglumine (Gastrografin, Bracco Diagnostics Inc, Princeton, NJ, USA) and 0.2% locust bean gum was better tolerated compared with bowel purgation in an asymptomatic screening population of 284 patients.[22] This did not translate into an overall patient preference for MRC compared with CC.[22] When 29 patients with inflammatory bowel disease (IBD) (17 with ulcerative colitis [UC]; 12 with Crohn disease [CD]) were surveyed after MRC with this tagging protocol and bowel catharsis with CC, Langhorst and colleagues[34] identified fecal tagging was preferred to bowel purgation. However, this also did not translate to overall acceptance of MRC, with 67% of patients with IBD preferring CC for future examinations. Achiam and colleagues[40] have also experimented with a thinner tagging combination of barium and ferumoxsil and have reported more promising tagging compliance, with most patients (66%) preferring MRC with tagging as a future screening method compared with CC (10%); 21% had no preference. The combination of ferumoxsil results in greater darkening of stool than barium alone. Thirty percent of patients still experienced nausea.[37] However, ferumoxsil itself can produce artifacts (Fig. 4) and more studies are necessary to determine if this protocol potentially obscures and reduces sensitivity of colonic lesions.[37,41]

Robust fecal tagging can depend on individual patient characteristics and timing of the MRC examination after tagging. Failures of uniform tagging have been seen in elderly patients[13] and patients with delayed colonic transit times of greater than 60 hours.[38] As more research is necessary for an optimal tagging regimen, the authors do not perform MRC with tagging at this time.

MRI TECHNIQUE

We prefer dark-lumen to bright-lumen MRC as a more robust method of colonic evaluation. Our protocol involves a cathartic preparation the previous day as described with PEG solution. An IV catheter is inserted and the patient is placed in the scanner in the supine position. Prone patient positioning is also acceptable. We administer

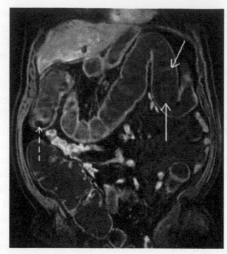

Fig. 4. MRC performed with fecal tagging. Supine coronal, dark-lumen MRC shows dark tagged fecal matter (*arrow*) and dark ferumoxsil artifact (*broken arrow*). (*From* Achiam MP, Logager V, Chabanova E, et al. Patient acceptance of MR colonography with improved fecal tagging versus conventional colonoscopy. Eur J Radiol 2008;73(1):146; with permission.)

0.5 mg of glucagon slowly via IV just before colonic distension via a warm tap-water enema (~2–2.5 L) through a rectal enema tube or large Foley catheter. A rapid, two-dimensional (2D) thick-slice, bright-lumen MRI sequence (ie, single-shot fast spin-echo sequence) is used to monitor filling with images acquired every 2 to 3 seconds until complete colonic distension is achieved (**Fig. 5**). A breath hold, oblique coronal volumetric (ie, 3D) bright-lumen sequence (ie, FIESTA) is performed (**Fig 6**). This sequence serves 3 major purposes: (1) to confirm complete filling and distension of the colon, (2) to facilitate image-acquisition planning of the dark-lumen sequences, and (3) to provide an additional image data set to confirm suspected pathology or pseudolesions on the dark-lumen images. Fat-suppressed, rapid T2-weighted axial or coronal imaging can be obtained for evaluation of colonic wall edema. A repeat dose of 0.5 mg of glucagon is administered just before acquisition of the dark-lumen 3D oblique coronal, fat-suppressed images. These images are obtained before

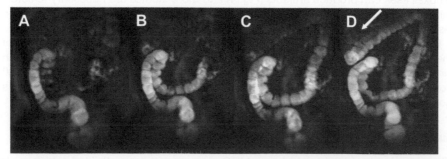

Fig. 5. Sequential, cine bright-lumen MRC technique used to monitor tap-water enema administration and distension of the colon to the mid-sigmoid (*A*), distal left colon (*B*), splenic flexure (*C*), and right colon/cecum (*D*) incidentally noted in the right upper quadrant (*arrow*).

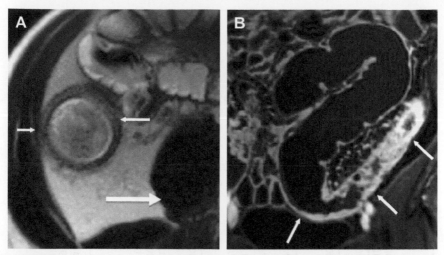

Fig. 6. Axial, T2-weighted image shows moderate wall thickening of the ascending colon with edema high signal changes (*small arrows*) relative to the psoas muscle (*large arrow*). Coronal, dark-lumen MRC after IV contrast administration showing marked enhancement of the sigmoid colon and descending colon (*arrows*) with mucosal irregularity compatible with ulcers and inflammatory pseudopolyps. (*From* Rimola J, Rodriguez S, Garcia-Bosch O, et al. Magnetic resonance for assessment of disease activity and severity in ileocolonic Crohn's disease. Gut 2009;58:1117; with permission.)

contrast and 75 seconds after contrast administration. Additional arterial (20-second) and equilibrium (180-second) phase imaging of the liver can also be considered.

MRC APPLICATIONS
Colorectal Screening: Lesion Detection Sensitivities

The reported sensitivities of MRC in detecting lesions (ie, polyps) have been variable. These studies have been performed at single institutions with technical differences that include variations in tagging protocol, cathartic preparation, magnetic field strength, and reader experience (**Table 1**). MRC sensitivities, like CTC, are dependent on lesion size. MRC is not sensitive in detecting diminutive polyps of 5 mm or less, with sensitivities at 1.5-T scanners ranging from 0% to 10.5%.[23,35,42,43] 3-T MRI scans offer faster scans with higher spatial resolutions. Saar and colleagues[10] achieved 3D resolutions of 1.6 × 1.0 × 1.5 mm^3 and reported a 50% sensitivity rate for detecting 0- to 5-mm lesions. MRC sensitivities vary from 25% to 100% for 6- to 9-mm polyps,[10,23,35,42,43] and similar to earlier CTC research, variability in protocols involving patient preparation, tagging, CT technique, and reader experience could have contributed to prior low sensitivities.[44,45] For example, Rodriguez Gomez and colleagues[23] achieved 25% sensitivity with barium tagging with air insufflation and inadequate colonic distension with severe imaging artifacts. This result led to discontinuation of this arm of the trial. Conversely, dark-lumen MRC with bowel purgation (PEG) achieved the highest sensitivities for 6- to 9-mm polyps at 84% to 100%.[10,42]

The advanced adenoma is typically defined as an adenoma measuring 10 mm or greater, having high-grade dysplasia, or having villous histology. Most would agree that colonoscopy with polypectomy is recommended when lesions 10 mm or greater are identified by VC.[46] MRC, in general, shows good sensitivities for lesions of 10 mm

Table 1
Dark-lumen MRC: MRI protocols and sensitivities compared with CC

Study (Year)	Tesla	Number of Patients	Population	Stool Tagging	Colonic Insufflation	Sensitivity[a] <6 mm	Sensitivity[a] 6–9 mm	Sensitivity[a] >10 mm	Comments
Saar et al (2008)[10]	3	34	CS, HR	None/(CP)	Water	50% (4/8)	100% (10/10)	100% (6/6)	No excluded patients
Hartmann et al (2006)[42]	1.5	100	CS, NR	None/(CP)	Water	(9%) 4/44[b] 18%[c]	78% (32/41)[b] 84%[c]	100% (22/22)	Excluded patients: claustrophobia (n = 2)/incomplete OC (n = 6)
Achiam et al (2008)[43]	1.5	56	First-time CC	B, F	Water	3.8%	71.4%	62.5%	Average performance of 2 readers. Excluded patients: vomiting (n = 2), incontinence (n = 1)
Kuehle et al (2007)[35]	1.5	315	NR	B, G, LBG	Water	10.5% 16/153[b] 37.5%[c]	57.6% 34/59[b] 84.6%[c]	73.9% 17/23[b] 81.3%[c]	Sizes ranges are <5, 5–10, >10 mm, respectively. Excluded patients: incontinence (n = 4), pain (n = 1)
Rodriguez Gomez et al (2008)[23]	1.5	54	CS, HR	B	Water	0% (0/36)	50% (6/12)	100% (8/8)	Excluded patients: poor tagging (n = 1), combined artifact and poor tagging (n = 1)
Rodriguez Gomez et al (2008)[23]	1.5	29	CS, HR	B	Air	7% (1/14)	25% (1/4)	100% (3/3)(2 CA, 1 polyp)	Excluded patients: poor tagging (n = 4), poor distension (n = 2), severe artifact (n = 4), thus remaining patients transfer to water enema

Abbreviations: B, barium; F, ferumoxsil; G, Gastrografin; LBG, locust bean gum; CS, clinical suspicion (rectal bleeding, + fecal occult blood test, altered bowel habits, abdominal pain, chronic diarrhea, cancer of unknown primary, anemia of unknown origin); HR, high risk (family history of colorectal cancer, history of polyps, previous polypectomies, ulcerative colitis); NR, normal risk; CP, cathartic preparation with PEG solution.
[a] Per polyp sensitivities.
[b] Includes hyperplastic polyps.
[c] Adenomatous polyp sensitivity (ie, disregarding hyperplastic polyps).

or greater, ranging from 81.3% to 100%.[10,35,42] As the highest sensitivities were achieved with a full cathartic preparation without stool tagging, we do not advocate stool tagging for MRC.

Hyperplastic polyps are not easily detectable by MRC.[10,42] Decreased sensitivity for hyperplastic polyps compared with adenomatous polyps has also been described with CTC.[47] Hyperplastic polyps tend to be smaller than adenomatous polyps and efface with air insufflation as described with VC and CC.[47,48] In addition, Hartmann and colleagues[42] also attribute the lack of hyperenhancement resulting from the similar vascular architecture of hyperplastic polyps with normal colonic mucosa as a possible cause of decreased sensitivity. Hyperplastic polyps have traditionally been believed to be benign; however, there is recent controversy regarding their clinical management and significance, especially of right colonic lesions.[49]

Inflammatory Bowel Disease

The absence of ionizing radiation with MRC is particularly appealing in chronic diseases like IBD, especially in the pediatric and young adult populations, in whom sensitivity to ionizing radiation is greater.[50] As opposed to CC, which is limited only to mucosal evaluation, MRC has the advantage of evaluating transmural and extraluminal disease (eg, fistula and abscess formation) as seen with CD. MR findings for CD include bowel wall thickening, wall edema, hyperenhancement after IV contrast administration (see **Fig. 6**), ulcerations, strictures, fistulas, phlegmons, abscesses, vascular engorgement, fibro-fatty proliferation, and enhancing mesenteric lymph nodes.[21,50–53]

There are few studies evaluating the performance of MRC in IBD, but the preliminary research is promising, with MRC able to detect active and relevant disease. For example, Rimola and colleagues[51] used combined MRC with MR enterography (MRE) to develop a method to correlate MR findings with CD activity. In a prospective study 50 patients with CD were investigated with dark-lumen MRC with additional ingestion of 1500 mL of PEG solution 45 minutes before scanning for small bowel evaluation. Ileocolonoscopy was the reference and MR findings of bowel wall thickness, bowel wall edema, relative contrast enhancement, and presence of ulcers (**Fig. 7**) were identified as independent predictors for disease activity as defined by the Crohn's Disease Endoscopic Index of Severity (CDEIS). Using these MR findings, the investigators derived a Magnetic Resonance Index of Activity (MRIA) to quantify segmental disease activity and achieved high accuracy for detecting active disease (receiver-operating characteristic [ROC] 0.891, sensitivity 0.81, and specificity 0.89) and ulcers (ROC 0.978, sensitivity 0.95, and specificity 0.91). These investigators also assessed global disease activity by summing each anatomic segmental (5 colonic segments and ileum) score. This assessment showed a significant correlation with CDEIS ($r = 0.78$, $P<.001$) (**Fig. 8**). Another dedicated dark-lumen MRC study of patients with UC and CD using scoring criteria that evaluated colonic wall enhancement, bowel wall thickening, lymph node number, and loss of haustral folds (**Fig. 9**) achieved sensitivity and specificity rates of 87% and 100%, respectively, for active disease using CC with histopathologic evaluation as the reference.[54]

As with MRC for colorectal cancer screening, eliminating cathartic preparation would be preferable for IBD evaluation but reduced inflammatory disease detection is a concern. Langhorst and colleagues[34] performed dark-lumen MRC with fecal tagging in 29 patients with IBD (17 with UC; 12 with CD) and compared findings with colonoscopy and biopsy. Analysis on a colonic segment basis showed a specificity rate of 88% but a poor sensitivity rate of 32%. Ergen and colleagues[55] studied a population with IBD (5 with CD, 6 with UC, 11 suspected IBD) with dark-lumen

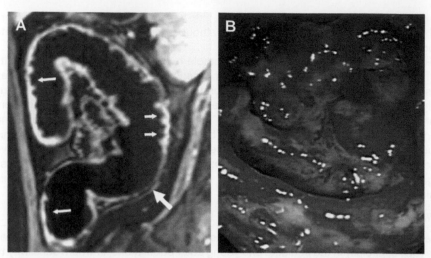

Fig. 7. Sagittal dark-lumen MRC (*A*) after IV contrast administration shows discontinuous lesions with segmental thickening of the colon wall and deep ulcers (*small arrows*) alternating with a segment without inflammatory changes (*large arrow*). Colonoscopy (*B*) shows the deep mucosal ulcers. (*From* Rimola J, Rodriguez S, Garcia-Bosch O, et al. Magnetic resonance for assessment of disease activity and severity in ileocolonic Crohn's disease. Gut 2009;58:1118; with permission.)

MRC and investigated bowel wall thickness/bowel distension ratios, signal intensity ratios before and after contrast administration, and vasa recta diameters. These investigators compared findings with endoscopic impressions of inflammation (without histopathology confirmation), and achieved sensitivity and specificity rates of 63%

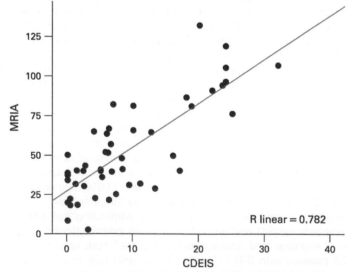

Fig. 8. Correlation between the CDEIS and the global MRIA. (*From* Rimola J, Rodriguez S, Garcia-Bosch O, et al. Magnetic resonance for assessment of disease activity and severity in ileocolonic Crohn's disease. Gut 2009;58:1119; with permission.)

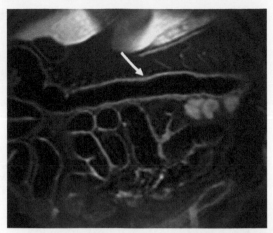

Fig. 9. Dark-lumen MRC showing loss of haustral folds with bowel wall thickening and increased contrast enhancement (*arrow*). Active moderate inflammation identified on subsequent endoscopy and biopsy. (*From* Ajaj W, Goyen M. MR imaging of the colon: technique, indications, results and limitations. Eur J Radiol 2007;61:418; with permission.)

and 80%, respectively. Although all subjects underwent a water enema, most of their subjects had fecal tagging (n = 16) compared with bowel purgation (n = 6).[55] Dinter and colleagues[56] performed MR examinations in patients with CD with only an enterography protocol without colonic catharsis and distension (ie, tap-water enema). Ileocolonic disease sensitivity and specificity rates compared with endoscopy were 64.4% and 81.1%, respectively.

MRC has also been used in patients with IBD who have undergone prior surgery. Specifically, in patients with CD who have undergone partial colonic resection, recurrent disease is common at the site of anastomosis.[57,58] In a small sample, MRC has been successful in detecting inflammation in patients with IBD who underwent end-to-end colonic anastomoses; MRC detected 9 of 11 cases of inflammation at the anastomosis (7 with CD and 2 with UC), missing 2 cases of mild inflammation.[21]

Incomplete Colonoscopies

Incomplete colonoscopies are not uncommon, occurring in 5% to 13% of examinations.[59–61] The most common causes are from colonic elongation, patient discomfort, stenosis (tumor or inflammatory), and endoscopist inexperience.[11,24,62,63] In patients with an obstructing colon cancer (**Fig. 10**) and incomplete CC, MRC can evaluate the primary tumor, the remaining colon for synchronous lesions (polyps, carcinoma), and for extracolonic disease (adenopathy and hepatic metastasis).[24,63–65] Identification of synchronous tumor requires extending the planned colonic resection, whereas simultaneous metastectomy may be considered if unsuspected metastatic disease is identified preoperatively.[21,24,65,66] Ajaj and colleagues[65] studied 37 patients with incomplete colonoscopies with MRC, and was able to evaluate 35 of them adequately. A total of 206 of 214 (96%) potential colonic segments were assessed. In comparison, CC failed in 127 segments (success of 40%) because of high-grade tumor stenosis (n = 12), high-grade inflammatory stenoses (n = 9), and colonic elongation and/or patient discomfort (n = 16). Prestenotic MRC evaluation identified 5 polyps (8–12 mm), colitis in 3 patients, and 2 suspicious synchronous carcinomas;

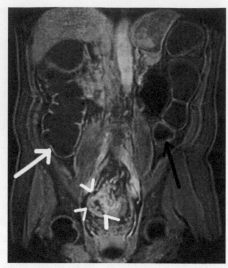

Fig. 10. Postcontrast, dark-lumen MRC showing obstructing lesion (*arrowheads*) with moderate (*black arrow*) and excellent (*white arrow*) distension of the sigmoid and cecum, respectively. (*From* Achiam MP, Andersen LPH, Klein M, et al. Differentiation between benign and malignant colon tumors using fast dynamic gadolinium-enhanced MR colonography; a feasibility study. Eur J Radiol 2009. doi:10.1016/j.ejrad.2009.03.033. p. 3; with permission.)

extracolonic findings included hepatic metastases in 3 patients. Another study by Wong and colleagues[24] investigated 51 patients with incomplete colonoscopies, and successfully performed air dark-lumen MRC without fecal tagging in all but 1 patient. Forty-four patients had obstructing tumors, in 2 of whom synchronous tumors were successfully identified in prestenotic segments with MRC. The remaining patients had incomplete CC as a result of excessive colonic elongation, and MRC identified 2 colonic tumors in the endoscopically inaccessible segments. [24]

OTHER USES OF MRC

MR evaluation of the colon has been applied in other situations. MRC was able to diagnose recurrent tumor at the site of colonic anastomosis (sizes of 17 and 22 mm) in patients with history of colorectal carcinoma status after end-to-end anastomosis.[21] Functional evaluation of the colon has been attempted with cine, real-time MRI.[67] Although not technically considered a classic MRC examination, small field of view MR imaging of the colon, specifically of the anorectal region, has also been used for preoperative rectal cancer staging[68] and perianal fistula evaluation for CD.[69]

MR ENTEROGRAPHY

Inflammatory bowel disease, small bowel tumors, gastrointestinal bleeding, and small bowel obstruction are just some of the major indications for small bowel imaging. Most patients referred for small bowel imaging are those with IBD, especially CD. Given the serious implications of the disease and its treatment, accurate diagnosis and close monitoring are important.[70,71] Small bowel imaging, because of anatomic and functional considerations, is challenging.[72] The small bowel is long, loops overlap, and motility is variable. For years, the only widely available technique was fluoroscopic examination with small bowel follow-through (SBFT) or conventional enteroclysis (CE). Yet, conventional fluoroscopic studies have a sensitivity of between 23% and 83% for the detection of CD.[73–75] The desire to improve small bowel visualization has led to technologic advances including ileocolonoscopy, wireless capsule endoscopy, and double-balloon and push enteroscopy. It is also increasingly recognized that cross-sectional techniques such as CT and MRE are complementary to these other examinations.[71,75] Whereas endoscopic methods assess the mucosa, cross-sectional techniques can evaluate the superficial and deep bowel wall, detect disease outside the range of the instrument, as well as evaluate extraintestinal structures.[75,76] Abnormalities detectable by MR include wall thickening, ulcerations, cobblestoning, fissures, stenoses, hyperenhancement, mesenteric hypervascularity, bowel wall edema, mesenteric inflammation, lymphadenopathy, fibrofatty proliferation (creeping fat) **(Fig. 11)**, as well as complications including sinus tracts, fistula, abscesses, and obstruction.[5,72] These examinations have evolved to be the standard of care in any state-of-the-art practice.

As mentioned earlier, increasing awareness of radiation exposure,[77] especially for younger patients with IBD who often undergo repeated examinations, has contributed to an interest in MR small bowel imaging. Improvements in temporal

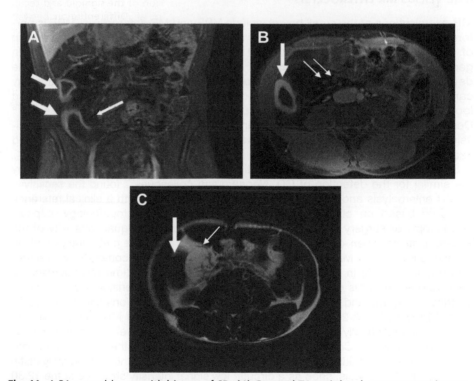

Fig. 11. A 31-year-old man with history of CD. (*A*) Coronal T1-weighted, postcontrast image shows abnormal wall thickening and hyperenhancement of the distal ileum (*large arrows*) with prominent mesenteric vessels (*small arrow*): the comb sign. (*B*). Axial T1-weighted post-IV contrast image shows wall thickening with hyperenhancement (*large arrow*), as well as mesenteric lymphadenopathy (*small arrows*). (*C*). Axial fat-sensitive image shows abundant high signal fibrofatty proliferation (*small arrow*) adjacent to the terminal ileum (*large arrow*).

and spatial resolution, improved bowel distending agents, superior soft tissue contrast, as well as multiplaner imaging capabilities have made MR increasingly desirable.[5,76,78,79] Furthermore, cine-MRI allows for functional evaluation of small bowel motility. Although CE has better spatial resolution than MRI and is better able to detect mild mucosal changes,[72,80–82] this difference is unlikely to be clinically relevant in practice.[83] MRI is preferable, largely because of the invaluable information it provides on the state of the entire bowel wall, as well as extraintestinal pathology.[72,76,84] In a recent retrospective analysis of more than 1000 cases at a single institution, 35% of MRE cases reported extraenteric findings that were classified as either highly or moderately significant, including abscesses, and extraintestinal tumors, metastases, or masses.[85] A recent prospective study using 2 independent readers that compared the accuracy of CT and MRE and SBFT for the detection of active CD showed that the 3 examinations had similar sensitivities for the detection of terminal ileal inflammation. However, CT and MRE had superior sensitivity for the detection of extraenteric complications (100% for CT and MR in both readers compared with 32% and 37% for SBFT in reader 1 and reader 2, respectively).[86]

MRE VERSUS MR ENTEROCLYSIS

MR examinations of the small bowel include MRE and MR enteroclysis. MRE is performed after the oral ingestion of enteric contrast. Enteroclysis entails administration of enteric contrast via a nasoduodenal or nasojejunal tube followed by MRI.[87] In general, MR enteroclysis is capable of superior luminal distention, critical for the detection of subtle lesions and morphologic changes. Similar to MRC, pathology can be obscured and missed in collapsed bowel. In addition, inadequately distended loops can show pseudothickening or pseudoenhancement, mimicking disease.[78] Despite the superior luminal distention and improved mucosal detail of MR enteroclysis compared with MRE,[88] controversy persists about which is the preferred examination.

Some studies have shown that sensitivities of MR enteroclysis and enterography are similar for the detection of CD. Negaard and colleagues[89] found the sensitivity of MR enteroclysis and enterography were 88% compared with a clinical reference standard based on clinical assessment, ileoscopy with histopathology, capsule endoscopy, or surgery. Schreyer and colleagues[80] showed equal sensitivity of the 2 examinations when compared with CE. However, a recent meta-analysis of 33 studies showed that MR enteroclysis had superior sensitivity compared with enterography ($P = .046$) in the evaluation of an IBD.[90] With real-time MR fluoroscopy, MRE and enteroclysis can provide information regarding distensibility of a stenosis so that high-grade and low-grade partial small bowel obstructions can be differentiated (Movie 1).[78,91] A 2008 study determined the sensitivity of MR enteroclysis and MRE to be statistically equivalent (100% and 89%, respectively) for the diagnosis of stenosis (Movie 1: Coronal single fast spin echo (SSFSE) of the abdomen demonstrates a hyperperistaltic loop of ileum in the right lower quadrant. Immediately distal is a high-grade stenosis, seen as a circular low signal intensity structure at the 12:30 clock position relative to the hyperperistaltic loop. This is a fibrotic stricture due to Crohn's disease.*) in patients with CD.[88] Drawbacks of MR enteroclysis include patient discomfort from nasoenteric intubation,[80] longer examination times, inconvenience in coordination of fluoroscopy and MRI, and cost.[71] Many prefer enterography for these reasons. The decision to perform one examination rather than another depends on the institution and the referring physician. Some perform MR enteroclysis as a first-line modality.[76] Others perform enterography for routine examinations and reserve enteroclysis for select cases such as low-grade small bowel obstruction.[89]

TECHNIQUE
Intraluminal Contrast Agents

Suboptimal small bowel distention at MR may be caused by several different factors. Fluid absorption along the length of small bowel, poor timing between contrast ingestion and scan acquisition, delayed gastric emptying, and insufficient volume of contrast ingestion by the patient can all be contributory. For these reasons, a variety of agents have been investigated with varying ingestion protocols.[92–96] These enteric contrast agents typically contain iso- or hyperosmolar ingredients to reduce fluid absorption or even draw fluid into the small bowel lumen.[94] With respect to MRI, 3 basic classes of agents are available: positive, negative, and biphasic. Positive contrast agents are high signal on T1- and T2-weighted sequences. Negative contrast agents, analogous to dark-lumen MRC, are low signal intensity on T1- and T2-weighted images. Biphasic agents are high signal intensity on one sequence and low signal intensity on the opposite.[5]

The most commonly used agents are biphasic, and most are high signal on T2-weighted sequences and low signal on T1-weighted sequences (**Fig. 12**). On T1-weighted images the low intraluminal signal intensity accentuates the contrast with an abnormally enhancing wall (**Fig. 13**A). High T2 intraluminal signal is helpful to visualize mural ulceration (**Fig. 13**B) as well as fistulas.[91] Water is one of several biphasic options, but its rapid absorption through the bowel mucosa bowel frequently results in suboptimal distention.[97] In a direct comparison of water with a low concentration barium (LCB) suspension (0.1% w/v) (VoLumen, E-Z-EM Inc, Lake Success, NY, USA), methylcellulose, and PEG, PEG and LCB produced the best bowel distention.[96] PEG was least preferred because of its taste and side effects, which include nausea, vomiting, and diarrhea. Methylcellulose, although as well tolerated as water, offered inferior distention compared with LCB.

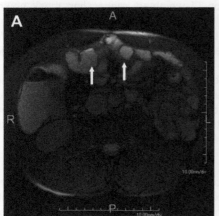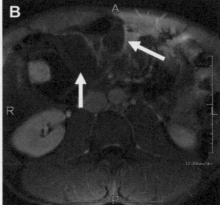

Fig. 12. MRE of the abdomen performed in a patient with CD who ingested LCB before the examination. (A) Axial T2-weighted sequence with fat saturation shows high intraluminal signal (*arrows*). (B) Axial T1-weighted image in the same patient shows low intraluminal signal.

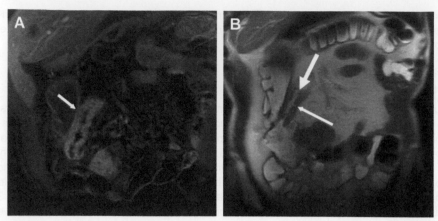

Fig. 13. Stricture in the neoterminal ileum in a 64-year-old patient with CD and prior ileal resection with ileocolonic anastomosis. Patient had recurrence of diarrheal symptoms. Coronal T1-weighted image (*A*) obtained 4 minutes after IV contrast administration shows abnormal enhancement of the irregularly thickened bowel wall (*arrow*). An additional area of inflammation is seen inferomedially. (*B*) Coronal T2-weighted image of the abdomen shows a short segment stenosis of the thickened neoterminal ileum (*large arrow*). Signal intensity is slightly increased when compared with the normal small bowel wall. A deep ulceration is identified (*small arrow*). This segment did not peristalse on MR fluoroscopy (See Movie 1).

The only commercially available negative contrast agent in the United States is a ferumoxsil oral suspension (GastroMark, Mallinckrodt Inc, St Louis, MO, USA). Because this reduces the signal intensity in the bowel lumen on T2-weighted images, contrast between low-intensity luminal contents and high signal bowel wall edema is accentuated.[5] As a result, other fluid-filled structures, such as abscesses, are more conspicuous. However, susceptibility artifacts, as mentioned earlier with MRC, are a drawback.

Positive contrast agents such as Gd are not so popular as biphasic and negative agents, mostly because a bright lumen on T1-weighted images can mask bowel wall enhancement.[5]

At our institution patients drink 1.35 L of LCB 1.5 hours before the examination. We do not administer water routinely as patients have difficulty ingesting such a large volume of liquid.

Rectal water enemas can be administered at the time of small bowel evaluation, and may improve visualization of the terminal ileum compared with oral contrast alone. It has been suggested that rectal enema in small bowel MRI be considered.[98] As mentioned earlier, an added benefit is the potential to simultaneously evaluate the colon with a combined MRC examination. We, however, do not administer rectal contrast.

Patient Positioning

MRI may be performed in either the supine or the prone position. Most centers perform the examination in the supine position, a more comfortable orientation for the patient, especially considering the potential length of the examination.[99] Some have advocated the prone position because of the benefits of abdominal autocompression. A decreased anteroposterior diameter can potentially improve separation of small bowel loops, allowing better mural visualization, as well as permitting fewer coronal acquisitions to be necessary.[78,88] A recent study showed that prone positioning improved small bowel distention, although no improvement in diagnostic performance was achieved.[99] We acquire images in the supine position only.

Antiperistaltics

Hyoscine-N-butylbromide (Buscopan, Boehringer Ingelheim Pharmaceuticals, Ingelheim, Germany) or glucagon can be administered to reduce peristalsis in an attempt to reduce motion artifacts.[78,79] We administer 1 mg of glucagon via a slow IV drip (rapid injection can cause nausea and vomiting) immediately before IV contrast administration. It is given near the end of the examination not only because of its short half-life but also because reduction of peristalsis may confound evaluation of small bowel motility when dynamic, cine-MRI evaluation is performed.

Pulse Sequences

A variety of pulse sequences have been used in the performance of MRE. In general, a premium is placed on methods that have high speed to freeze out bowel motion and produce sharp images, as well as to keep examination time to a minimum. After obtaining images to localize the position of the bowel, coronal cine-MR (fluoroscopic) images are obtained to visualize bowel peristalsis. Next, stacks of rapid 2D fluid sensitive sequences are obtained in axial and coronal planes. At that point, 1 mg of glucagon is administered intravenously. Then IV contrast is administered followed by volumetric (ie, 3D) acquisition designed to detect regions of increased IV contrast uptake. These images can then be reformatted in any plane for analysis after the patient has left the MRI suite.

For enteroclysis, a nasojejunal tube is placed under fluoroscopy, and the patient is taken to the MR scanner. The infusion of contrast is performed while the patient is supine. Baseline scans are performed before beginning the infusion. Filling can be monitored every 2 minutes until contrast fills the ileum. At this point multiplaner sequences are obtained. When contrast reaches the colon, glucagon and then IV contrast are administered.

IV Contrast

IV contrast administration is crucial to identify active wall inflammation.[100,101] Loops of inflamed bowel enhance more avidly than unaffected loops. With IV contrast, MRI can also help differentiate inflammatory from fibrostenotic strictures.[91] With both of these types of strictures, bowel wall thickening can be observed. However, a finding of preserved mural stratification with enhancing mucosa, low-intensity submucosa, and enhancing muscularis and serosa on IV contrast-enhanced MRI can indicate potential reversibility. Mural stratification is lost in long-standing disease if transmural fibrosis has occurred. Sinus tracts and fistulas, as well as abscesses, are made more discernible by rim enhancement.[91] Peak bowel wall enhancement occurs in normal patients at approximately 60 to 70 seconds.[102] However, peak enhancement in CD has been shown to vary,[103] and this unpredictability necessitates multiphasic post-contrast acquisitions.[5] We typically obtain 3 to 4 phases after contrast administration.

MRE for the Diagnosis of CD

MRI has excellent sensitivity for the diagnosis of CD.[71,78,81,84,87] A recent, blinded, prospective study assessing the accuracy of MRE for detecting small bowel CD compared MRE with CT enterography (CTE) and a clinical reference standard. Although image quality was higher for CTE, the sensitivities of the 2 were similar (both more than 90%). Both provided information which was complementary to that gained at ileocolonoscopy with biopsy. For example, 24% of the patients who were ultimately diagnosed as having active small bowel inflammation had normal appearing mucosa ileocolonoscopically but abnormal CT and MR findings.[71]

MRI has also been shown to provide more than just anatomic information; it also correlates with pathologic findings. A recent retrospective study of 55 patients with CD reported that patients with imaging findings of segmental hyperenhancement and mild wall thickening on MRI were more likely to respond to medical therapy than patients with luminal narrowing and functional obstruction. Of the 17 patients who underwent surgery, pathologic findings of fibrosis and the severity of inflammation correlated well with MRI findings. The investigators suggest that MRE may be of prognostic use in CD patients.[104]

New Techniques

Higher field strength 3T magnets are more commonly used for neuroradiology and musculoskeletal imaging but protocols are evolving for abdominal/pelvic applications. They offer improved spatial and temporal resolution,[72] but at the cost of increased air-related artifacts. Diffusion-weighted imaging is currently being investigated, and was recently shown to be feasible in identifying inflammation in a small trial of patients with CD.[105]

Certain mural hemodynamic parameters derived from dynamic contrast-enhanced MRI can be quantified, and have been shown to correlate with disease chronicity and angiogenesis in patients with CD. These parameters could be a valuable adjunct to clinical and histologic markers of inflammation.[106] Quantitative assessment of bowel wall contrast agent concentration has also been shown to be feasible using T1 mapping and calculation of Gd values in CD. These values correlate positively with more active disease.[107]

MRC AND MRE CONCLUSION

In light of the recent decision by the Centers for Medicare and Medicaid Services not to reimburse CTC for asymptomatic colorectal cancer screening,[108] MRC as the other method to perform VC is far from consideration as a wide spread screening modality. Similar to CTC, an optimized protocol (eg, tagging, field strength) must be designed with subsequent validation through a prospective multicenter trial. In addition, minimizing cost and increasing patient compliance to show economic feasibility by cost-effectiveness analysis are also necessary.

Minimizing scan time is necessary to reduce cost, and an optimized MRC protocol can be performed in 12 to 15 minutes, with a total of 30 minutes of MRI suite time.[40] Because no postprocedure monitoring is necessary compared with CC when sedation is used, MRC has the potential to be a highly time-efficient screening modality. However, as with CTC, 1 of the main disadvantages of MRC is the lack of tissue sampling and treatment options compared with CC in which biopsy and polypectomy can be performed. Reduced or even elimination of a cathartic preparation with improved accuracy rates by stool tagging are current goals of MRC research.

The clear advantage of MRI of the colon and small bowel, MRC and MRE is the ability to examine the colon and small bowel noninvasively without exposure to ionizing radiation. This advantage is particularly appealing in pediatric and young adult populations with inflammatory bowel disease in whom a decrease in the cumulative radiation dose from multiple CT or fluoroscopic examinations is highly desirable. The potential of evaluating bowel function and motility through dynamic, cine-MRI is useful in the identification and evaluation of IBD stenoses and bowel obstructions. The role of MRC and MRE in the management of patients with IBD is still evolving but clear strengths of these techniques compared with endoscopic evaluations include the ability to evaluate transmural and extraluminal disease. In addition, preliminary studies of MRI for noninvasively identifying active disease and inflammation in IBD are promising.

ACKNOWLEDGMENTS

Special thanks to Shreyas Vasanawala for his assistance in editing.

REFERENCES

1. Jemal A, Siegel R, Ward E, et al. Cancer statistics, 2009. CA Cancer J Clin 2009; 59:225–49.
2. Johnson CD, Chen MH, Toledano AY, et al. Accuracy of CT colonography for detection of large adenomas and cancers. N Engl J Med 2008;359:1207.
3. Kim DH, Pickhardt PJ, Taylor AJ, et al. CT colonography versus colonoscopy for the detection of advanced neoplasia. N Engl J Med 2007;357:1403.
4. Pickhardt PJ, Choi JR, Hwang I, et al. Computed tomographic virtual colonoscopy to screen for colorectal neoplasia in asymptomatic adults. N Engl J Med 2003;349:2191.
5. Siddiki H, Fidler J. MR imaging of the small bowel in Crohn's disease. Eur J Radiol 2009;69:409.
6. Sodickson A, Baeyens PF, Andriole KP, et al. Recurrent CT, cumulative radiation exposure, and associated radiation-induced cancer risks from CT of adults. Radiology 2009;251:175.
7. Griffey RT, Sodickson A. Cumulative radiation exposure and cancer risk estimates in emergency department patients undergoing repeat or multiple CT. AJR Am J Roentgenol 2009;192:887.
8. Huang B, Law MW, Khong PL. Whole-body PET/CT scanning: estimation of radiation dose and cancer risk. Radiology 2009;251:166.
9. Morrin MM, Pedrosa I, McKenzie CA, et al. Parallel imaging enhanced MR colonography using a phantom model. J Magn Reson Imaging 2008;28: 664.
10. Saar B, Gschossmann JM, Bonel HM, et al. Evaluation of magnetic resonance colonography at 3.0 Tesla regarding diagnostic accuracy and image quality. Invest Radiol 2008;43:580.
11. Rimola J, Rodriguez S, Garcia-Bosch O, et al. Role of 3.0-T MR colonography in the evaluation of inflammatory bowel disease. Radiographics 2009;29:701.
12. Lauenstein TC, Saar B, Martin DR. MR colonography: 1.5T versus 3T. Magn Reson Imaging Clin N Am 2007;15:395.
13. Luboldt W, Bauerfeind P, Steiner P, et al. Preliminary assessment of three-dimensional magnetic resonance imaging for various colonic disorders. Lancet 1997; 349:1288.
14. Ajaj W, Pelster G, Treichel U, et al. Dark lumen magnetic resonance colonography: comparison with conventional colonoscopy for the detection of colorectal pathology. Gut 2003;52:1738.
15. Schreyer AG, Scheibl K, Heiss P, et al. MR colonography in inflammatory bowel disease. Abdom Imaging 2006;31:302.
16. Morrin MM, Hochman MG, Farrell RJ, et al. MR colonography using colonic distention with air as the contrast material: work in progress. AJR Am J Roentgenol 2001;176:144.

17. Saar B, Heverhagen JT, Obst T, et al. Magnetic resonance colonography and virtual magnetic resonance colonoscopy with the 1.0-T system: a feasibility study. Invest Radiol 2000;35:521.

18. Zhang S, Peng JW, Shi QY, et al. Colorectal neoplasm: magnetic resonance colonography with fat enema–initial clinical experience. World J Gastroenterol 2007;13:5371.

19. Hagspiel KD, Altes TA, Mugler JP 3rd, et al. MR virtual colonography using hyperpolarized (3)He as an endoluminal contrast agent: demonstration of feasibility. Magn Reson Med 2000;44:813.

20. Florie J, Birnie E, van Gelder RE, et al. MR colonography with limited bowel preparation: patient acceptance compared with that of full-preparation colonoscopy. Radiology 2007;245:150.

21. Ajaj W, Goyen M, Langhorst J, et al. MR colonography for the assessment of colonic anastomoses. J Magn Reson Imaging 2006;24:101.

22. Kinner S, Kuehle CA, Langhorst J, et al. MR colonography vs. optical colonoscopy: comparison of patients' acceptance in a screening population. Eur Radiol 2007;17:2286.

23. Rodriguez Gomez S, Pages Llinas M, Castells Garangou A, et al. Dark-lumen MR colonography with fecal tagging: a comparison of water enema and air methods of colonic distension for detecting colonic neoplasms. Eur Radiol 2008;18:1396.

24. Wong TY, Lam WW, So NM, et al. Air-inflated magnetic resonance colonography in patients with incomplete conventional colonoscopy: comparison with intraoperative findings, pathology specimens, and follow-up conventional colonoscopy. Am J Gastroenterol 2007;102:56.

25. Lomas DJ, Sood RR, Graves MJ, et al. Colon carcinoma: MR imaging with CO_2 enema–pilot study. Radiology 2001;219:558.

26. Ajaj W, Lauenstein TC, Pelster G, et al. MR colonography: how does air compare to water for colonic distention? J Magn Reson Imaging 2004;19:216.

27. Lauenstein TC, Goehde SC, Debatin JF. Fecal tagging: MR colonography without colonic cleansing. Abdom Imaging 2002;27:410.

28. Luboldt W, Bauerfeind P, Wildermuth S, et al. Colonic masses: detection with MR colonography. Radiology 2000;216:383.

29. Knopp MV, Giesel FL, Radeleff J, et al. Bile-tagged 3d magnetic resonance colonography after exclusive intravenous administration of gadobenate dimeglumine, a contrast agent with partial hepatobiliary excretion. Invest Radiol 2001; 36:619.

30. Lauenstein T, Holtmann G, Schoenfelder D, et al. MR colonography without colonic cleansing: a new strategy to improve patient acceptance. AJR Am J Roentgenol 2001;177:823.

31. Kinner S, Lauenstein TC. MR colonography. Radiol Clin North Am 2007;45:377.

32. Weinreb JC, Kuo PH. Nephrogenic systemic fibrosis. Magn Reson Imaging Clin N Am 2009;17:159.

33. Lauenstein TC, Goehde SC, Ruehm SG, et al. MR colonography with barium-based fecal tagging: initial clinical experience. Radiology 2002;223:248.

34. Langhorst J, Kuhle CA, Ajaj W, et al. MR colonography without bowel purgation for the assessment of inflammatory bowel diseases: diagnostic accuracy and patient acceptance. Inflamm Bowel Dis 2007;13:1001.

35. Kuehle CA, Langhorst J, Ladd SC, et al. Magnetic resonance colonography without bowel cleansing: a prospective cross sectional study in a screening population. Gut 2007;56:1079.

36. Weishaupt D, Patak MA, Froehlich J, et al. Faecal tagging to avoid colonic cleansing before MRI colonography. Lancet 1999;354:835.
37. Achiam MP, Chabanova E, Logager VB, et al. MR colonography with fecal tagging: barium vs. barium ferumoxsil. Acad Radiol 2008;15:576.
38. Savoye-Collet C, Thoumas D, Savoye G, et al. Colonic transit time and MR colonography. AJR Am J Roentgenol 2002;179:435.
39. Goehde SC, Descher E, Boekstegers A, et al. Dark lumen MR colonography based on fecal tagging for detection of colorectal masses: accuracy and patient acceptance. Abdom Imaging 2005;30:576.
40. Achiam MP, Chabanova E, Logager V, et al. Implementation of MR colonography. Abdom Imaging 2007;32:457.
41. Achiam MP, Logager V, Chabanova E, et al. Patient acceptance of MR colonography with improved fecal tagging versus conventional colonoscopy. Eur J Radiol 2010;73:143-7.
42. Hartmann D, Bassler B, Schilling D, et al. Colorectal polyps: detection with dark-lumen MR colonography versus conventional colonoscopy. Radiology 2006; 238:143.
43. Achiam MP, Logager VB, Chabanova E, et al. Diagnostic accuracy of MR colonography with fecal tagging. Abdom Imaging 2009;34:483-90.
44. Rockey DC, Paulson E, Niedzwiecki D, et al. Analysis of air contrast barium enema, computed tomographic colonography, and colonoscopy: prospective comparison. Lancet 2005;365:305.
45. Cotton PB, Durkalski VL, Pineau BC, et al. Computed tomographic colonography (virtual colonoscopy): a multicenter comparison with standard colonoscopy for detection of colorectal neoplasia. JAMA 2004;291:1713.
46. van Dam J, Cotton P, Johnson CD, et al. AGA future trends report: CT colonography. Gastroenterology 2004;127:970.
47. Fenlon HM, Nunes DP, Schroy PC 3rd, et al. A comparison of virtual and conventional colonoscopy for the detection of colorectal polyps. N Engl J Med 1999; 341:1496.
48. Bertoni G, Sassatelli R, Conigliaro R, et al. Visual "disappearing phenomenon" can reliably predict the nonadenomatous nature of rectal and rectosigmoid diminutive polyps at endoscopy. Gastrointest Endosc 1994;40:588.
49. O'Brien MJ. Hyperplastic and serrated polyps of the colorectum. Gastroenterol Clin North Am 2007;36:947.
50. Paolantonio P, Ferrari R, Vecchietti F, et al. Current status of MR imaging in the evaluation of IBD in a pediatric population of patients. Eur J Radiol 2009;69:418.
51. Rimola J, Rodriguez S, Garcia-Bosch O, et al. Magnetic resonance for assessment of disease activity and severity in ileocolonic Crohn's disease. Gut 2009; 58:1113.
52. Gourtsoyianni S, Papanikolaou N, Amanakis E, et al. Crohn's disease lymphadenopathy: MR imaging findings. Eur J Radiol 2009;69:425.
53. Rottgen R, Herzog H, Lopez-Haninnen E, et al. Bowel wall enhancement in magnetic resonance colonography for assessing activity in Crohn's disease. Clin Imaging 2006;30:27.
54. Ajaj WM, Lauenstein TC, Pelster G, et al. Magnetic resonance colonography for the detection of inflammatory diseases of the large bowel: quantifying the inflammatory activity. Gut 2005;54:257.
55. Ergen FB, Akata D, Hayran M, et al. Magnetic resonance colonography for the evaluation of colonic inflammatory bowel disease: correlation with conventional colonoscopy. J Comput Assist Tomogr 2008;32:848.

56. Dinter DJ, Chakraborty A, Brade J, et al. Endoscopy and magnetic resonance imaging in patients with Crohn's disease: a retrospective single-centre comparative study. Scand J Gastroenterol 2008;43:207.

57. Hashemi M, Novell JR, Lewis AA. Side-to-side stapled anastomosis may delay recurrence in Crohn's disease. Dis Colon Rectum 1998;41:1293.

58. Tersigni R, Alessandroni L, Barreca M, et al. Does stapled functional end-to-end anastomosis affect recurrence of Crohn's disease after ileocolonic resection? Hepatogastroenterology 2003;50:1422.

59. Shah HA, Paszat LF, Saskin R, et al. Factors associated with incomplete colonoscopy: a population-based study. Gastroenterology 2007;132:2297.

60. Anderson JC, Gonzalez JD, Messina CR, et al. Factors that predict incomplete colonoscopy: thinner is not always better. Am J Gastroenterol 2000;95:2784.

61. Marshall JB, Barthel JS. The frequency of total colonoscopy and terminal ileal intubation in the 1990s. Gastrointest Endosc 1993;39:518.

62. Dafnis G, Granath F, Pahlman L, et al. The impact of endoscopists' experience and learning curves and interendoscopist variation on colonoscopy completion rates. Endoscopy 2001;33:511.

63. Hartmann D, Bassler B, Schilling D, et al. Incomplete conventional colonoscopy: magnetic resonance colonography in the evaluation of the proximal colon. Endoscopy 2005;37:816.

64. Meier C, Wildermuth S. Feasibility and potential of MR-colonography for evaluating colorectal cancer. Swiss Surg 2002;8:21.

65. Ajaj W, Lauenstein TC, Pelster G, et al. MR colonography in patients with incomplete conventional colonoscopy. Radiology 2005;234:452.

66. Abdalla EK, Vauthey JN, Ellis LM, et al. Recurrence and outcomes following hepatic resection, radiofrequency ablation, and combined resection/ablation for colorectal liver metastases. Ann Surg 2004;239:818.

67. Buhmann S, Kirchhoff C, Wielage C, et al. [Visualization and quantification of large bowel motility with functional cine-MRI]. Rofo 2005;177:35 [in German].

68. Taylor FG, Swift RI, Blomqvist L, et al. A systematic approach to the interpretation of preoperative staging MRI for rectal cancer. AJR Am J Roentgenol 2008;191:1827.

69. Szurowska E, Wypych J, Izycka-Swieszewska E. Perianal fistulas in Crohn's disease: MRI diagnosis and surgical planning: MRI in fistulazing perianal Crohn's disease. Abdom Imaging 2007. [Epub ahead of print].

70. Gourtsoyiannis N, Papanikolaou N, Grammatikakis J, et al. Assessment of Crohn's disease activity in the small bowel with MR and conventional enteroclysis: preliminary results. Eur Radiol 2004;14:1017.

71. Siddiki HA, Fidler JL, Fletcher JG, et al. Prospective comparison of state-of-the-Art MR enterography and CT enterography in small-bowel Crohn's disease. Am J Roentgenol 2009;193:113.

72. Frøkjaer JB, Larsen E, Steffensen E, et al. Magnetic resonance imaging of the small bowel in Crohn's disease. Scand J Gastroenterol 2005;40:832.

73. Marmo R, Rotondano G, Piscopo R, et al. Capsule endoscopy versus enteroclysis in the detection of small-bowel involvement in Crohn's disease: a prospective trial. Clin Gastroenterol Hepatol 2005;3:772.

74. Triester SL, Leighton JA, Leontiadis GI, et al. A meta-analysis of the yield of capsule endoscopy compared to other diagnostic modalities in patients with non-stricturing small bowel Cohn's disease. Am J Gastroenterol 2006;101:954.

75. Solem CA, Loftus EV Jr, Fletcher JG, et al. Small-bowel imaging in Crohn's disease: a prospective, blinded, 4-way comparison trial. Gastrointest Endosc 2008;68:255.

76. Masselli G, Gualdi G. Evaluation of small bowel tumors: MR enteroclysis. Abdom Imaging 2010;35:23–30.
77. Brenner DJ, Hall EJ. Computed tomography–an increasing source of radiation exposure. N Engl J Med 2007;357:2277.
78. Gourtsoyiannis N, Papanikolaou N, Grammatikakis J, et al. MR enteroclysis: technical considerations and clinical applications. Eur Radiol 2002; 12:2651.
79. Fidler J. MR imaging of the small bowel. Radiol Clin North Am 2007;45:317.
80. Schreyer AG, Seitz J, Feuerbach S, et al. Modern imaging using computer tomography and magnetic resonance imaging for inflammatory bowel disease (IBD) AU1. Inflamm Bowel Dis 2004;10:45.
81. Prassopoulos P, Papanikolaou N, Grammatikakis J, et al. MR enteroclysis imaging of Crohn disease. Radiographics 2001;21(Spec No):S161.
82. Gourtsoyiannis N, Grammatikakis J, Papamastorakis G, et al. Imaging of small intestinal Crohn's disease: comparison between MR enteroclysis and conventional enteroclysis. Eur Radiol 2006;16:1915.
83. Ryan E, Heaslip I. Magnetic resonance enteroclysis compared with conventional enteroclysis and computed tomography enteroclysis: a critically appraised topic. Abdom Imaging 2008;33:34.
84. Rieber A, Wruk D, Potthast S, et al. Diagnostic imaging in Crohn's disease: comparison of magnetic resonance imaging and conventional imaging methods. Int J Colorectal Dis 2000;15:176.
85. Herfarth HH, Grunert M, Klebl F, et al. Frequency and nature of incidental extra-enteric lesions found on magnetic resonance enterography (MR-E) in patients with inflammatory bowel diseases (IBD). PLoS One 2009;4:e4863.
86. Lee SS, Kim AY, Yang SK, et al. Crohn disease of the small bowel: comparison of CT enterography, MR enterography, and small-bowel follow-through as diagnostic techniques. Radiology 2009;251:751.
87. Umschaden HW, Szolar D, Gasser J, et al. Small-bowel disease: comparison of MR enteroclysis images with conventional enteroclysis and surgical findings. Radiology 2000;215:717.
88. Masselli G, Casciani E, Polettini E, et al. Comparison of MR enteroclysis with MR enterography and conventional enteroclysis in patients with Crohn's disease. Eur Radiol 2008;18:438.
89. Negaard A, Paulsen V, Sandvik L, et al. A prospective randomized comparison between two MRI studies of the small bowel in Crohn's disease, the oral contrast method and MR enteroclysis. Eur Radiol 2007;17:2294.
90. Horsthuis K, Bipat S, Bennink RJ, et al. Inflammatory bowel disease diagnosed with US, MR, scintigraphy, and CT: meta-analysis of prospective studies. Radiology 2008;64:247.
91. Masselli G, Vecchioli A, Gualdi GF. Crohn disease of the small bowel: MR enteroclysis versus conventional enteroclysis. Abdom Imaging 2006;31:400.
92. Maccioni F, Viscido A, Broglia L, et al. Evaluation of Crohn disease activity with magnetic resonance imaging. Abdom Imaging 2000;25:219.
93. Lauenstein TC, Schneemann H, Vogt FM, et al. Optimization of oral contrast agents for MR imaging of the small bowel. Radiology 2003;228:279.
94. Ajaj W, Goehde SC, Schneemann H, et al. Oral contrast agents for small bowel MRI: comparison of different additives to optimize bowel distension. Eur Radiol 2004;14:458.
95. Gourtsoyiannis N, Papanikolaou N, Grammatikakis J, et al. MR enteroclysis protocol optimization: comparison between 3D FLASH with fat saturation after

intravenous gadolinium injection and true FISP sequences. Eur Radiol 2001;11: 908.

96. Young BM, Fletcher JG, Booya F, et al. Head-to-head comparison of oral contrast agents for cross-sectional enterography: small bowel distention, timing, and side effects. J Comput Assist Tomogr 2008;32:32.

97. Lomas DJ, Graves MJ. Small bowel MRI using water as a contrast medium. Br J Radiol 1999;72:994.

98. Waleed A, Thomas CL, Jost L, et al. Small bowel hydro-MR imaging for optimized ileocecal distension in Crohn's disease: should an additional rectal enema filling be performed? J Magn Reson Imaging 2005;22:92.

99. Cronin CG, Lohan DG, Mhuircheartaigh JN, et al. MRI small-bowel follow-through: prone versus supine patient positioning for best small-bowel distention and lesion detection. Am J Roentgenol 2008;191:502.

100. Low RN, Sebrechts CP, Politoske DA, et al. Crohn disease with endoscopic correlation: single-shot fast spin-echo and gadolinium-enhanced fat-suppressed spoiled gradient-echo MR imaging. Radiology 2002;222:652.

101. Sempere GA, Martinez Sanjuan V, Medina Chulia E, et al. MRI evaluation of inflammatory activity in Crohn's disease. AJR Am J Roentgenol 2005;184:1829.

102. Lauenstein TC, Ajaj W, Narin B, et al. MR imaging of apparent small-bowel perfusion for diagnosing mesenteric ischemia: feasibility study. Radiology 2005;234:569.

103. Florie J, Wasser MN, Arts-Cieslik K, et al. Dynamic contrast-enhanced MRI of the bowel wall for assessment of disease activity in Crohn's disease. AJR Am J Roentgenol 2006;186:1384.

104. Lawrance IC, Welman CJ, Shipman P, et al. Correlation of MRI-determined small bowel Crohn's disease categories with medical response and surgical pathology. World J Gastroenterol 2009;15:3367.

105. Oto A, Zhu F, Kulkarni K, et al. Evaluation of diffusion-weighted MR imaging for detection of bowel inflammation in patients with Crohn's disease. Acad Radiol 2009;16:597.

106. Taylor SA, Punwani S, Rodriguez-Justo M, et al. Mural Crohn Disease: correlation of dynamic contrast-enhanced MR imaging findings with angiogenesis and inflammation at histologic examination–pilot study. Radiology 2009;251:369.

107. Karin H, Aart JN, Marijn-Willem de F, et al. Mapping of T1-values and Gadolinium-concentrations in MRI as indicator of disease activity in luminal Crohn's disease: a feasibility study. J Magn Reson Imaging 2009;29:488.

108. Centers for Medicare & Medicaid Services decision memo for screening computed tomography colonography (CTC) for colorectal cancer (CAG-00396N). Available at: https://www.cms.hhs.gov/mcd/viewdecisionmemo.asp?id=220. Updated April 2009. Accessed August 18, 2009.

CT Enterography

Giulia A. Zamboni, MD[a],*, Vassilios Raptopoulos, MD[b]

KEYWORDS

- Computed tomography • CT enterography • Crohn disease
- Gastrointestinal bleeding • Neoplasm

Imaging the small bowel has always been a challenge: conventional radiologic and endoscopic evaluations are often limited by the length, caliber, and motility of the small bowel loops. Computed tomography (CT) is used extensively in the abdomen for a variety of indications, but imaging evaluation of the bowel, especially the bowel wall, can be limited because of its length and orientation, the difficulty in sustaining distension and homogeneity of the oral contrast column, and variability in intravenous (IV) contrast enhancement. The development of new multidetector-row CT scanners, with faster scan times and isotropic spatial resolution, allows high-resolution multiphasic and multiplanar assessment of the bowel, bowel wall, and lumen. Conventional positive (high) attenuation oral contrast material shows mucosal detail while neutral attenuation oral contrast allows assessment of mucosal enhancement.

CT Enterography (CTE) is a variant of routine abdominal scanning, geared toward more sustained bowel filling with oral contrast material, and the use of multiplanar images, that can enhance gastrointestinal (GI) tract imaging.

TECHNIQUE

The goal of CTE is to discriminate the bowel, distend the lumen, visualize the intestinal wall, identify the vessels supplying the bowel loops, and assess the mesentery. While oral gastrointestinal luminal contrast material is required, the use of IV contrast material is also very helpful and should be encouraged unless there are contraindications. The amount and timing of oral contrast administration affect the degree of distension of the bowel, while the timing and injection rate of IV contrast administration determine the degree of bowel wall enhancement.

Data are acquired with volumetric techniques using thin collimation. Prone positioning can help disperse the bowel loops but is rarely used.

Oral Contrast Agents: Positive and Neutral Attenuation

The small bowel must be adequately distended to perform CTE, because collapsed or poorly distended loops can obscure existing pathologic processes, or mimic

[a] Istituto di Radiologia, Policlinico GB Rossi, P.le L.A. Scuro 10, 37134 Verona, Italy
[b] Department of Radiology, Beth Israel Deaconess Medical Center, Harvard Medical School, 330 Brookline Avenue, Boston, MA 02215, USA
* Corresponding author.
E-mail address: gzamboni@hotmail.com

Gastrointest Endoscopy Clin N Am 20 (2010) 347–366
doi:10.1016/j.giec.2010.02.017
1052-5157/10/$ – see front matter © 2010 Elsevier Inc. All rights reserved.
giendo.theclinics.com

pathology. To achieve optimal small bowel distension, a large volume of oral contrast must be administered within a short time. Two types of oral contrast agents can be used for CTE: positive and neutral (**Fig. 1**). High-attenuation, or positive, contrast agents are routinely used in CT, and were used in the initial descriptions of CTE. Neutral, or near-water attenuation contrast, has been proposed as an alternative medium as it allows assessment of mucosal enhancement.

Positive oral contrast

For CTE, 1600 mL of 2% barium-based or 2% to 2.5% water-soluble iodine-based oral contrast are administered over 1 to 2 hours before scanning.[1] This dose is 1.5 to 2 times that used for abdominal CT.[2] High-attenuation oral contrast is helpful in patients with Crohn disease to evaluate for fistula and sinus tracks, or in those with suspected abscess. In suspected partial obstruction, high-attenuation oral contrast can be used in conjunction with low-dose sequential scanning. This technique may provide indirect information on bowel motility and degree of obstruction. Variations to this regimen are used, all with very good results. The authors routinely administer 400 to 600 mL over an interval of 40 to 60 minutes before scanning and another 200 to 400 mL in the last 20 minutes.[3]

The use of positive contrast agents provides excellent background for detecting intraluminal filling defects, for example polyps, and depiction of mucosal detail. However, the high attenuation can impair detection of the mural features of the GI tract, identification of sources of obscure GI bleeding, and assessment of mucosal enhancement.

In a randomized controlled trial, Erturk and colleagues[4] compared high-attenuation and low-attenuation oral contrast agents in 90 patients without small bowel disease, and concluded that neutral (low-attenuation) contrast agents provide equal or superior distension and bowel wall visualization compared with high-attenuation contrast media.

For CTE, most investigators nowadays favor the use of neutral oral contrast agents, but all agree that positive oral contrast is preferable when intravenous contrast

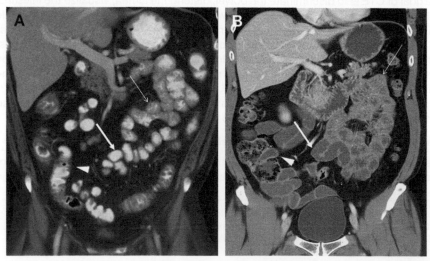

Fig. 1. Coronal image from CTE with positive contrast (*A*; barium) and neutral contrast (*B*; VoLumen) show findings in the normal bowel: the jejunum has a feathery pattern (*thin arrow*), while the ileum has a smooth surface (*thick arrow*). The normal terminal ileum is also depicted (*arrowhead*).

material cannot be administered. In addition, a modified CTE technique[5] can be used instead for routine abdominal or emergency scanning, in which 1 L of oral contrast (2% barium suspension + 5 mL of Gastrografin) is given as tolerated, 40 to 50 min before scanning. This modification is well tolerated by patients with abdominal pain, and provides satisfactory and consistent filling and homogeneity of intestinal lumen from duodenum to cecum in the majority of studies.

Neutral oral contrast

Several neutral enteric contrasts with near-water attenuation (0 HU) are available: water, whole milk (4% fat), polyethylene glycol (PEG), 12.5% corn-oil emulsion, and methylcellulose. Recently a low-attenuation barium solution with sorbitol (0.1% weight per volume barium sulfate suspension; VoLumen, E-ZEM) has gained popularity and is considered the neutral oral agent of choice. Sorbitol minimizes water resorption in the small bowel, improving lumen distension.[3]

Young and colleagues[6] and Kuehle and colleagues[7] compared different neutral contrast agents, and concluded that water provides the poorest distension because it is absorbed more readily than the other agents, while VoLumen provided the best distension. Megibow and colleagues[8] demonstrated that VoLumen significantly improved distension in all bowel segments compared with water and methylcellulose solution. Finally, Koo and colleagues[9] compared milk and VoLumen without observing significant differences in bowel distension.

Several slight variations in oral contrast administration protocols have been proposed in the literature.

Fasting before the examination is generally advised to reduce the possibility of misinterpreting ingested hyperattenuating debris such as enhancing lesions or bleeding.[10]

Kuehle and colleagues[7] showed that the best bowel distension was achieved with 1350 mL of low-attenuation barium suspension with sorbitol, and that increasing the volume to 1800 mL did not improve distension, but led to a lower patient acceptance and a higher rate of side effects.

Tochetto and Yaghmai[11] and Paulsen and colleagues[3] propose the administration of 1350 mL of neutral enteric contrast over 60 minutes: 450 mL in the first 20 minutes, 450 mL in the second 20 minutes, 225 mL in the third 20 minutes, and 225 mL on the CT table. A similar protocol has been proposed by Huprich and Fletcher.[12]

Optimal distension of the terminal ileum is achieved 45 to 60 minutes after the ingestion of oral contrast.[6,13] The intake of oral contrast should be continuous and well timed. It is therefore advisable that patients are monitored by technologists or nurses while ingesting contrast, to avoid the risk of a poor study.

Positive versus neutral attenuation oral contrast media

Positive oral contrast agents are better bowel markers and can assess obstruction more accurately. In addition, they provide mucosal detail and can depict intraluminal defects, strictures, ulcers, perforation, and abscess. Neutral agents provide more consistent bowel dilation and are unique in assessing mucosal enhancement, which is associated with exacerbation of chronic inflammatory bowel disease. In addition, they depict mucosal folds and can be used in imaging of GI bleed.

CT Enteroclysis

Enteroclysis is performed after insertion of a nasoduodenal tube just beyond the ligament of Treitz and administration of more than 2000 mL (60–100 mL/min) of enteric contrast with an automatic pump. Previous preparation of the bowel is advised. As described by Maglinte and colleagues,[14,15] this technique provides superior distension of the small bowel. However, placement of a nasoenteric tube is associated with patient discomfort and longer examination times.

IV Contrast

The combination of high iodine concentration and relatively fast injection rates produces excellent and consistent vascular, intestinal wall, and organ enhancement.

Most often, CTE includes single-phase scanning known as the "enteric phase." Schindera and colleagues[16] examined the attenuation of the aorta and the small bowel wall at 5-second intervals after injection of contrast medium at 5 mL/s, and observed peak small bowel wall enhancement 50 seconds after the start of the contrast medium injection. Wold and colleagues[17] did not observe significant differences between arterial and venous phase images in patients with Crohn disease, which supports single-phase imaging.

The authors vary the amount of IV contrast between 120 mL and 150 mL of IV depending on patient weight (under or over 75 kg, respectively). The authors routinely use a 320 mgI/mL solution. For patients who weigh more than 90 kg, 350 mgI/mL solution is used. Nonionic contrast is now universally used, and is preferred in order to avoid nausea or vomiting in patients with gastrointestinal tracts already overdistended by oral contrast. The authors use a split-bolus injection and single, combined-phase scanning regimen: first, 40 mL of contrast is injected at 2 mL/s. After a delay of 2 to 3 minutes, 80 mL is injected at 2 to 3 mL/s. For patients heavier than 75 kg, 50 mL is injected first, followed by 100 mL. Scanning starts 60 seconds after the beginning of the second dose. This split-bolus injection regimen results in a combined phase with good enhancement of the bowel wall, the solid organs, the mesenteric and retroperitoneal vessels, as well as the kidneys and ureters.[5] Other regimens are also effective, and one may not need to change the general IV contrast regimen used for routine abdominal scanning in the particular institution.

For the evaluation of occult GI bleeding, a multiphasic CTE protocol has been proposed by Huprich,[18] based on a bolus triggering technique. The first "arterial" phase is triggered automatically when aortic attenuation reaches 150 HU after contrast injection by placing a cursor over the descending aorta 2 cm above the diaphragm. The second, "enteric" and third, "delayed," phases are acquired 20 to 25 seconds and 70 to 75 seconds, respectively, after the beginning of the injection. However, this repeated scanning is associated with high radiation dose and should be used only when other methods have failed.

Scanning Techniques

The abdomen is scanned from the dome of the diaphragm to below the symphysis pubis. Volumetric isotropic scanning with thin collimation (0.5 or 0.625 mm) is important so that meaningful multiple projection reformatted (MPR) images can be obtained. To improve quality and decrease image glut, thicker slices are used for image interpretation: 3- to 5-mm thick axial and MPR images, reconstructed from thin overlapping slices.

Multiplanar reformations

Jaffe and colleagues[19] showed that, with regard to the presence of intra-abdominal abnormalities, coronal reformations from isotropic voxels (same resolution in all planes) are equivalent to transverse scans in terms of interpretation time and reader agreement. Similarly, Sebastian and colleagues[20] have demonstrated that the use of coronal reformats increases reader confidence, and these investigators suggest that coronal views could be used for primary interpretation. Coronal images are useful for quantifying the length of involved bowel and improve visualization of the terminal ileum,[21] whereas sagittal reformations are useful in evaluating the rectum and the presacral area, as well as the mesenteric vessels.[11]

Multiplanar CTE Versus CT Enteroclysis

As with conventional fluoroscopic enteroclysis, CT enteroclysis provides a consistent and high degree of bowel distension. The resultant studies are of superb quality and can provide the fine mucosal and luminal detail comparable to conventional double-contrast fluoroscopic enteroclysis.[10,16,17] CT enteroclysis is contraindicated in patients with suspected bowel perforation or small bowel obstruction; however, it is very helpful in patients with partial small bowel obstruction and Crohn disease. Despite high image quality, CT enteroclysis may be uncomfortable for the patient and the cost is increased because of the tubing, the pump, and the longer use of the CT room. The risk of complications is also increased because, in contrast to fluoroscopic techniques, the bowel is filled without visual monitoring. Thus, the additional information provided may not be worth the effort in the majority of indications. In the past few years magnetic resonance (MR) enteroclysis techniques have been developed, providing an alternative to CT enteroclysis and CTE.[13,14,18,19] In addition, these studies can provide real-time functional information allowing assessment of peristalsis.

Although multiplanar oral CTE provides less distension of the bowel, this may be more physiologic than the unnaturally overdistended small bowel achieved with CT enteroclysis. Furthermore, the examination is more comfortable to the patients and requires less preparation and room/equipment use. Although the fine anatomic mucosal details fall behind fluoroscopic studies, other signs that help characterize small bowel disease are available, including wall enhancement patterns, extraluminal abnormalities, and assessment of the mesentery.[1,5] Therefore, the authors favor the use of CTE with high-attenuation oral contrast, which they use as a routine protocol for CT evaluation of gastrointestinal abnormalities, including acute abdominal pain. The authors use neutral attenuation CTE selectively for occult GI bleeding and for evaluation of active inflammatory bowel disease.

CLINICAL APPLICATIONS

Bowel evaluation may be difficult because of the length of the small bowel (about 7 m), its convoluted course, and physiologic peristaltic motion. Even the relatively shorter colon, about 1.5 m, with its predictable course from the right lower quadrant to the rectum, has multiple variations, including the location of the cecum, the ileocecal valve or the appendix, and the undulation of the hepatic or splenic flexures and the sigmoid colon. Multiplanar CTE can help recognize bowel components, localize abnormalities, and show the extent of disease.[1]

The stomach is usually easily distended: the gastric folds are delineated well, and their thickness or disruption on axial and MPR images should be considered abnormal. The duodenum has a very active peristalsis: milk reduces duodenal peristalsis, and appears to be particularly helpful in evaluating the pancreas and duodenum.[22] The jejunum is rich in folds, and the plicae circularis may mimic a thickened wall, especially if poorly distended. The ileum shows less internal architecture, having a relatively smoother wall with occasional folds.

In general, normal small bowel loops appear similar to the next, and are pliable in relation to each other. In thin patients with little or no mesenteric fat, the shape of the bowel loops is interdependent, whereas in patients with more mesenteric fat they separate, and appear round or oval. In contrast, abnormal bowel with a thickened wall appears stiff with loss of curvature or undulation. The terminal ileum and ileocecal valve can always be recognized in multiplanar CTE. Evaluation of the colon may be hindered by fecal material, and if not distended it may be considered abnormal. On occasion, 100 to 300 mL of rectal contrast (water, or 2% barium suspension or water-soluble iodinated solution) may be helpful. Most frequently, however, colon abnormalities are associated with other findings in the adjacent mesentery, making the use of enema rarely necessary.

Interactive multiplanar viewing is helpful in identifying normal structures or bowel abnormalities, in assessing extent of disease, and in evaluating postoperative anatomy and anastomoses.

Increased thickness of the bowel wall is a nonspecific but important finding. Because of peristalsis, considerable variations have been observed. Normal distended small bowel wall thickness is 1 to 2 mm, whereas nondistended bowel may be as thick as 4 mm, especially the jejunum.[2,23] For the differential diagnosis between collapsed bowel and pathologic narrowing, it is useful to compare the attenuation of the thickened bowel loops with the distended bowel loops of the same segment[3]: normal, undistended bowel loops will be isoattenuating to the other loops in the same segment, whereas diseased loops will appear hyperenhancing (due to hyperemia) or hypoenhancing (due to edema).

Attenuation and IV contrast enhancement patterns of the wall may aid in the differential diagnosis. Wittenberg and colleagues[24] described 5 different patterns of bowel wall enhancement (**Table 1**): (1) homogeneous bright enhancement (white) can be seen in shock bowel, ischemia, inflammatory bowel disease, adhesions, and occasionally in tumor; (2) hypoenhancing (gray) wall may be seen in inflammatory bowel disease and tumor; (3) water attenuation (water halo or target pattern) is seen in ischemia, inflammatory bowel disease, acute infection, radiation, and occasionally in tumor; (4) fat attenuation (fat halo) is seen in inflammatory bowel disease (usually chronic disease) such as Crohn or ulcerative colitis, and chronic radiation enteritis; (5) pneumatosis can be seen in trauma (blunt or iatrogenic), ischemia, and acute infection.

CROHN DISEASE

The American College of Radiology Appropriateness Criteria (2008) defined CTE as the most appropriate radiologic method in evaluating the initial presentation of, or

Table 1 Common enhancement patterns of bowel wall abnormalities	
Homogeneous enhancement (white)	Shock bowel, ischemia, inflammatory bowel disease (IBD), adhesion, tumor (uncommon)
Hypoattenuation	IBD, tumor
Water attenuation (water halo or target)	Ischemia, IBD, tumor (uncommon), acute infection, radiation
Fat attenuation (fat halo)	IBD (usually chronic): Crohn and ulcerative colitis; radiation (chronic)
Pneumatosis	Trauma, ischemia, acute infection

Data from Wittenberg J, Harisinghani MG, Jhaveri K, et al. Algorithmic approach to CT diagnosis of the abnormal bowel wall. Radiographics 2002;22:1093–107.

known Crohn disease with acute exacerbation or known complication, in both adults and children.[25]

CT can demonstrate bowel involvement, bowel length and distribution, and extraintestinal manifestations. Bowel involvement in Crohn disease is transmural, segmental, and usually discontinuous. The small bowel is involved in up to 80% of cases, and the terminal ileum is the most commonly involved segment, in excess of 50% of cases.[11] CTE can differentiate between active and chronic disease (**Table 2**), an important distinction because the treatment is different.

Active Crohn Disease

The classic CTE features of active small bowel Crohn disease include bowel wall thickening, mural hyperenhancement, mural stratification, increased attenuation of the mesenteric fat, and engorged vasa recta.

Mucosal hyperenhancement is best seen with neutral attenuation oral contrast and is a sensitive sign of activity (**Fig. 2**). Booya and colleagues[26] observed that terminal ileal attenuation was higher in patients with active Crohn disease than in patients without Crohn disease, and that terminal ileal attenuation was higher than normal-appearing distended ileum attenuation in patients with active Crohn disease. According to radiological assessment, the most sensitive visual CT finding of Crohn disease activity was mural hyperenhancement (73%–80%).[26] Baker and colleagues[27] have studied the efficacy of relative attenuation (highest absolute attenuation of the bowel wall divided by arterial attenuation), absolute attenuation, and wall thickness in distinguishing normal from active inflammatory Crohn disease of the terminal ileum. These investigators observed that, when taking into account wall thickness, relative attenuation appears to be the equivalent of absolute enhancement in differentiating between normal bowel and active inflammatory Crohn disease of the terminal ileum. When the bowel wall is thicker than 3 mm, a relative attenuation cutoff of 0.5 is reliable for distinguishing normal terminal ileum from active inflammatory Crohn disease.[27]

Aphthous ulcers are specific findings of activity but are uncommonly seen (best with high positive attenuation contrast) (**Fig. 3**). Small bowel thickening is a sensitive finding of Crohn disease (**Figs. 4 and 5**).[28–31] Normal small bowel loops, when distended, are up to 3 mm thick. When thickness is greater than 3 mm, the loop is considered abnormal. Mural thickening is the most frequently observed finding in patients with Crohn disease. Del Campo and colleagues[30] and Choi and colleagues[29] have suggested that the thickness of the small bowel is correlated to disease activity, with bowel wall thicker in active than in chronic disease.

Mural hyperenhancement is the most sensitive finding of active Crohn disease,[26] and significantly correlates with histologic[26,28] and clinical findings[30] of active disease. When using a mural attenuation threshold of 109 HU and an abnormal-to-normal loop enhancement ratio of more than 1.3, CTE correlates well with histologic findings of

Table 2 Findings in active and chronic Crohn disease	
Active Disease	**Chronic Disease**
Mural thickening	Submucosal fat deposition
Mural and mucosal hyperenhancement	Sacculations
Mural stratification	Fibrofatty proliferation
Edema of mesenteric fat	Strictures
Engorgement of the vasa recta ("comb sign")	

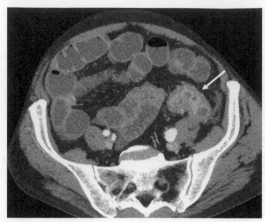

Fig. 2. Axial image from neutral contrast CTE (PEG) shows thickened matted ileal loops (*arrow*) with increased attenuation of the mesenteric fat in a patient affected by Crohn disease.

active disease.[28] However, visual assessment is more specific than quantitative measurements: 69% for quantitative versus 82% for visual assessment.[28]

Mural stratification after IV contrast administration is another sign of active Crohn disease. The bowel wall shows alternating layers of hyper- and hypoenhancement, the latter representing edema between bowel wall layers.[26,32] Choi and colleagues[29] demonstrated that it is more likely to indicate histologically active disease than a homogeneously enhancing bowel wall. Different mural stratification patterns can be observed. Most commonly, edematous bowel wall has a trilaminar "target sign" appearance, with an internal ring of mucosal enhancement, an external ring of serosal and muscular enhancement, and decreased intramural enhancement.[3,11]

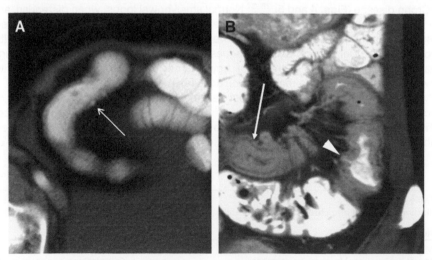

Fig. 3. Positive contrast CTE shows fine mucosa detail. Shallow (aphthous like) ulcers (*arrow in A*) are depicted in a small bowel loop. Coronal image (*B*) shows an intramural sinus (*arrowhead*), and striated enhancement of bowel loops, better noted in a loop not filled with positive oral contrast (*arrow*).

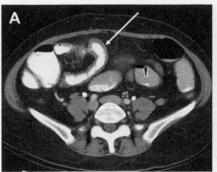
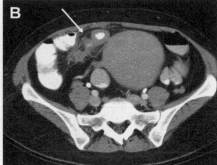

Fig. 4. Axial images from positive contrast CTE show the terminal ileum with a thickened wall and loss of undulation (*arrow in A*); matted loops with a small bowel stricture are also depicted (*arrow in B*).

The most common extraenteric findings in active Crohn disease include fibrofatty proliferation of the mesentery due to edema and engorgement of the vasa recta. Engorged and prominent vasa recta that penetrate the bowel wall perpendicular to the lumen create the "comb sign," a very specific finding of active Crohn disease (**Fig. 6**).[33–35] Lee and colleagues[34] showed that patients with prominent mesenteric vasculature were more likely to be admitted to the hospital and receive aggressive treatment than patients with Crohn disease without prominent vasculature.

Chronic Crohn Disease

The chronic signs of Crohn disease include submucosal fat deposition, sacculations or dilated amorphous bowel loops, fibrofatty proliferation, and strictures (**Fig. 7**).[32] Submucosal fat deposition may mimic the mural stratification of active disease.[36]

Sacculations are the consequence of asymmetric fibrosis: inflammation involves preferentially the mesenteric border of the bowel, which eventually leads to

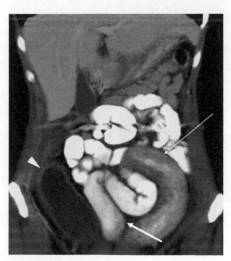

Fig. 5. Positive contrast CTE shows a small bowel loop with a thickened wall and irregular ulcers of the mucosa (*thin arrow*). An amorphous small bowel loop with diluted contrast (*thick arrow*) is seen in the pelvis, where the appendix is also involved (*arrowhead*).

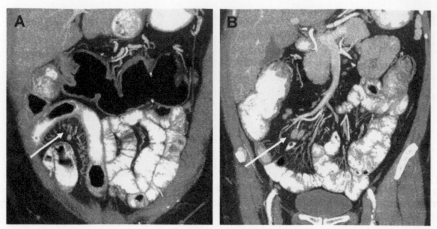

Fig. 6. Coronal images from positive contrast CTE show thickened terminal ileum wall and engorged vasa recta ("comb sign," *arrow in A*) in a patient with relapsing Crohn disease. Prominent mesenteric nodes are also noted (*arrow in B*).

asymmetric fibrosis that, combined with the increased intraluminal pressure during peristalsis, causes sacculations of the antimesenteric wall.[3]

Fibrofatty proliferation extends from the mesenteric attachment of the bowel and partially covers the chronically inflamed bowel loop seen in chronic disease. However, when it is associated with engorged perpendicular distal mesenteric vessels (comb sign), it is considered surgically pathognomonic for the disease, and highly specific for active Crohn disease.[28] Strictures and fistulas are other manifestations of chronic Crohn disease.

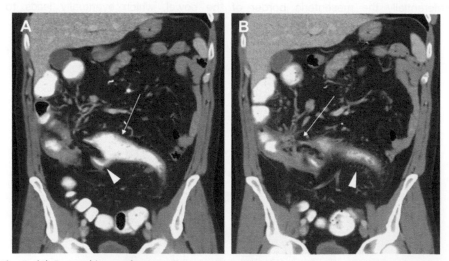

Fig. 7. (*A*) Coronal image from positive contrast CTE depicts a flaccid appearing amorphous bowel loop, with thickened wall, irregular mucosa (*arrow*) and a fistula (*arrowhead*). (*B*) Fibrofatty proliferation is seen, with matted bowel loops in the right lower quadrant (*arrow*). The thickened bowel loop is surrounded by fatty proliferation and engorged vasa recta (*arrowhead*).

Complications of Crohn Disease

The most common complications of Crohn disease include strictures, fistulas, and abscesses. The cumulative risk of developing fistulas for patients with Crohn disease is 33% after 10 years and 50% after 20 years,[37] with perianal fistulas being the most common type. Fistulas usually are hyperenhancing tracts, with the exception of perianal fistulas, which might be isoattenuating and can be present without signs of inflammation. When CT is performed to identify fistulas, the administration of positive oral contrast is preferred over neutral attenuation agents (see **Fig. 7**).

Abscesses are often connected to inflamed bowel loops by sinus tracts, and are most commonly seen in the retroperitoneum or in the mesentery (**Fig. 8**).[32]

Strictures and matted loops of bowel are associated with bowel wall thickening and fistulas; they may progress to bowel obstruction and may require bowel resection.[38]

Performance of CTE in Crohn Disease

Wold and colleagues[17] showed the superiority of CTE compared with small bowel follow-through (SBFT): CTE had 78% sensitivity and 83% specificity, whereas SBFT had 62% sensitivity and 90% specificity. Although the difference was not significant, CTE was more sensitive in detecting abscesses and fistulas.

Solem and colleagues[39] prospectively and blindly compared CTE, capsule endoscopy, ileoscopy, and SBFT in 41 patients with Crohn disease, using clinical consensus as a gold standard. Capsule endoscopy and CTE had equal sensitivities for active Crohn disease (82%–83%), but CTE was more specific (89% vs 53%). Hara and colleagues[40] retrospectively evaluated the use of CTE to monitor Crohn disease activity, comparing CTE findings with disease progression or regression based on symptoms and clinical follow-up. These investigators observed that imaging changes between CTE examinations have excellent potential for reliably monitoring Crohn disease progression and regression.

As Crohn disease is a chronic condition with repeated flares of active disease, repeated imaging studies are often necessary. The major concern in repeating CTE

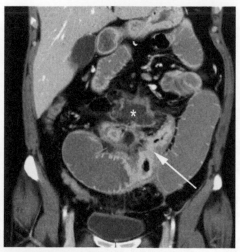

Fig. 8. Coronal image from neutral contrast CTE (VoLumen) depicts a thickened bowel loop with a stricture (*arrow*): the enhancement of mucosa indicates activity. The use of neutral contrast makes it difficult to distinguish the abscess (*asterisk*) from abnormal bowel loop.

for evaluation of Crohn disease is increased radiation exposure, which can be greater than 15 mSv or up to 5 times higher than with SBFT.[41] The situation is further underscored by these patients often being young. This fact favors the use of MR enterography, especially in younger patients (**Fig. 9**). MR enterography moreover provides excellent depiction of perianal fistulas and allows assessment of bowel motility.[42] The benefit/risk ratio should be evaluated in each patient undergoing CTE. CTE is indicated for initial diagnosis, and in patients with known Crohn disease and suspicion of complications. MR enterography may be preferred in younger patients, especially for follow-up, although Siddiki and colleagues[43] have recently demonstrated that a low-dose CTE technique has equivalent diagnostic value to conventional CTE.

OBSCURE GASTROINTESTINAL BLEEDING

As defined by the American Gastroenterological Association, obscure gastrointestinal bleeding (OGIB) is a persistent or recurring condition of unknown origin after negative upper and lower endoscopies.

The cause of OGIB has been described to exist in the small bowel in 5% to 10% up to 27% of patients.[44,45] Wireless endoscopy is the most sensitive examination for detecting sources of OGIB, with reported sensitivities ranging from 42% to 80%.[46,47] However, this method is not able to show submucosal or serosal abnormalities, and has long reporting times. Multiphasic CTE is less invasive and quicker to perform than capsule endoscopy, and allows assessment of the entire bowel wall and extraintestinal findings. Neutral attenuation oral contrast is required, and the enhancement phases include arterial (around 20–30 seconds) and enteric (around 55 seconds) phases. Some investigators advocate delayed phase scanning, 90 seconds after injection. Arterial phase is best achieved with automatic bolus triggering by sequential monitoring of the aorta and starting to scan when attenuation reaches 250 to 300 HU. The enteric phase follows 45 seconds after the start of the arterial phase.

Most cases of OGIB are due to benign vascular abnormalities, such as angiodysplasia. A vascular tuft is frequently seen in the arterial phase, with an early draining

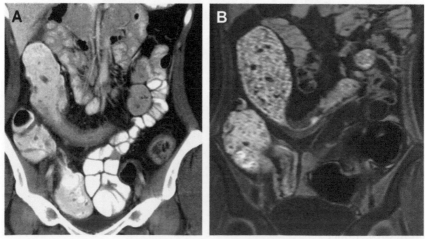

Fig. 9. A 25-year-old woman with Crohn disease. Coronal CTE (*A*) and MRE (*B*) images show excellent correlation in depiction of the thickened bowel loop.

mesenteric vein. Small bowel tumors most commonly present with frank bleeding, but may also cause OGIB. The most common neoplastic causes of OGIB are leiomyomas and stromal tumors (**Fig. 10**). Active bleeding will appear as progressive accumulation of contrast medium in the dependent portion of the lumen during multiphasic scanning. Kuhle and Sheiman[48] found in a swine model that helical CT can detect active GI hemorrhage at rates of less than 4 mL/s.

Data from angiographic experience suggest that arterial phase and delayed scans are required to detect small bowel angiodysplasias, the most common abnormalities causing OGIB; therefore, CTE protocols for evaluating OGIB require multiphase scanning.[18] The scan phases must be carefully examined in multiple planes. Angiodysplasias enhance most intensely in the enteric phase, appearing as nodular or plaquelike lesions.[18]

Huprich compared multiphasic CTE with capsule and traditional endoscopy, surgery, and angiography for the diagnosis of OGIB.[18] CTE was positive for bleeding source in 10 of 22 patients (45%), and correctly identified 3 lesions undetected at capsule endoscopy. Huprich concluded that multiphasic multiplanar CTE may have a role in the evaluation of OGIB. Multiphase scanning should be used sparingly as radiation is 2 to 3 times that of conventional CTE, and the risk benefit should always be

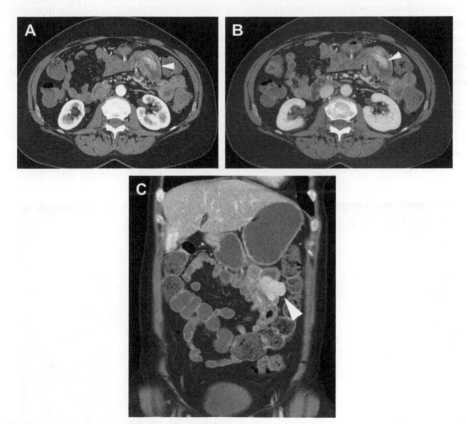

Fig. 10. Axial unenhanced (*A*), and axial (*B*) and coronal (*C*) images from multiphasic neutral contrast CTE performed for occult GI bleed shows a large, well-enhancing tumor in a small bowel loop, consistent with a gastrointestinal stromal tumor (*arrowheads*) (*Courtesy of Martin Smith, MD, Beth Israel Deaconess Medical Center, Boston, MA.*)

considered before ordering a study. Split-bolus CTE with neutral attenuation oral contrast and a single combined-phase scan may be a more sensible technique.

TUMORS

Small bowel tumors are uncommon, and represent a minority of all gastrointestinal tumors. Because of the liquid content of the small bowel, obstruction occurs late and when the masses are large, and the diagnosis is delayed.[49] The most common tumors are gastrointestinal stromal tumors, adenocarcinoma, lymphoma, and carcinoid.[50,51] At diagnosis, stromal tumors are usually large, most commonly located in the upper tract, and appear homogeneous on nonenhanced scan, with variable enhancement on enhanced scans. A little less than half of them are localized in the stomach with about half in the small bowel.[52] Small bowel lymphomas are large, usually ulcerated masses, most commonly located in the distal small bowel (**Fig. 11**). Carcinoid tumors may produce mesenteric reaction with retractile and often calcified mesenteric mass. Bowel wall edema and mural nodularity are other signs, probably secondary to peptide excretion by the tumor (**Fig. 12**).[53] Multiplanar CTE has a role in treatment planning and in the detection of extraintestinal extension, and can be used for a full survey of the abdomen. The origin of the tumor and its local extension, mesenteric lymphadenopathy, as well as distant metastasis to the liver and peritoneum can be evaluated in one single examination. To detect small bowel tumors, multiphasic CTE protocols are suggested, similar to those employed in GI bleeding,[49] although there are no large studies in the literature on the efficacy of CTE in detecting small bowel tumors. Pilleul and colleagues[49] report an accuracy of 84.7% in depicting small bowel tumors for CT enteroclysis.

ACUTE ABDOMINAL PAIN

Rosen and colleagues[54] have shown the impact of CT on the diagnosis and management of patients with acute abdominal pain. CT is especially useful in patients without previous history of abdominal disease. In this group, the sensitivity of CT was 90%

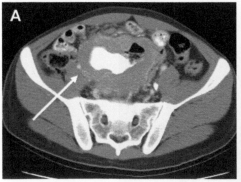
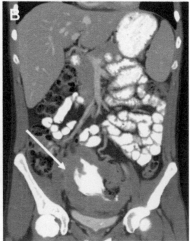

Fig. 11. Axial (*A*) and coronal (*B*) CTE images show a markedly thickened small bowel loop (*arrows*) in the lower quadrants, which proved to be lymphoma.

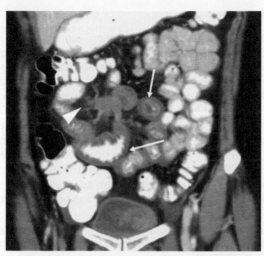

Fig. 12. Coronal CTE image from a patient with carcinoid tumor extending to mesenteric root as spiculated mass (*arrowhead*). Desmoplastic process tethers adjacent bowel loops toward the mass. Edema and mural modularity (*arrows*) are secondary signs of carcinoid probably secondary to peptides excreted by the tumor and edema from mechanical effect of fibrosis on mesenteric vessels. *Data from* Macari M, Balthazar EJ. CT of bowel wall thickening: significance and pitfalls of interpretation. AJR Am J Roentgenol 2001;176:1105–16.

compared with 47% of initial clinical assessment, and CT changed therapeutic plans in 22 of 59 (37%) patients studied.[55]

The abnormal appendix is usually easily recognized on axial images, but in many cases visualization of a normal appendix is difficult. Although nonvisualization of the appendix on CT can exclude acute appendicitis,[56] confidence increases when the appendix is visualized. Routine multiplanar (axial, coronal, and sagittal) and, occasionally, interactive multiplanar viewing may increase confidence in absence of disease. Similarly, the addition of MPR images facilitates visualization of the uterus and ovaries. Diagnosis of conditions other than those of small bowel origin, such as cholecystitis, ulcerative colitis, diverticulitis, and abdominal abscess is enhanced by the multiplanar CTE technique.[5]

Gourtsoyianni and colleagues[5] reviewed 165 consecutive Emergency Department patients presenting with nontraumatic acute abdominal pain examined with a modified split-bolus CTE protocol: ingestion, as tolerated, of 900 to 1200 mL of 2% barium suspension + 5 mL of Gastrografin over 45 min, and administration of 150 mL of IV contrast given in 2 boluses (50 and 100 mL) 3 minutes apart (split-bolus injection protocol). With this modified CTE protocol, a cause for abdominal pain was identified in 81 patients (intestinal in 54 and extraintestinal in 27). Oral contrast reached the cecum in 76% of patients; the small bowel was well distended and opacified. There was good mucosa detail that correlated significantly with bowel opacification and distension for both jejunum and ileum. A combined nephrographic and excretory phase was achieved, and the great vessels were well opacified, allowing for vascular evaluation. The investigators conclude that modified CTE is well tolerated by patients with acute nontraumatic abdominal pain, and can be used routinely as a noninvasive examination, informative of bowel, vessel, and organ pathology in Emergency Department patients.

BOWEL OBSTRUCTION

CT is accurate in detecting small bowel obstruction, with sensitivity reported between 80% and 100%.[57] Because peristalsis cannot be assessed, the CT diagnosis of bowel obstruction relies on changes of bowel caliber and identification of a transitional zone.[23] Multiplanar images may be very helpful in detecting the site of obstruction.[58] The transition point can be recognized and the cause of obstruction identified. Small bowel is considered dilated if its caliber is greater than 2.5 cm.[59] Dilated obstructed bowel must be differentiated from focal or generalized adynamic ileus. Oral contrast may be contraindicated in patients with nausea or already overdistended bowel loops. On the other hand, even when oral contrast is tolerated, it may not reach the site of obstruction for hours. Initial scanning 1 hour after oral contrast ingestion may be diagnostic in most cases. In the remainder, follow-up scanning with low-dose technique after a 4- to 6-hour delay may be reasonable to assess the degree or progress of obstruction.

Hong and colleagues[60] have assessed the value of 3-dimensional (3D) CTE using oral Gastrografin in patients with small bowel obstruction, comparing the results with axial images and SBFT. All patients tolerated the ingestion of Gastrografin. 3D CTE significantly improved diagnostic confidence for interpretation of the level, cause of small bowel obstruction, and the assessment of the interpretability of each image as compared with the use of axial CT images, and was superior to SBFT.

The most common cause of small bowel obstruction is adhesions, followed by hernia.[57,61] Multiplanar viewing of axial and coronal images is helpful in identifying the site of transition, and adhesions might be seen as enhancing bands. Similarly, MPR images may be helpful in closed loop obstruction. Imaging findings include a C- or U-shaped dilated bowel loop, adjacent collapsed loops, conversion of mesenteric vessels, and beak or whirl signs.[61,62] MPR images also help to evaluate for cecal or sigmoid volvulus. After adhesions, hernias are another frequent cause of obstruction. Hernias can be external, through the abdominal wall, or internal, through bowel mesenteries or peritoneal bands. Hernias can be spontaneous or traumatic, including

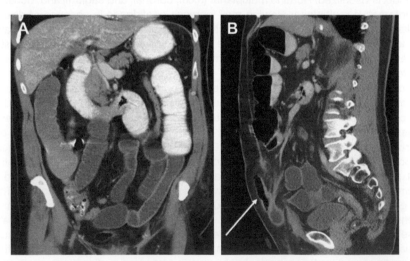

Fig. 13. Coronal (*A*) and sagittal (*B*) images from CTE show small bowel occlusion due to ventral hernia (*arrow in B*), with dilated small bowel loops and slow progress of the positive oral contrast

iatrogenic (eg, incisional). The diagnosis of external hernia is simple with CT, and depending on the orientation, MPR images can be helpful (**Fig. 13**). Internal hernias are less obvious and should be suspected when bowel loops are in nonconventional regions[63] such as in the lesser sac, to the right of the duodenum, or lateral to ascending or descending colon. If a large portion of jejunum appears on the right side of the abdominal cavity without other evidence of malrotation, consider the possibility of internal hernia.

CTE may also enhance the diagnostic confidence in all the other possible causes of small bowel obstruction, including tumors, abscess and hematomas, inflammatory lesions, radiation or ischemic enteritis, trauma, intussusceptions, and foreign bodies.

Finally, small bowel obstruction may cause ischemia. On multiplanar CTE, strangulating (ischemic) obstruction may be recognized with a combination of findings relating to obstruction and ischemia, including transition zone with proximal bowel dilation, hyper- or hypoenhancement of the bowel wall, pneumatosis, edema, or fluid in the mesentery.[64]

REFERENCES

1. Raptopoulos V, Schwartz RK, McNicholas MM, et al. Multiplanar helical CT enterography in patients with Crohn's disease. AJR Am J Roentgenol 1997;169:1545–50.
2. Raptopoulos V. Technical principles in CT evaluation of the gut. Radiol Clin North Am 1989;27:631–51.
3. Paulsen SR, Huprich JE, Hara AK. CT enterography: noninvasive evaluation of Crohn's disease and obscure gastrointestinal bleed. Radiol Clin North Am 2007;45:303–15.
4. Erturk SM, Mortele KJ, Oliva MR, et al. Depiction of normal gastrointestinal anatomy with MDCT: comparison of low- and high-attenuation oral contrast media. Eur J Radiol 2008;66:84–7.
5. Gourtsoyianni S, Zamboni GA, Romero JY, et al. Routine use of modified CT enterography in patients with acute abdominal pain. Eur J Radiol 2009;69:388–92.
6. Young BM, Fletcher JG, Booya F, et al. Head-to-head comparison of oral contrast agents for cross-sectional enterography: small bowel distention, timing, and side effects. J Comput Assist Tomogr 2008;32:32–8.
7. Kuehle CA, Ajaj W, Ladd SC, et al. Hydro-MRI of the small bowel: effect of contrast volume, timing of contrast administration, and data acquisition on bowel distention. AJR Am J Roentgenol 2006;187:W375–85.
8. Megibow AJ, Babb JS, Hecht EM, et al. Evaluation of bowel distention and bowel wall appearance by using neutral oral contrast agent for multi-detector row CT. Radiology 2006;238:87–95.
9. Koo CW, Shah-Patel LR, Baer JW, et al. Cost-effectiveness and patient tolerance of low-attenuation oral contrast material: milk versus VoLumen. AJR Am J Roentgenol 2008;190:1307–13.
10. Macari M, Megibow AJ, Balthazar EJ. A pattern approach to the abnormal small bowel: observations at MDCT and CT enterography. AJR Am J Roentgenol 2007;188:1344–55.
11. Tochetto S, Yaghmai V. CT enterography: concept, technique, and interpretation. Radiol Clin North Am 2009;47:117–32.
12. Huprich JE, Fletcher JG. CT enterography: principles, technique and utility in Crohn's disease. Eur J Radiol 2009;69:393–7.

13. Fletcher JG. CT enterography technique: theme and variations. Abdom Imaging 2009;34:283–8.
14. Maglinte DD, Sandrasegaran K, Lappas JC. CT enteroclysis: techniques and applications. Radiol Clin North Am 2007;45:289–301.
15. Maglinte DD, Sandrasegaran K, Lappas JC, et al. CT enteroclysis. Radiology 2007;245:661–71.
16. Schindera ST, Nelson RC, DeLong DM, et al. Multi-detector row CT of the small bowel: peak enhancement temporal window—initial experience. Radiology 2007;243:438–44.
17. Wold PB, Fletcher JG, Johnson CD, et al. Assessment of small bowel Crohn disease: noninvasive peroral CT enterography compared with other imaging methods and endoscopy—feasibility study. Radiology 2003;229:275–81.
18. Huprich JE. Multi-phase CT enterography in obscure GI bleeding. Abdom Imaging 2009;34:303–9.
19. Jaffe TA, Martin LC, Miller CM, et al. Abdominal pain: coronal reformations from isotropic voxels with 16-section CT-reader lesion detection and interpretation time. Radiology 2007;242:175–81.
20. Sebastian S, Kalra MK, Mittal P, et al. Can independent coronal multiplanar reformatted images obtained using state-of-the-art MDCT scanners be used for primary interpretation of MDCT of the abdomen and pelvis? A feasibility study. Eur J Radiol 2007;64:439–46.
21. Yaghmai V, Nikolaidis P, Hammond NA, et al. Multidetector-row computed tomography diagnosis of small bowel obstruction: can coronal reformations replace axial images? Emerg Radiol 2006;13:69–72.
22. Thompson SE, Raptopoulos V, Sheiman RL, et al. Abdominal helical CT: milk as a low-attenuation oral contrast agent. Radiology 1999;211:870–5.
23. Balthazar EJ. CT of the gastrointestinal tract: principles and interpretation. AJR Am J Roentgenol 1991;156:23–32.
24. Wittenberg J, Harisinghani MG, Jhaveri K, et al. Algorithmic approach to CT diagnosis of the abnormal bowel wall. Radiographics 2002;22:1093–107 [discussion: 1107–9].
25. American College of Radiology. ACR appropriateness criteria 2005. Available at: http://acsearch.acr.org/TopicList.aspx?topic_all=&topic_any='%22crohn*%22'&connector=+And+&cid=0. Accessed February 18, 2010.
26. Booya F, Fletcher JG, Huprich JE, et al. Active Crohn disease: CT findings and interobserver agreement for enteric phase CT enterography. Radiology 2006; 241:787–95.
27. Baker ME, Walter J, Obuchowski NA, et al. Mural attenuation in normal small bowel and active inflammatory Crohn's disease on CT enterography: location, absolute attenuation, relative attenuation, and the effect of wall thickness. AJR Am J Roentgenol 2009;192:417–23.
28. Bodily KD, Fletcher JG, Solem CA, et al. Crohn disease: mural attenuation and thickness at contrast-enhanced CT enterography—correlation with endoscopic and histologic findings of inflammation. Radiology 2006;238:505–16.
29. Choi D, Jin Lee S, Ah Cho Y, et al. Bowel wall thickening in patients with Crohn's disease: CT patterns and correlation with inflammatory activity. Clin Radiol 2003; 58:68–74.
30. Del Campo L, Arribas I, Valbuena M, et al. Spiral CT findings in active and remission phases in patients with Crohn disease. J Comput Assist Tomogr 2001;25: 792–7.

31. Maccioni F, Bruni A, Viscido A, et al. MR imaging in patients with Crohn disease: value of T2- versus T1-weighted gadolinium-enhanced MR sequences with use of an oral superparamagnetic contrast agent. Radiology 2006;238: 517–30.
32. Paulsen SR, Huprich JE, Fletcher JG, et al. CT enterography as a diagnostic tool in evaluating small bowel disorders: review of clinical experience with over 700 cases. Radiographics 2006;26:641–57 [discussion: 657–62].
33. Colombel JF, Solem CA, Sandborn WJ, et al. Quantitative measurement and visual assessment of ileal Crohn's disease activity by computed tomography enterography: correlation with endoscopic severity and C reactive protein. Gut 2006;55:1561–7.
34. Lee SS, Ha HK, Yang SK, et al. CT of prominent pericolic or perienteric vasculature in patients with Crohn's disease: correlation with clinical disease activity and findings on barium studies. AJR Am J Roentgenol 2002;179:1029–36.
35. Meyers MA, McGuire PV. Spiral CT demonstration of hypervascularity in Crohn disease: "vascular jejunization of the ileum" or the "comb sign". Abdom Imaging 1995;20:327–32.
36. Jones B, Fishman EK, Hamilton SR, et al. Submucosal accumulation of fat in inflammatory bowel disease: CT/pathologic correlation. J Comput Assist Tomogr 1986;10:759–63.
37. Schwartz DA, Loftus EV Jr, Tremaine WJ, et al. The natural history of fistulizing Crohn's disease in Olmsted County, Minnesota. Gastroenterology 2002;122: 875–80.
38. Cheung O, Regueiro MD. Inflammatory bowel disease emergencies. Gastroenterol Clin North Am 2003;32:1269–88.
39. Solem CA, Loftus EV Jr, Fletcher JG, et al. Small-bowel imaging in Crohn's disease: a prospective, blinded, 4-way comparison trial. Gastrointest Endosc 2008;68:255–66.
40. Hara AK, Alam S, Heigh RI, et al. Using CT enterography to monitor Crohn's disease activity: a preliminary study. AJR Am J Roentgenol 2008;190:1512–6.
41. Jaffe TA, Gaca AM, Delaney S, et al. Radiation doses from small-bowel follow-through and abdominopelvic MDCT in Crohn's disease. AJR Am J Roentgenol 2007;189:1015–22.
42. Froehlich JM, Patak MA, von Weymarn C, et al. Small bowel motility assessment with magnetic resonance imaging. J Magn Reson Imaging 2005;21: 370–5.
43. Siddiki H, Fletcher JG, Bruining D, et al. Performance of lower-dose CT enterography for detection of inflammatory Crohn's disease. Chicago: RSNA; 2007.
44. Lahoti S, Fukami N. The small bowel as a source of gastrointestinal blood loss. Curr Gastroenterol Rep 1999;1:424–30.
45. Lewis BS. Small intestinal bleeding. Gastroenterol Clin North Am 2000;29: 67–95, vi.
46. Magnano A, Privitera A, Calogero G, et al. The role of capsule endoscopy in the work-up of obscure gastrointestinal bleeding. Eur J Gastroenterol Hepatol 2004; 16:403–6.
47. Pennazio M, Santucci R, Rondonotti E, et al. Outcome of patients with obscure gastrointestinal bleeding after capsule endoscopy: report of 100 consecutive cases. Gastroenterology 2004;126:643–53.
48. Kuhle WG, Sheiman RG. Detection of active colonic hemorrhage with use of helical CT: findings in a swine model. Radiology 2003;228:743–52.

49. Pilleul F, Penigaud M, Milot L, et al. Possible small-bowel neoplasms: contrast-enhanced and water-enhanced multidetector CT enteroclysis. Radiology 2006; 241:796–801.
50. Horton KM, Kamel I, Hofmann L, et al. Carcinoid tumors of the small bowel: a multitechnique imaging approach. AJR Am J Roentgenol 2004;182:559–67.
51. Minardi AJ Jr, Zibari GB, Aultman DF, et al. Small-bowel tumors. J Am Coll Surg 1998;186:664–8.
52. Burkill GJ, Badran M, Al-Muderis O, et al. Malignant gastrointestinal stromal tumor: distribution, imaging features, and pattern of metastatic spread. Radiology 2003;226:527–32.
53. Macari M, Balthazar EJ. CT of bowel wall thickening: significance and pitfalls of interpretation. AJR Am J Roentgenol 2001;176:1105–16.
54. Rosen MP, Siewert B, Sands DZ, et al. Value of abdominal CT in the emergency department for patients with abdominal pain. Eur Radiol 2003;13:418–24.
55. Siewert B, Raptopoulos V, Mueller MF, et al. Impact of CT on diagnosis and management of acute abdomen in patients initially treated without surgery. AJR Am J Roentgenol 1997;168:173–8.
56. Ganguli S, Raptopoulos V, Komlos F, et al. Right lower quadrant pain: value of the nonvisualized appendix in patients at multidetector CT. Radiology 2006;241: 175–80.
57. Furukawa A, Yamasaki M, Takahashi M, et al. CT diagnosis of small bowel obstruction: scanning technique, interpretation and role in the diagnosis. Semin Ultrasound CT MR 2003;24:336–52.
58. Caoili EM, Paulson EK. CT of small-bowel obstruction: another perspective using multiplanar reformations. AJR Am J Roentgenol 2000;174:993–8.
59. Fukuya T, Hawes DR, Lu CC, et al. CT diagnosis of small-bowel obstruction: efficacy in 60 patients. AJR Am J Roentgenol 1992;158:765–9 [discussion: 771–2].
60. Hong SS, Kim AY, Kwon SB, et al. Three-dimensional CT enterography using oral gastrografin in patients with small bowel obstruction: comparison with axial CT images or fluoroscopic findings. Abdom Imaging 2009. [Epub ahead of print].
61. Balthazar EJ, George W. Holmes lecture. CT of small-bowel obstruction. AJR Am J Roentgenol 1994;162:255–61.
62. Balthazar EJ, Bauman JS, Megibow AJ. CT diagnosis of closed loop obstruction. J Comput Assist Tomogr 1985;9:953–5.
63. Blachar A, Federle MP, Brancatelli G, et al. Radiologist performance in the diagnosis of internal hernia by using specific CT findings with emphasis on transmesenteric hernia. Radiology 2001;221:422–8.
64. Balthazar EJ, Liebeskind ME, Macari M. Intestinal ischemia in patients in whom small bowel obstruction is suspected: evaluation of accuracy, limitations, and clinical implications of CT in diagnosis. Radiology 1997;205:519–22.

The Role of CT Colonography in a Colorectal Cancer Screening Program

Klaus Mergener, MD, PhD

KEYWORDS

- Computed tomography • Colonography • Colon cancer
- Screening • Colonoscopy • Endoscopy

Colorectal cancer (CRC) remains the third most commonly diagnosed cancer and the second leading cause of cancer death in the United States. In 2009, an estimated 146,970 new cases of CRC were diagnosed, and approximately 49,920 people died of the disease.[1] The average lifetime risk of developing CRC is 6%, with men and women almost equally affected. CRCs typically develop from adenomatous polyps which progress from small to large (>1 cm) size, and then to high-grade dysplasia and cancer. This progression from adenoma to carcinoma is believed to take at least 10 years.[2] The slow transition from polyps to CRC in most patients allows opportunities to prevent cancer by removing polyps, and to prevent cancer death by finding and removing early cancers. Several screening tests are available and well established, each with advantages and limitations. Although stool-based tests improve disease prognosis mainly by detecting early stage cancers, endoscopic and radiologic tests that visualize the bowel mucosa have the potential to also prevent cancer by detecting polyps that can be removed before malignant transformation. This article discusses the potential role of computed tomographic colonography (CTC) in a CRC screening program by first providing a brief review of current screening recommendations and traditional screening options, followed by a discussion of specific CTC test characteristics, economics and implementation issues that may affect the adoption and positioning of CTC within the overall framework of CRC screening.

CRC SCREENING: PREVALENCE AND BARRIERS

Despite considerable evidence supporting the effectiveness of CRC screening and the availability of various screening tests, half of the US population aged 50 years

Digestive Health Specialists, 3209 South 23rd Street, Suite 340, Tacoma, WA 98405, USA
E-mail address: klausmergener@aol.com

Gastrointest Endoscopy Clin N Am 20 (2010) 367–377
doi:10.1016/j.giec.2010.02.008
1052-5157/10/$ – see front matter © 2010 Elsevier Inc. All rights reserved.

and older is still not undergoing CRC screening according to 2005 estimates from the National Health Interview Survey.[3] This compares with more than 80% of eligible women participating in breast cancer screening programs. The prevalence rates for CRC screening are lower among people aged 50 to 64 years and especially low among individuals who are nonwhite, have fewer years of education, lack health insurance coverage, and are recent immigrants. These low rates cannot be attributed to any single factor (such as fear of undergoing colonoscopy) but are related to a variety of issues including lack of public knowledge about the importance of screening and testing options, lack of time, fear of being diagnosed with cancer, embarrassment, unpleasantness of the test, as well as concerns about costs. Health insurance barriers such as insurance status and coverage limitations are also significant factors. Although the addition of new and potentially less invasive screening tests such as CTC may overcome some of these barriers, they are unlikely to resolve all of them. Their effect on overall screening rates and the costs of screening can therefore not be easily predicted and need to be carefully studied and evaluated over time.

CURRENT RECOMMENDATIONS FOR CRC SCREENING

For more than 2 decades, CRC screening guidelines have been independently developed and updated by multiple organizations. Recently, 2 new sets of guidelines were published. One was developed by the American Cancer Society, the US Multisociety Task Force on Colorectal Cancer (a consortium representing the American College of Gastroenterology, the American Society of Gastrointestinal Endoscopy, the American Gastroenterological Association, and representation from the American College of Physicians), and the American College of Radiology (ACS-MSTF-ACR).[4] The other guideline was developed by the US Preventive Services Task Force (USPSTF).[5] The recommendations from these 2 guidelines are detailed in **Table 1**. Although their conclusions are similar, they differ in several specific recommendations, especially as they relate to CTC. To put these recommendations into the appropriate context, the traditional CRC screening tests are briefly reviewed.

Fecal Occult Blood Tests

Fecal occult blood testing (FOBT) is most commonly performed using a guaiac-based test that detects peroxidase activity of heme in small stool samples. These tests can be performed at home, are noninvasive, have a low initial cost, and require few specialized resources. Colonoscopy should be recommended if FOBT is positive, and testing should be done annually if the results are negative. One-time testing (3 samples) with a standard guaiac test has a sensitivity for advanced neoplasia of only 33% to 50%,[4] whereas a more sensitive guaiac test (Hemoccult Sensa) has a sensitivity of 50% to 75%.[6,7] The Minnesota Colorectal Cancer Control Trial showed that individuals who were screened with FOBT on an annual basis experienced a 33% reduction in CRC mortality with 38% of these individuals undergoing colonoscopy at some point during the 13-year study.[8]

Immunochemical-based FOBT tests use antibodies against human hemoglobin or other blood components and are therefore more specific for human blood. Their sensitivity for detecting cancer ranges from 60% to 85% but the performance of different commercially available tests has varied considerably leaving many questions with regard to the optimal test and the required number of stool samples.[9]

Stool DNA testing is based on the detection of specific mutations associated with CRC in DNA which is excreted in stool. Advantages include the potential for high

Table 1
US colorectal cancer screening guidelines 2008

Screening Test	ACS-MSTF-ACR	USPSTF	Recommended Interval for Rescreening
Sensitive guaiac fecal occult blood test	Recommended if >50% sensitivity for CRC	Recommended	1 y
Fecal immunochemical test	Recommended if >50% sensitivity for CRC	Recommended, high-sensitivity test only	1 y
Stool DNA test	Recommended if >50% sensitivity for CRC	Not recommended (insufficient evidence to assess sensitivity and specificity of fecal DNA)	Uncertain
Flexible sigmoidoscopy	Recommended if sigmoidoscope is inserted to 40 cm of the colon or to the splenic flexure	Recommended; with guaiac fecal occult blood test every 3 y	5 y
Barium enema examination	Recommended, but only if other tests not available	Not recommended	5 y
Colonoscopy	Recommended	Recommended	10 y
CTC	Recommended, with referral for colonoscopy if polyps ≥6 mm in diameter detected	Not recommended (insufficient evidence to determine risk-benefit ratio)	5 y

ACS-MSTF-ACR, American Cancer Society, US Multisociety Task Force on Colorectal Cancer, and American College of Radiology; USPSTF, US Preventive Services Task Force.
Data from Lieberman, DA. Screening for colorectal cancer. N Engl J Med 2009;361:1179–87.

test accuracy, the theoretic ability to detect cancers proximal to the colon, and the relative noninvasiveness of the test. However, the lack of data from screening populations, and the high cost of the currently available versions of the test limit its usefulness at this time.[10]

Barium Enema

Double contrast barium enema (DCBE) is no longer a recommended CRC screening modality according to the USPSTF guideline, and is only noted as a secondary modality in the ACS-MSTF-ACR guideline. DCBE identifies most late-stage cancers but cannot detect clinically important precursor lesions with any accuracy. It is rarely used as a screening tool in today's practice.

Sigmoidoscopy

Sigmoidoscopy allows for direct visualization of the bowel lumen and the ability to take a biopsy or remove lesions at the time of the procedure. Adenomas found during sigmoidoscopy often prompt full colonoscopy with subsequent detection of premalignant or malignant lesions in the portion of the colon not seen with the sigmoidoscope.

It is estimated that approximately half of all polyps and cancers are within reach of a flexible sigmoidoscope and that the prevalence of advanced proximal neoplasia in patients without distal adenomas is around 2% to 5%. An often-quoted case-control study found a 59% reduction in CRC mortality for cancers within the reach of the sigmoidoscope but no benefit of sigmoidoscopy with respect to mortality from cancers beyond the reach of the instrument.[11] A large randomized controlled trial found no reduction in the incidence of colorectal cancer among individuals assigned to screening sigmoidoscopy, and in an intention-to-treat analysis, there was only a nonsignificant reduction in mortality at 6 years among these individuals compared with controls.[12] Sigmoidoscopy requires a bowel preparation, an office visit, and it is not well reimbursed relative to the required resources. For many patients and physicians, colonoscopy has therefore become a more appealing option.

Colonoscopy

Colonoscopy is an attractive screening tool because it offers the ability to visualize the entire colon in most patients and to detect, take a biopsy, and/or remove mucosal lesions in 1 setting. Colonoscopy is also the final common pathway for the evaluation of other positive screening tests. The American College of Gastroenterology guidelines for CRC screening list colonoscopy as the preferred screening modality.[13] The sensitivity and specificity of colonoscopy are difficult to measure because colonoscopy is often considered to be the gold standard. However, tandem colonoscopy studies have shown that 0% to 6% of large polyps ($\geq$1 cm) are missed and up to 27% of smaller lesions are missed.[14] Several large cohort studies have shown the feasibility and safety of colonoscopy as a primary screening test.[15–17] These studies show that among patients at average risk who undergo screening colonoscopy, 0.5% to 1% have colon cancer and 5% to 10% have advanced neoplasia that can be removed. No randomized controlled trials have compared the outcomes of colonoscopy with those of other forms of screening. In case-control studies, colonoscopy is associated with reductions in the incidence of and mortality from CRC. The recommended 10-year interval for repeat examination is based on case-control studies.[18,19]

GUIDELINE RECOMMENDATIONS RELATED TO CTC

Although the USPSTF and the ACS-MSTF-ACR reviewed the same evidence and similar decision models, these consensus groups reached different conclusions with regard to CTC (see **Table 1**). A commentary accompanying the USPSTF publication suggests that subtle differences in emphasis may underlie the differing conclusions. The USPSTF judged the evidence for CTC to be insufficient to evaluate its benefits and harms. This guideline put more emphasis on the unknown effects of radiation exposure and the potential for harm caused by the evaluation of extracolonic findings, taking a more longitudinal perspective. In contrast, the ACS-MSTF-ACR guidelines include CTC as a recommended screening option with a suggested interval of testing every 5 years. They focus on the capability of CTC to detect large polyps in a single screening visit and as such favor screening technologies with superior single screening detection characteristics over less sensitive tests, based in part on the presumption that the availability of additional methods of screening will improve compliance.

FACTORS INFLUENCING THE ADOPTION OF CTC AS A SCREENING TOOL

If CTC can be demonstrated to be effective, safe, and economically viable, and if it increases patients' acceptance of CRC screening, its addition to the list of screening options will be a positive development from a public health perspective. Whether CTC will be widely adopted as a screening tool is not entirely clear at the time of this writing and will depend, among other factors, on the demonstration of its accuracy outside of tertiary referral centers, the availability of testing facilities and trained readers, a proven safety record of the test itself and the follow-up studies it triggers, its associated costs, and coverage determinations by insurance carriers. Some of these issues are reviewed in the following sections.

Accuracy of CTC

The performance of CTC relative to colonoscopy is discussed in greater detail in other articles in this issue. Early studies of CTC typically involved smaller numbers of individuals at higher risk for colorectal disease and did not always control well for interpreter experience and technical factors. Initial, large, multicenter trials yielded variable results with regard to the sensitivity for polyp detection.[20–22] CTC technology and techniques have since evolved at a rapid pace and it is not appropriate to simply combine results from those older studies with newer ones.

The largest study of a screening population, the American College of Radiology Imaging Network (ACRIN) trial, was recently published and showed favorable results.[23] The primary aim of the trial was to evaluate the sensitivity of CTC compared with colonoscopy, for detecting individuals with a clinically significant lesion, defined as larger than 10 mm. The study found a 90% sensitivity and an 86% specificity of CTC for polyps 10 mm or larger. The positive and negative predictive values were 23% and 99%, respectively. Many of the current conclusions about the potential role of CTC as a screening tool rely on the generalizability of this trial to general screening populations and community radiologists. Important features of the trial included large number of enrolled individuals (>2500), multiple institutions (n = 15), minimum 16-slice CT scanner, stool tagging, and comparison of several commonly used bowel preparation regimens. It should be noted that the ACRIN trial featured a strict training and operator qualifying examination component. Each participating radiologist was required to submit confirmation of having interpreted at least 500 CTC examinations or having participated in a specialized 1.5-day CTC training session. In addition, all participating radiologists were required to complete a qualifying examination in which they achieved a detection rate of 90% or more for polyps measuring 10 mm or more in diameter in a reference image set. The importance of adequate training of CTC readers for the effectiveness of the technique has now been widely acknowledged,[24,25] and it remains to be seen if similar high reading performance can be achieved in everyday clinical practice.

Translating this diagnostic sensitivity to an inference of effectiveness for preventing colon cancer mortality requires the same chain of logic that supports colonoscopy as an effective screening test. Thus, it can be assumed that a test that approaches the sensitivity of colonoscopy for the detection of clinically relevant polyps should logically approach the clinical effectiveness of colonoscopy as well. However, several other differences between colonoscopy and CTC regarding comfort, convenience, screening intervals, and other ancillary health outcomes are difficult to quantify. Although they may be viewed as minor, patients should be adequately informed of these differences, as these may influence the ultimate choice of the screening procedure.

Patient Preference

How CTC is perceived and tolerated will play an important role in its ultimate acceptance as a screening tool. Studies on patient preference for various colon imaging procedures have yielded mixed results with some studies showing a preference for CTC and others concluding that colonoscopy is the preferred test.[20–22,26,27] Current CTC techniques require meticulous bowel preparation analogous to that required for colonoscopy. Feasibility studies are being performed to evaluate if electronically subtractable fecal markers could be used to allow detection of polyps without a colon preparation. The elimination of the need for a purgative preparation would certainly further enhance the appeal of CTC, but these techniques are not currently ready for widespread use.[28,29] Although it requires a full bowel cleansing similar to that required for colonoscopy, CTC is usually done without sedation, may be faster to perform than colonoscopy and might therefore be more attractive to some patients. To what degree these differences will serve to enhance screening compliance remains to be determined. Presumably, the availability of same-day colonoscopy, if needed to remove polyps found on CTC, will be important to individuals who do not want to undergo a second colon preparation on a separate day. As outlined in the article by Cash in this issue, the number of cases requiring same-day colonoscopy can be anticipated to be small, but close coordination between radiology and gastroenterology units will be required. According to the ACRIN trial, 12% of patients would be referred for colonoscopy if the lesion threshold was 6 mm or larger (as recommended in the ACS-MSTF-ACR guideline), with approximately 4% of individuals exhibiting lesions of 10 mm or larger.[23]

Safety

CTC is well tolerated. Colon insufflation has been associated with a small risk of perforation, but most of these complications occurred in symptomatic patients who underwent manual air insufflation as opposed to automated low-pressure carbon dioxide insufflation.[30,31] The International Working Group on Virtual Colonoscopy reported no perforations in more than 11,000 screening CTC examinations and 1 perforation in 22,000 screening and diagnostic CTC examinations.[32]

Another risk associated with CTC relates to radiation exposure, especially in patients who are obese and in those undergoing repeated examinations to follow up on small polyps left in situ.[33] A routine CT scan of the abdomen administers a radiation dose of approximately 15 milliSievert (mSv). The dose of a CTC is less, but estimating the precise risk to the individual is difficult. In one model that used typical current scanner techniques, an approximately 0.14% increased lifetime cancer risk was calculated for a 50-year-old patient undergoing a single CTC.[33] Imaging techniques using lower-dose radiation are currently being studied.[34,35] Highly publicized studies on the potential hazards and uncertain risk-benefit ratios of ionizing radiation exposure during medical imaging[36] may well contribute to the reluctance on the part of the public and some health professionals to consider screening modalities based on x-rays.

Effect of Extraluminal Findings

CTC can detect extracolonic lesions of varying importance (eg, calcifications, gallstones, hernias, bone lesions, abdominal aortic aneurysms, and benign and malignant tumors).[37–39] The effect of these extraluminal findings has not fully been assessed, nor has its effect on cost-effectiveness. Although the opportunity to find and treat serious problems such as abdominal aortic aneurysms, renal cancers, and ovarian cancers in asymptomatic patients may be important, it is unclear if these discoveries change mortality (except for aortic aneurysms). Flicker and colleagues[40] suggested that the incremental cost may be minimal if strict parameters are implemented for triggering additional evaluations, but further studies are needed to better understand the effect of these extracolonic findings as well as the benefits and costs of their work-up.

Cost-effectiveness

Cost-effectiveness assessments for screening tests are complex and need to include the costs associated with the original test, as well as the costs associated with the evaluation of positive test results, surveillance, complications, and the costs of cancers not avoided. Several cost-effectiveness models have been developed for screening CTC.[41–45] Although some studies have found CTC to be a cost-effective screening strategy, others have suggested that it will not be as cost-effective as colonoscopy. These models are sensitive to CTC performance characteristics, presumed costs of various interventions, and the threshold for referring patients for colonoscopy. Many were based on older CTC studies and are now outdated. As screening CTC becomes more widely adopted, additional analyses using more up-to-date inputs will be needed to more accurately assess the cost-effectiveness of CTC.

Insurance Coverage

Reimbursement for CTC in general, and coverage of screening CTC in particular, remains highly variable but payor decisions are increasingly favorable. In May 2009, the Center for Medicare and Medicaid Services (CMS) issued a noncoverage decision stating that "the evidence is inadequate to conclude that CT colonography is an appropriate colorectal cancer screening."[46] This noncoverage decision by the largest US payor undoubtedly slowed the adoption of CTC as a screening test. The CMS decision notwithstanding, many health insurance plans are now covering CTC for screening and/or for a variety of other indications. To some degree, coverage by private payors is driven by state laws, now in place in 26 States and the District of Columbia,[47] mandating coverage for CRC screening services.

The Blue Cross/Blue Shield Technology Evaluation Center (TEC), a group of research scientists and medical advisors who provide comprehensive evaluations of the clinical effectiveness and appropriateness of medical procedures, devices or drugs, recently revised its initial negative assessment and concluded that CTC for the purpose of colon cancer screening meets their TEC criteria.[48] The California Technology Assessment Forum (CTAF), a public service forum spearheaded by the Blue Shield of California Foundation, which assesses new and emerging medical technologies, concluded in their March 2009 assessment of CTC that "...despite the exciting results of the ACRIN trial, several important questions remain before CTC can be recommended for widespread use. First, how well would it perform in a setting where the radiologists were not so highly trained. Second, what is the clinical impact of the possible harms of the procedure, including radiation risk (especially with CTC repeated periodically) and the high incidence of extracolonic findings? Thus, despite its diagnostic accuracy, because the impact of the potential harms is not currently known, CTC is not currently recommended for screening asymptomatic individuals for CRC."[49]

The Current Procedural Terminology (CPT) Panel of the American Medical Association established category I CPT codes for CT colonography in January 2010. CPT 74263 now describes screening CTC, and CPT 74261 and CPT 74262 are to be used to describe diagnostic CTC without and with contrast, respectively. The existence of category I CPT codes does not immediately equate to insurance coverage and payment for these services, but their existence facilitates reporting of a service, indicates to third parties that a service has become more established, and as such often prompts carriers to reevaluate previous coverage decisions.

IMPLEMENTATION ISSUES

Before CTC can be implemented as a screening tool on a more widespread basis, several additional pragmatic and logistical issues have to be addressed.[50] The first relates to the number of centers and qualified readers required to perform CTC on a widespread basis. With some 40 to 60 million Americans eligible for a colon cancer screening examination and in excess of 10 million colonoscopies performed each year, there is a high demand for screening services. It has been estimated that although the number of multidetector CT facilities in the United States may be adequate, there are currently no more than a few hundred highly trained readers; there will be a demand for several thousand readers if this screening volume is to be met.[50]

Another issue has to do with whether and how to report polypoid lesions at the time of CTC. Should small lesions (<5–6 mm) be ignored and not reported as some have suggested?[45] Although the rate of malignancy in such small lesions is likely very small, it is not zero, and leaving small polyps in place and following these patients with serial CTC examinations would represent a fundamental departure from current screening paradigms. The optimal surveillance protocol for this situation has not been established, and cumulative costs, procedural risks, and radiation exposure from serial CTC examinations would have to be considered. More research is needed in these areas, especially as it relates to flat lesions, right colonic hyperplastic polyps, and certain types of serrated adenomas where size alone may not be the key determinant of neoplastic risk.[51] It remains unclear whether patients and providers would accept a practice in which patients are given a choice as to whether or not to remove certain lesions or leave them in place and follow them on a regular basis. Studies of this issue have yielded conflicting results.[52,53]

The potential effects of CTC adoption on colonoscopy rates has been hotly debated. Is CTC attractive enough as a new screening modality to increase the proportion of those being screened, or will it simply divert those who are already being screened from one test to another? Will it lead to a decrease in the number of colonoscopies being performed or increase the number of therapeutic examinations being done for removal of polyps that were detected on CTC? To some degree, the answer to the latter question depends on the threshold set for triggering a colonoscopy[50]; although a polyp size threshold of greater than 10 mm might lead to fewer follow-up colonoscopies, a reduced polyp size threshold, if coupled with an increased number of individuals recruited for CRC screening, would likely lead to a significant demand for follow-up colonoscopies.

As mentioned previously, any implementation of a CTC screening program will benefit from a close collaboration between radiologists and gastroenterologists with regard to triaging individuals to the various available screening methods, arrangements for same-day colonoscopy if required, patient education about test results, and follow-up arrangements.

SUMMARY

In summary, CTC has become well established as a new technology for large bowel imaging. Following favorable results in recent large-scale trials, CTC is gaining acceptance among patients, clinicians, professional societies, and third party payors as a viable option for CRC screening. It remains to be determined, however, whether CTC will ultimately become a preferred screening tool or play a secondary role within CRC screening programs. High test accuracies need to be replicated in community practice settings, and additional testing facilities and highly trained readers are required to meet demand. Various patient and provider concerns still need to be addressed with regard to safety issues, and optimal management algorithms need to be determined for lesions found on CTC. Additional favorable coverage determinations and reimbursement decisions from third party payors will also further promote the widespread adoption of CTC as a screening tool.

REFERENCES

1. Jemal A, Siegel R, Ward E, et al. Cancer statistics, 2009. CA Cancer J Clin 2009; 59:225–49.
2. Winawer SJ, Fletcher RH, Miller L, et al. Colorectal cancer screening: clinical guidelines and rationale. Gastroenterology 1997;112:594–642.
3. Centers for Disease Control and Prevention, National Center for Health Statistics. 2005 National Health Interview Survey. Public Use Data File. Available at: http://wonder.cdc.gov/wonder/sci_data/surveys/nhis/type_txt/nhis2005/NHIS2005.asp. Accessed March 1, 2010.
4. Levin B, Lieberman DA, McFarland B, et al. Screening and surveillance for the early detection of colorectal cancer and adenomatous polyps, 2008: a joint guideline from the American Cancer Society, the US Multi-Society Task Force on Colorectal Cancer, and the American College of Radiology. CA Cancer J Clin 2008;58:130–60.
5. U.S. Preventive Services Task Force. Screening for colorectal cancer: U.S. preventive services task force recommendation statement. Ann Intern Med 2008;149:627–37.
6. Lieberman DA. Screening for colorectal cancer. N Engl J Med 2009;361:1179–87.
7. Allison JE, Sakoda LC, Levin TR, et al. Screening for colorectal neoplasms with new fecal occult blood tests: update on performance characteristics. J Natl Cancer Inst 2007;99:1462–70.
8. Mandel JS, Bond JH, Church TR, et al. Reducing mortality from colorectal cancer by screening for fecal occult blood. Minnesota Colon Cancer Control Study. N Engl J Med 1993;328:1365–71.
9. Hundt S, Haug U, Brenner H. Comparative evaluation of immunochemical fecal occult blood tests for colorectal adenoma detection. Ann Intern Med 2009;150: 162–9.
10. Levin B, Brooks D, Smith RA, et al. Emerging technologies in screening for colorectal cancer. CA Cancer J Clin 2003;53:44–55.
11. Selby JV, Friedman GD, Quesenberry CP Jr, et al. A case-control study of screening sigmoidoscopy and mortality from colorectal cancer. N Engl J Med 1992;326:653–7.
12. Hoff G, Grotmol T, Skoulund E, et al. Risk of colorectal cancer seven years after flexible sigmoidoscopy screening: randomized controlled trial. BMJ 2009;338: 1846–57.
13. Rex DK, Johnson DA, Anderson JC, et al. American College of Gastroenterology guidelines for colorectal cancer screening 2008. Am J Gastroenterol 2009;104: 739–50.
14. Rex DK, Cutler CS, Lemmel GT, et al. Colonoscopic miss rates of adenomas determined by back-to-back colonoscopies. Gastroenterology 1997;112:24–8.
15. Lieberman DA, Weiss DG, Bond JH, et al. Use of colonoscopy to screen asymptomatic adults for colorectal cancer. N Engl J Med 2000;343:162–8.
16. Imperiale TF, Wagner DR, Lin CY, et al. Risk of advanced proximal neoplasms in asymptomatic adults according to the distal colorectal findings. N Engl J Med 2000;343:169–74.

17. Regula J, Rupinski M, Kraszewska E, et al. Colonoscopy in colorectal cancer screening for detection of advanced neoplasia. N Engl J Med 2006;355: 1863–72.
18. Lieberman DA, Weiss DG, Harford WV, et al. Five year colon surveillance after screening colonoscopy. Gastroenterology 2007;133:1077–85.
19. Imperiale TF, Glowinski EA, Lin-Cooper C, et al. Five-year risk of colorectal neoplasia after negative screening colonoscopy. N Engl J Med 2008;359: 1218–24.
20. Pickhardt PJ, Choi JR, Hwang I, et al. Computed tomographic virtual colonoscopy to screen for colorectal neoplasia in asymptomatic adults. N Engl J Med 2003;349:2191–200.
21. Cotton PB, Durkalski VL, Pineau BC, et al. Computed tomographic colonography (virtual colonoscopy): a multicenter comparison with standard colonoscopy for detection of colorectal neoplasia. JAMA 2004;291:1713–9.
22. Rockey DC, Paulson E, Niedzwiecki D, et al. Analysis of air contrast barium enema, computed tomographic colonography, and colonoscopy: prospective comparison. Lancet 2005;365:305–11.
23. Johnson CD, Chen MH, Toledano AY, et al. Accuracy of CT colonography for detection of large adenomas and cancers. N Engl J Med 2008;359:1207–17.
24. McFarland EG, Fletcher JG, Pickhardt PJ, et al. ACR colon cancer committee white paper: status of CT colonography 2009. J Am Coll Radiol 2009;6: 756–72.
25. Johnson CD. CT colonography: coming of age. AJR Am J Roentgenol 2009;193: 1239–42.
26. Van Gelder RE, Birnie E, Florie J, et al. CT colonography and colonoscopy: assessment of patient preference in a 5-week follow-up study. Radiology 2004; 233:328–37.
27. Bosworth HB, Rockey DC, Paulson EK, et al. Prospective comparison of patient experience with colon imaging tests. Am J Med 2006;119:791–9.
28. Iannaccone R, Laghi A, Catalano C, et al. Computed tomographic colonography without cathartic preparation for the detection of colorectal polyps. Gastroenterology 2004;127:1300–11.
29. Zalis ME, Perumpillichira JJ, Magee C, et al. Tagging-based, electronically cleansed CT colonography: evaluation of patient comfort and image readability. Radiology 2006;239:149–59.
30. Burling D, Halligan S, Slater A, et al. Potentially serious adverse events at CT colonography in symptomatic patients: national survey of the United Kingdom. Radiology 2006;239:464–71.
31. Sosna J, Blanchar A, Amitai M, et al. Colonic perforation at CT colonography: assessment of risk in a multicenter large cohort. Radiology 2006;239:457–63.
32. Pickhardt PJ. Incidence of colonic perforation at CT colonography: review of existing data and implications for screening of asymptomatic adults. Radiology 2006;239:313–6.
33. Brenner DJ, Georgsson MA. Mass screening with CT colonography: should the radiation exposure be of concern? Gastroenterology 2005;129:328–37.
34. Iannaccone R, Laghi A, Catalano C, et al. Feasibility of ultra-low-dose multislice CT colonography for the detection of colorectal lesions: preliminary experience. Eur Radiol 2003;13:1297–302.
35. Vogt C, Cohnen M, Beck A, et al. Detection of colorectal polyps by multislice CT colonography with ultra-low-dose technique: comparison with high-resolution videocolonoscopy. Gastrointest Endosc 2004;60:201–9.

36. Fazel R, Krumholz HM, Wang Y, et al. Exposure to low-dose ionizing radiation from medical imaging procedures. N Engl J Med 2009;361:849–57.
37. Gluecker TM, Johnson CD, Wilson LA, et al. Extracolonic findings at CT colonography: evaluation of prevalence and cost in a screening population. Gastroenterology 2003;124:911–6.
38. Pickhardt PJ, Taylor AJ. Extracolonic findings identified in asymptomatic adults at screening CT colonography. AJR Am J Roentgenol 2006;186:718–28.
39. Tolan DJ, Armstrong EM, Chapman AH. Replacing barium enema with CT colonography in patients older than 70 years: the importance of detecting extracolonic abnormalities. AJR Am J Roentgenol 2007;189:1104–11.
40. Flicker MS, Tsoukas AT, Hazra A, et al. Economic impact of extracolonic findings at computed tomographic colonography. J Comput Assist Tomogr 2008;32:497–503.
41. Hassan C, Zullo A, Laghi A, et al. Colon cancer prevention in Italy: cost-effectiveness analysis with CT colonography and endoscopy. Dig Liver Dis 2007;39: 242–50.
42. Vijan S, Hwang I, Inadomi J, et al. The cost-effectiveness of CT colonography in screening for colorectal neoplasia. Am J Gastroenterol 2007;102:380–90.
43. Hur C, Chung DC, Schoen RE, et al. The management of small polyps found by virtual colonoscopy: results of a decision analysis. Clin Gastroenterol Hepatol 2007;5:237–44.
44. Pickhardt PJ, Hassan C, Laghi A, et al. Small and diminutive polyps detected at screening CT colonography: a decision analysis for referral to colonoscopy. AJR Am J Roentgenol 2008;190:136–44.
45. Pickhardt PJ, Hassan C, Laghi A, et al. Cost-effectiveness of colorectal cancer screening with computed tomography colonography: the impact of not reporting diminutive lesions. Cancer 2007;109:2213–21.
46. Centers for Medicare and Medicaid Services. Decision memo for screening computed tomography colonography (CTC) for colorectal cancer (CAG-00396N). Available at: https://www.cms.hhs.gov/mcd/viewdecisionmemo.asp?id=220. Accessed January 26, 2010.
47. American Cancer Society. Colorectal cancer facts & figures 2008–2010. American Cancer Society; 2008. Available at: http://www.cancer.org/downloads/STT/F861708_finalforweb.pdf. Accessed January 26, 2010.
48. Blue Cross Blue Shield Association Technology Evaluation Center. CT colonography ("virtual colonoscopy") for colon cancer screening. Available at: http://www.bcbs.com/blueresources/tec/vols/24/24_01.pdf. Accessed January 26, 2010.
49. California Technology Assessment Forum. Computed tomographic colonography (virtual colonoscopy) for colorectal cancer screening in average risk individuals. Available at: http://www.ctaf.org/files/989_file_VC_final_W.pdf. Accessed January 26, 2010.
50. Rockey DC. Computed tomographic colonography: current perspectives and future directions. Gastroenterology 2009;137:7–17.
51. Soetikno RM, Kaltenbach T, Rouse RV, et al. Prevalence of nonpolypoid (flat and depressed) colorectal neoplasms in asymptomatic and symptomatic adults. JAMA 2008;299:1027–35.
52. Pickhardt PJ, Taylor AJ, Kim DH, et al. Screening for colorectal neoplasia with CT colonography: initial experience from the 1st year of coverage by third-party payers. Radiology 2006;241:417–25.
53. Shah JP, Hynan LS, Rockey DC. Management of small polyps detected by screening CT colonography: patient and physician preferences. Am J Med 2009;122(687):e1–9.

Establishing a CT Colonography Service

Brooks D. Cash, MD[a,b,c,*]

KEYWORDS

• CT colonography • Medical practice • Colon cancer screening

Computed tomographic colonography (CTC) has been recommended by the American Cancer Society, the Multi-Society Task Force on Colorectal Cancer (MSTF), and the American College of Radiology as an appropriate first-line preventative screening test for people at average risk of developing colorectal cancer (CRC).[1] However, the debate regarding the merits of this form of CRC screening continues to rage, pitting several of the gastroenterological professional societies at odds with various radiological societies and with different recommendations from various guideline issuers such as the MSTF and the United States Preventive Services Task Force (USPSTF). In their entirety, the clinical trial data comparing CTC to colonoscopy in patients undergoing CRC screening are mixed, but the most recent and methodologically rigorous trials have concluded that CTC is comparable to colonoscopy for the detection of polyps 10 mm in diameter or larger.[2–5] Proponents of CTC point to these trials as well as national CRC screening adherence rates that hover around 50%, as reasons to promote screening with CTC as an equivalent option to existing modalities. Opponents of CTC cite the more variable performance characteristics of CTC compared with colonoscopy for the detection of polyps of less than 10 mm and a myriad of other unknowns that are inherent to CTC, such as the potential impact of extracolonic findings, radiation exposure, and cost-effectiveness, to bolster their argument that CTC is not ready for widespread adoption as a first-line CRC screening option.[6]

The opinions and assertions contained herein are the sole views of the authors and should not be construed as official or as representing the views of the US Navy, Department of Defense, or Department of Veteran Affairs.

[a] Department of Medicine, Uniformed Services University of the Health Sciences, 4301 Jones Bridge Road, Bethesda, MD, USA

[b] Gastroenterology Service, National Naval Medical Center, 8901 Wisconsin Avenue, Building 9, Bethesda, MD, USA

[c] Department of Medicine, Walter Reed Army Medical Center, 6900 Georgia Avenue, NW, Washington, DC 20307, USA

* Gastroenterology Service, National Naval Medical Center, 8901 Wisconsin Avenue, Building 9, Bethesda, MD 20889.

E-mail address: brooks.cash@med.navy.mil

Gastrointest Endoscopy Clin N Am 20 (2010) 379–398
doi:10.1016/j.giec.2010.02.016
1052-5157/10/$ – see front matter. Published by Elsevier Inc.

giendo.theclinics.com

Over the past 12 months several decisions pertaining to the practice of CTC were made that promise to have wide-ranging effects on the practice of CTC in the future. The first was the decision of the Centers for Medicare and Medicaid (CMS) to deny coverage for screening CTC under Medicare rules.[7] The rationale for this decision was the relative lack of outcomes data for Medicare aged patients undergoing screening CTC as well as many of the unknowns cited above.[8] Efforts are currently underway to provide this evidence in the hope that this decision will ultimately be reversed. During 2009, the American Gastroenterological Association (AGA) and the American College of Radiology (ACR) jointly submitted a request to the American Medical Association (AMA) current procedural terminology (CPT) Editorial Panel to establish category I CPT codes for screening and diagnostic CTC, and provided physician work and practice expense recommendations to CMS through the AMA/Specialty Society RBRVS Update Committee (AMA RUC). The details of this decision were released in November 2009. CTC was assigned 3 category I CPT codes, 2 for diagnostic CTC and 1 for screening CTC. Diagnostic CTC without contrast (74261) was assigned 2.4 relative value units (RVU), diagnostic CTC with contrast (74262) was assigned 2.5 RVU, and screening CTC (74263) was assigned 2.28 RVU. It should be noted that CMS disagrees with the AMA RUC–recommended values and believes the diagnostic CTC code without contrast should be comparable to the CTC screening code. CMS notes that the image post processing virtually has the same description of work-, pre-, intra-, and postservice time for which the AMA RUC recommended 2.28 work RVUs. Therefore CMS has assigned 2.28 work RVUs to CPT code 74261. CMS also notes that screening CTC is a noncovered service because it does not have the statutory authority that has been provided for mammography, diabetes, and CRC screening; this means that legislative action will be necessary to get the status of CTC screening changed to a covered service.

Finally, an updated version of the Blue Cross/Blue Shield Technology Evaluation Center (TEC) analysis of CTC was recently issued.[9] In the previous analysis from 2004, the TEC concluded that CTC did not meet their criteria to determine that there was adequate evidence to demonstrate that CTC screening is effective in reducing mortality from CRC. In the current analysis, bolstered by the data from several additional studies of screening and diagnostic CTC, the TEC concluded that CTC meets the criteria for a CRC screening test. The components of the TEC criteria are: (1) the technology must have final approval from the appropriate governmental regulatory bodies; (2) the scientific evidence must permit conclusions concerning the effect of the technology on health outcomes; (3) the technology must improve the net health outcome; (4) the technology must be as beneficial as any established alternatives; and (5) the improvement must be attainable outside investigational settings. Based on current evidence, it appears clear that the question is no longer if or when CTC is ready for prime time, but rather how CTC will be deployed into routine clinical practice in the United States. This article discusses the issues surrounding the intricacies of setting up a CTC practice.

ESTABLISHING A CTC PRACTICE: THE NNMC EXPERIENCE

The Colon Health Initiative (CHI) at the National Naval Medical Center (NNMC) was created in 2004 on the heels of the seminal article on CRC screening with CTC by Pickhardt and colleagues.[2] This study of more than 1200 patients compared primary CRC screening with CTC and subsequent blinded colonoscopy on the same day, and showed that CTC had statistically equivalent sensitivity to colonoscopy for adenomas 8 mm or larger. Shortly after publication of this article, investigators at NNMC received an appropriation from the US Congress to establish a CRC screening center with the goal of providing screening to all eligible beneficiaries (>250,000 eligible adults $\geq$ age 50 years) in the National Capitol Area (NCA). It was abundantly clear that the supply of qualified endoscopists at NNMC and the other military medical treatment facilities within the NCA were insufficient to meet this mandate, so the decision was made to support their efforts by offering what was thought to be the closest alternative to colonoscopy, CTC. Thus the CHI was born, with the plan to offer screening CTC as an alternative to colonoscopy in average-risk adults undergoing CRC screening.

The CHI hired and trained 2 experienced radiologists and purchased 2 multidetector computed tomography (CT) scanners. Dedicated CTC nurses and CT technicians were also hired and additional endoscopy unit nursing staff and endoscopists were hired in the expectation that colonoscopy volume would increase as the practice of CTC became more ingrained in the lexicons of patients and referring providers. From the outset, the CHI was incorporated as a division of the gastroenterology service at NNMC, due to the facts that patients were scheduled and educated regarding their CRC screening options and preparation within the gastroenterology spaces by gastroenterology nursing personnel and that CRC screening results in subsequent surveillance examinations in a substantial proportion of individuals. It was felt that the gastroenterology service had the requisite experience and content expertise to effect seamless follow-up in terms of CTC-generated colonoscopies as well as maintenance of surveillance recommendations and schedules for all patients undergoing CRC screening at NNMC. Finally, the potential research applications of this technology were recognized, and efforts to maximize the research yield of introducing screening CTC were concentrated within the gastroenterology service.

One of the first steps required in setting up this service was to convince the referring primary care providers that CTC was an acceptable alternative to colonoscopy for their patients. These efforts included advertising with articles about CRC screening and CTC in the hospital newspaper, a CHI Web site,[10] patient-oriented pamphlets strategically placed in the primary care spaces and pharmacy waiting area, aggressive signage at high-volume areas of the medical center, and scholarly activities such as grand rounds presentations and "road trips" to satellite care sites to explain the new center and referral rules. To this end, the process of scheduling CRC screening procedures was changed from a referral-based process to an open-access system whereby individuals could discuss their screening options with a scheduler on demand, either in person or over the telephone, without the requirement of a referral from their primary care provider. Finally, the decision for which form of CRC screening was put into the hands of the patient, with guidance from the schedulers based on algorithms devised collaboratively by the gastroenterology and radiology staff. Thus, even if the primary care provider explicitly stated that they preferred the patient to undergo colonoscopy, if a patient was eligible for CTC and elected to undergo this test rather than colonoscopy, a CTC was performed. This last practice was somewhat controversial when it was initiated, and the unique practice environment of our military medical system may preclude such an approach in the referral-based civilian world. Over time, however, this has become a nonissue and the acceptance of referring providers regarding the accuracy and value of screening CTC at the author's institution is now established after 5 years of operation.

CHI STANDARD OPERATING PROCEDURE

Obtaining CRC screening at the NNMC begins with patient exposure (either via consultation of self-referral) to the nursing staff in the scheduling office. The schedulers take accurate medical histories from patients and employ an algorithm developed jointly by gastroenterologists and radiologists that is largely based on the ACS-MSTF recommendations of 2008 to educate patients regarding their CRC screening options.[1] The schedulers recognize that not every patient, based on personal or family history, should undergo CTC and route patients to colonoscopy when it is judged to be the more appropriate screening test. By locating the scheduling personnel within the gastroenterology clinical spaces, questions regarding the appropriateness of CTC or colonoscopy can be immediately answered by deference to an on-site physician. **Fig. 1** depicts the current CRC screening algorithm in place at NNMC. The algorithm is a dynamic document that has changed over time based on specialists' experience and clinical confidence in CTC as a CRC screening modality. The most significant change has been the inclusion of patients undergoing polyp surveillance who have a personal history of nonadvanced adenomas (size <10 mm,

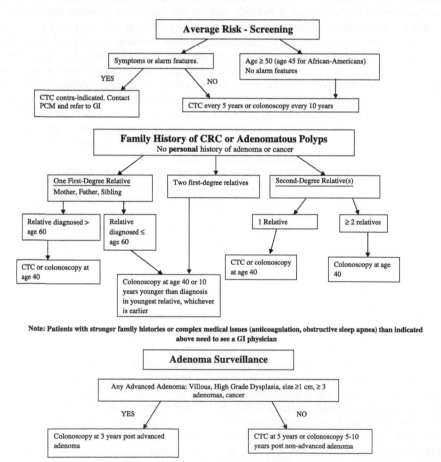

Fig. 1. CHI algorithm to determine eligibility for CTC. GI, gastrointestinal; PCM, primary care manager.

absence of villous, high-grade, or cancerous histology) found on previous examinations.

On arrival at the CHI, patients are escorted to the CTC spaces by one of the nurses. The nurse reviews the patient history and checks the electronic medical record for prior CRC screening examinations. Significant prior medical history is denoted for the radiologist, with special attention to absolute and relative contraindications to CTC screening, such as presentation within 6 weeks of the completion of antibiotics for diverticulitis. The nurse reiterates the specifics of the procedure, answers any questions the patient may have, and obtains informed consent for the procedure. Patients are given the option of undergoing colonoscopy, if clinically indicated, on the same day as the CTC or at a future date, based on their desires and schedules. For "same-day colonoscopy" CTC examinations, the radiologists interpret the CTC images real-time and patients receive their results within 15 to 20 minutes after completion of the CTC. If the results of the CTC interpretation are such that a colonoscopy is indicated, the presence of available escorts for transport home post colonoscopy are verified. The threshold for referral to colonoscopy is the presence of any polypoid or flat lesion suspicious for a polyp that is 6 mm or larger in diameter at its widest point as measured by electronic calipers. Nondiagnostic CTC examinations (largely avoidable with appropriate CTC technique) occur in approximately 1% of screening CTC in the author's experience.

Once the scan is completed, the nurse verifies that the patient is clinically stable. Patients who have not elected the same-day colonoscopy option are discharged. The CTC radiologists interpret images from these CTC examinations later in the day, once they have completed their interpretations of the same-day colonoscopy examinations. Once interpreted, all CTC results (intracolonic and extracolonic) are dictated into the hospital's radiology dictation system for subsequent transcription and viewing by other medical personnel within the hospital's electronic medical record. Results are transmitted to patients using a retrievable, server-based voice recording system that patients may access with a unique personalized identification number (PIN) that they are issued on a laminated card. This card also includes a contact number for the CHI personnel, in the event that patients have any postprocedure questions regarding their CTC or results. Finally, a hard copy of the CTC report is mailed to the patient with a cover letter reemphasizing recommendations resulting from the CTC. Any findings that require an additional study are documented in the electronic medical record based on the CTC reporting and data system (C-RADS) scheme,[11] the radiologist or nursing personnel contact the patients' primary care provider to ensure that potentially important findings are communicated.

Patients who do not wait for their results and who are found to require polypectomy are subsequently offered colonoscopy by CHI personnel with follow-up phone calls. Intracolonic findings concerning for prevalent malignancy are reported directly to the gastroenterology staff physician on duty, who contacts the patient to explain the CTC findings and need for colonoscopy. Because the clinical history has already been obtained in preparation of the CTC, colonoscopy for these patients is typically arranged without an intervening office visit, although patients with specific clinical issues pertaining to colonoscopy (sedation concerns or those requiring anticoagulation management) may be required to see a gastroenterologist before the colonoscopy is scheduled.

Approximately 10% of patients undergoing screening CTC receive a recommendation to proceed to colonoscopy. Among those patients, approximately 40% to 50% elect to undergo the procedures on the same day as the CTC. Thus, with a full schedule capacity of 25 to 30 patients undergoing CTC, the maximum number of colonoscopies that would typically need to be incorporated into the endoscopy schedule is 2 to 3 per day. Because the actual average number of patients undergoing CTC is closer to 15 to 20 per day, the endoscopy schedule remains largely unaffected. Standard procedure, however, is for the attending gastroenterology staff on duty to be available to perform any same-day colonoscopies. These colonoscopies are performed on a space-available basis, typically after the completion of morning procedures in a previously booked endoscopy room, in an unbooked endoscopy room when available, or over the lunch hour. The author has found that performing CTC from 6:30 AM to 12:30 PM is most popular with patients as well as endoscopy personnel, as this schedule permits the rapid disposition of CTC patients in the endoscopy suite prior to the afternoon and concentration of the latter part of the day for add-on inpatient or outpatient cases. The gastroenterology service uses the same PIN-based service for communication of laboratory and pathology results as well as subsequent recommendations arising from the colonoscopy. Sensitivity regarding the use of such a message retrieval system is emphasized to the clinical staff, and findings with serious implications (such as advanced neoplasia or frank CRC) are discussed one-on-one between the clinician and patient. All patients undergoing CRC screening at NNMC are entered into a CRC screening database for subsequent screening or surveillance scheduling in accordance with clinic guidelines.

As with intracolonic findings suggestive of malignancy, patients who are found to have concerning extracolonic findings referable to the digestive system are discussed immediately with a staff gastroenterologist. This discussion provides expeditious evaluation and close coordination of subsequent diagnostic testing (radiologic or otherwise), and likely helps to alleviate the concerns of the patient and the primary care provider regarding delay in the follow-up of these findings. The author believes that this process may prove to optimize clinical outcomes in some cases by minimizing the time between the discovery of extracolonic processes and eventual therapeutic interventions, although data to that effect are lacking and difficult to ascertain. In the author's experience, potentially significant extracolonic findings occur in 5% to 7% of patients undergoing CTC. The cost related to additional studies recommended as a result of these findings is between $20 and $30, and is kept low by comparing findings on the 2-dimensional (2D) CT images to prior examinationss when available and by adherence to the C-RAD reporting scheme[11] whereby further evaluation is recommended only for E3 or E4 findings. That CTC images are low-radiation, are not designed to evaluate regions of the body outside of the colon, and may miss important extracolonic lesions is included within the informed consent document that all patients undergoing CTC sign before the examination.

EQUIPMENT SPECIFICATIONS

Colonic insufflation is performed before image acquisition using air or carbon dioxide, which may reduce postprocedure cramping.[12] Colonic insufflation with automated insufflators results in improved colonic distention compared with manual insufflation.[13] Automatic insufflators may also be safer owing to preset ramped flow rates and automatic venting at predetermined intracolonic pressures.[14]

CT SCANNERS

Multislice CT scanners have several advantages over single-slice helical scanners for CTC. Faster tube rotation times and an increased number of detectors permit faster table speeds, so that a patient can be scanned in less time than on single-slice machines. Faster scanning is important because the patient is required to hold his or her breath during image acquisition, and may experience some discomfort as the colon is maximally inflated or produce respiratory artifacts with slower, single-slice helical CT scanners.[15] In addition, most multislice CT scanners are equipped with automatic exposure control, which varies the x-ray tube current over the body region as the patient travels through the scanner as well as the projection angle, resulting in significant dose savings for average-sized patients.[16,17]

While submillimeter slice thicknesses are now possible with newer CT systems, utilization of such slice thicknesses results in datasets of thousands of images, increases image noise, and will result in increased radiation dose if noise is held constant. Numerous phantom experiments have demonstrated that polyps 6 mm or greater in size can be detected using slice thicknesses of 3 mm or less, with narrower slice thicknesses potentially increasing lesion conspicuity.[18–20] Several large patient studies employing 2.5- or 3-mm slice thickness have demonstrated acceptable performance for detecting polyps 6 to 9 mm in size.[2,21,22]

CT images should be sent to a dedicated CT workstation for interpretation and should be archived as part of the medical record for future comparison purposes. Adequate CTC workstations permit the viewing of enlarged 2D images in multiple planes, 3-dimensional (3D) endoluminal navigation and interrogation, simultaneous viewing of 2D and 3D images, simultaneous viewing of supine and prone images, and variation of window/level settings and field of view size to examine intralesional attenuation and extracolonic tissues.[23] There are multiple software packages available for CTC display, and at the current time one cannot be stridently recommended over others. The choice of which CTC software package to employ will necessarily be based on professional and economic realities that will be unique to each practice setting.

TRAINING

CTC is currently indicated as a primary screening modality for CRC in asymptomatic adults, the evaluation of the colon proximal to an obstructing lesion, and after failure of colonoscopy advance to adequately complete CRC screening. For these reasons, proactive education and training of physicians in CTC is essential. Because published studies like the ACRIN trial[3] are technological comparisons performed by experts, there is a valid concern that if the relative sensitivity of CTC compared with colonoscopy is 90% in the hands of experts, it may be lower when the procedures are performed by "everyday" specialists. Certification criteria for participation in the ACRIN trial required that each participating radiologist submit confirmation of having interpreted at least 500 CTC examinations, or having participated in a specialized 1.5-day training course in CTC performance and interpretation. In addition, all participating radiologists in this trial were required to complete a qualifying examination in which they achieved a detection rate of at least 90% for polyps measuring 10 mm or greater in diameter in a reference image set.[3]

Because the health benefit of CTC screening depends on the skills of the individuals performing and interpreting the procedure, requirements for training and developing expertise have been formulated.[24] In one such evaluation of standardized CTC training, 7 novices (6 medical students and 1 abdominal imaging fellow) received intensive training that included 1 day of training similar to that provided to staff radiologists as well as computer self-assessment modules, reading assignments, expert observation, and independent evaluation of CTC training cases.[25] Post-training evaluation documented performance similar to that reported in the

CTC clinical trials noted earlier.[2-5] Another recent report also demonstrated that gastroenterologists can also read CTC with accuracy comparable to CTC trained radiologists, but their CTC interpretation in this study was limited to the intracolonic portion of CTC and the most accurate gastroenterology readers had undergone formal training in CTC, underscoring the value of such training.[26]

Minimum training in CTC requires the following: (1) formal hands-on training on CTC interpretation, (2) supervision with a CTC trained physician serving as a double-reader, and/or (3) correlation of CTC and endoscopy findings in patients who undergo both procedures. It has been proposed that CTC training for radiologists should include interpretation of 75 to 100 cases, along with the standardized training as outlined above, with subsequent proctoring and quality assessment.[27] Persistent learning for ongoing practical experience in CTC interpretation is required to maintain clinical competence, although the annual numbers required to maintain competence have not yet been specified.

The AGA summary recommendations found in the previous report, "Standards for Gastroenterologists for Performing and Interpreting Diagnostic Computed Tomographic Colonography," outlined the vision for gastroenterologist training to perform and interpret CTC.[28] Key Task Force recommendations related to basic requirements that gastroenterologists should meet included the following: interpretation of at least 75 endoscopically confirmed cases within 2 separate educational settings; participation in a mentored CTC training program through physical presence on site for 1 week involving direct observation of CTC data acquisition and interpretation; ongoing training, and self-assessment via formal CME-accredited CTC courses; and collaboration with radiologists to review the extracolonic portion of the CTC examination. There are also cognitive skills that are required for competence in CTC: knowledge of the physics of CT and radiation generation and exposure; the scanning principles and scanning modes for contrast-enhanced colonic imaging; the principles of colonic preparation and contrast administration for optimal CTC; the principles 2D and 3D colonic image interpretation; clinical guidelines for CRC screening in high- and low-risk patient populations; the natural history and clinical importance of small and large colorectal polyps; and familiarity with the range of extracolonic findings encountered during CTC.

At present, the ACR and AGA both offer CTC training courses. The AGA courses, directed toward gastroenterologists, consist of 2 meetings. The first is a beginner's course in which participants are exposed to 50 to 70 cases over 2 to 3 days. Education is enhanced by didactics and a post-test that is completed at the conclusion of the course. Students are also directed to 10 to 15 carefully selected manuscripts covering subjects critical to CTC, such as small polyps, current CRC screening guidelines, extracolonic findings, and cost-effectiveness analyses. This phase is followed by attendance at an advanced course (ideally occurring within 16 weeks of the beginner's CTC course) where participants are exposed to 50 to 70 additional cases that they review with more autonomy. A post-test is also completed after this 2-day course. Subsequent to these didactic and hands-on courses, mentored learning with at least 5 days of on-site observation of CTC data acquisition and interpretation is encouraged.

Due to the portable nature of CTC images, it is entirely conceivable that this training could be accomplished via Web-based learning. Such training could also allow for evaluation of competing software platforms as well as ongoing training and self-assessment. Finally, participation in a CTC data registry such as the one developed by the ACR[29] will likely be important for data acquisition regarding CTC utilization and outcomes in the community, and is also encouraged.

REGULATORY CONSIDERATIONS OF A CTC PRACTICE

Several regulatory issues affect the decision to perform CTC, including who can perform the service, who can interpret the images and bill for that service, and the need for risk management considerations.

Who can Perform CTC: Implications of Stark Laws

The first consideration with regard to who is allowed to perform CTC centers around the concept of self-referral. Concern that self-referral could corrupt the professional judgment of referring physicians and result in overuse or unnecessary use of items and services led to the 1972 Federal Anti-kickback Law.[30] Since its creation, the original anti-kickback statute has been revised to allow more than 20 exceptions or "safe harbors," such as for investments in group practices, small health care joint ventures, as well as space and equipment rental. In 1989 Congress passed the "Stark I" law, prohibiting a physician from referring Medicare patients to an entity for clinical laboratory services if the physician (or their imme-diate family member) has a financial relationship with that entity. In 1993, "Stark II" expanded the Medicare self-referral ban to prohibit physicians from referring "designated health services" to an entity with which the physician has a financial relationship, unless that financial relationship meets an exception.[31] The definition of "designated health services" is vitally important and includes, among other things, imaging services such as ultrasound, CT, magnetic resonance imaging, and nuclear medicine.[32] Sanctions for violating the Stark statutes are severe, including refunds to the Medicare program, civil monetary penalties, and even exclusion from the Medicare and Medicaid programs. Because CMS has decided not to cover screening CTC,[7] the practice is not currently subject to the Stark regulations, although prudence would dictate that individuals considering owner-ship and operation of a CTC center be familiar with the statutes in the event that CMS does elect to cover screening CTC in the future.

According to the Stark statute, "referral" includes the request by a physician for an item or service. When he or she personally performs a service, a physician does not make a referral. If, however, the service is provided by any other person, including the physician's employees, independent contractors, or other group practice members, a referral has been made. Stark prohibits referrals only if the physician has a financial relationship with the entity to which the referral is made. A financial relationship may consist of an ownership, investment interest, or compensation arrangement, which can be direct or indirect. An indirect financial relationship could arise, for example, if a physician has a contract with, or ownership in, an entity such as an imaging center that has a contract with a hospital to which the physician refers. The Stark regulations clarify that an indirect ownership interest will trigger Stark sanctions only if the entity furnishing the designated health services has actual knowledge of, or acts in reckless disregard or deliberate ignorance of, the fact that the referring physician (or an immediate family member) has some ownership or investment interest in the entity.[33]

Interpretation and Billing for Services

CTC evaluation can be divided into the following 2 steps: (1) a primary search for suspicious colonic lesions and (2) lesion characterization. The primary search can be achieved using either an initial 2D search strategy, in which enlarged 2D images are evaluated sequentially from rectum to cecum[34–36] or a primary 3D search, in which the endoluminal surface of the colon is reviewed, similar to a colonoscopy.[37] Performing a primary 3D search in addition to a primary 2D search may increase sensitivity by about 10%,[38] but requires additional interpretation time.[39] Use of a primary 3D search has been cited as a reason for the high sensitivity achieved in some studies,[2] but smaller studies employing primary 2D searches have also achieved similar results.[21,40] Flat lesions, which can appear as cigar-shaped, plaquelike, focal regions of soft tissue attenuation, are best seen using 2D images.[41] Given the advantage of primary 2D and 3D searches, optimal performance likely involves both search methods. Lesion morphology is assessed by correlation of 2D and 3D images to distinguish polyps from folds or fecal matter. Lesion density is determined by visual interrogation of intralesional attenuation (to differentiate stool from neoplasia or lipoma). Lesion mobility is judged by comparison of the lesion position on supine and prone images. When a polyp or cancer is identified it should be measured on 2D images with lung window settings or by using 3D endoluminal views and electronic calipers.[42,43]

At the CHI, several of the gastroenterologists have been trained to interpret the intracolonic CTC images and can interpret them with similar accuracy as CTC trained radiologists.[26] These specialists do not, however, have the requisite knowledge, training, or credentials needed to interpret the extracolonic CTC images. The author prefers the partnership arrangement with his radiology colleagues whereby they interpret and report the findings on CTC. The radiologists can read these images faster, with greater reproducible accuracy and attention to problem-solving and detail, and have the appropriate skill set to recommend additional testing for extracolonic lesions if necessary. Split interpretation, the situation whereby a nonradiologist (such as a gastroenterologist) furnishes the interpretation of the intracolonic images and a radiologist furnishes the interpretation of the extracolonic findings, is a complicated issue for billing purposes. The most applicable safe harbor for a compensation arrangement between the nonradiologist and the radiologist in a split-interpretation scenario is the personal services and management agreements safe harbor.[44] This is an agreement, made in advance, between 2 physicians that specifies the schedule and precise length of work to be furnished, and the aggregate compensation paid over the term of the agreement. In developing such an agreement, the nonradiologist and radiologist should consult with legal counsel and ensure that the agreement includes at least (1) a specific timeframe, (2) the specifics of reimbursement, (3) the parameters of each physician's responsibility, (4) the basis for splitting the interpretation, (5) which physician is responsible for recommending additional diagnostic tests or consultations with other specialists, and (6) which physician is responsible for communicating the interpretation results to the patient and for managing the patient's course of treatment.

Risk Management

Split interpretations raise a risk management issue as to whether a nonradiologist is clinically competent to read intracolonic and/or extracolonic images without assistance from a radiologist, and whether either could be held liable for the errors or omissions of the other in connection with their respective interpretations of the CTC source images. The premise that a split interpretation is medically necessary, and indeed clinically preferable, is based on 2 assumptions, The first is that whereas the radiologist is presumptively qualified to provide an interpretation of all source images, the gastroenterologist may be qualified to interpret the intracolonic images, and is arguably the more appropriate professional to conduct that portion of the review based on that physician's training and clinical knowledge of the particular patient. The second assumption is that although the gastroenterologist may be competent in interpreting the intracolonic images, he or she may not be best qualified to interpret the extracolonic images without specialized training and experience akin to that of a radiologist. Other major risk management questions posed by a split-interpretation arrangement include whether the gastroenterologist could be held liable for an incorrect or incomplete interpretation by the radiologist, or whether the physician who signs the report is affirming the other physician's interpretation and is therefore assuming any liability associated with that interpretation. A gastroenterologist who agrees to a split-interpretation arrangement should prospectively consult with his or her malpractice carrier to obtain guidance from the carrier concerning limitations of coverage relating to such services, and whether such limitations could be different in a split-interpretation versus an over-read arrangement.

BUSINESS PLAN

One of the initial steps in determining if the establishment of a CTC program makes economic sense for a gastroenterology practice is to develop a business plan. Fajardo and colleagues[45] described their business plan process at the University of Iowa in an article published in 2006. The first step that these investigators described was the establishment of a multidisciplinary panel comprising radiology personnel, gastroenterologists, marketing experts, and business operations staff. This panel began by analyzing the available clinical data regarding the effectiveness of CTC as a first-line CRC screening test as well as the historical effectiveness of alternative CRC screening tests such as colonoscopy, flexible sigmoidoscopy, fecal occult blood testing, and fecal DNA analysis. Once they concluded that CTC had acceptable performance characteristics compared with the alternative tests, they assessed the local environment and opportunity data through a variety of marketing tools, taking into account specific characteristics of their population and its adherence to current CRC screening recommendations. Fajardo and colleagues determined that there was substantial room to increase the penetration of CRC screening in their local area and that these increases would continue to grow over the ensuing years after introduction of a test such as CTC, which could, in all likelihood, be expected to recruit CRC screening-eligible patients who objected to more invasive screening modalities such as colonoscopy. The next step in the development of their business plan was to estimate the potential demand and use of CTC screening as well as to model the potential impact of this new service on existing clinical capabilities. Using best estimates from various modeling studies, they concluded that there was significant uncertainty regarding the uptake of CTC and that the central component to success would likely be a concerted and collaborative effort by both radiology and gastroenterology specialists. Similarly, with regard to the potential impact on current practices and capabilities, these investigators recognized that the introduction of CTC could potentially decrease the demand for colonoscopy early on, but that over time colonoscopy demand, especially therapeutic colonoscopy with a view to performing polypectomy due to CTC findings, would likely increase. In addition, they evaluated the current wait time for colonoscopy screening and determined that the introduction of CTC screening would have the additional benefit of shortening the period of time from referral to actual CRC screening, thus potentially increasing patient and referring clinician satisfaction while also increasing patient throughput and organizational revenue streams. The final steps in their business plan were to compute the costs of a CTC program in terms of capital equipment, personnel, space, and other resources and to estimate the potential return on investment of these expenditures. One of the key features of their plan was a pilot, IRB-sanctioned program to demonstrate efficacy of the model, which if satisfactory, could be used to justify the potential economic merits to third-party payers. With this plan in place, net positive revenue could be expected within 4 years of the establishment of the program. If third-party payment was already in place, pilot programs such as the one described by Fajardo and colleagues could potentially be eschewed, thus potentially hastening the return on investment and revenue stream.

REIMBURSEMENT FOR CTC

The issue of reimbursement for CTC remains unsettled. There are few data regarding the market value of this test, but prices vary between $600 and $1000. At present 19 states as well as the District of Columbia mandate that insurers cover the costs of tests endorsed by the American Cancer Society, so theoretically CTC should be a covered benefit in these locales. The first area in the United States where CTC was covered by a third-party payer was in Madison, Wisconsin. In a unique scenario, a single practice at the University of Wisconsin received reimbursement for screening CTC from the 3 leading local third-party payers. In their summary of the first year's experience involving approximately 1200 patients, Pickhardt and colleagues[46] reported a per-patient positive predictive value of CTC of 91.5%, no CTC-related complications, a test-positive rate (referral to colonoscopy) of 10.8%, and no decrement in colonoscopy volume. Over the ensuing 5 years multiple other third-party payers have covered screening CTC. The updated BC/BS TEC referred to previously, though not a guarantee of future coverage determination or policy, also signals the acknowledgment of the potential of CTC to decrease CRC morbidity and mortality by third-party payer organizations.

Multiple cost-effective analyses of CTC have been performed, with varying conclusions.[47–49] In general, most of these analyses have determined that CTC approaches the cost-effectiveness of colonoscopy for CRC screening and is well within acceptable ranges for society ($40,000–$50,000 per quality-adjusted life year). The recent simulation modeling performed for the Medicare Evidence Development & Coverage Advisory Committee (MEDCAC) by the Agency for Healthcare Research and Quality determined that the cost of CTC needed to be around $205 to $250 to dominate colonoscopy.[50] It should be realized, however, that due to the inherent differences between the 2 testing modalities, it is very unlikely that CTC will dominate colonoscopy. The value of CTC is much more likely to derive from its ability to supplement colonoscopy screening and increase CRC screening adherence rates.

In the past, 2 Category III CPT codes were used for CTC, 1 for screening studies and 1 for diagnostic CTC (typically secondary to incomplete colonoscopy). Category III codes are temporary codes that are used to track emerging technologies, services, and procedures.[51] Because Medicare does not set specific reimbursement criteria for these codes, payment for a Category III code is up to the discretion of the specific carriers.[52] The reader is directed to the excellent article by Knechtges and colleagues[53] for a more detailed description of the CPT process and public/private coverage scenarios throughout the United States, although it should be realized that this is a rapidly evolving topic. Case in point, several category I CPT codes were recently established for diagnostic and screening CTC and the details regarding these codes was highlighted earlier in this article.

QUALITY CONTROL
Procedural Quality Control

All intracolonic findings on CTC should be examined, and any segment not adequately evaluated should be documented. All large masses and lesions that compromise luminal caliber should be communicated. The size and location of colorectal lesions should be reported, with appropriate images annotated or described. Descriptive features of polyps and masses should include morphologic features (sessile, pedunculated, flat), location (anatomic and distance from the anus), and lesion attenuation (soft tissue attenuation and fat).

General agreement exists that all polyps 10 mm or larger should be reported and the patient referred to endoscopic polypectomy, because 10% to 25% of these lesions may harbor high-grade dysplasia or cancer.[6] However, full consensus relating to the reporting or management of subcentimeter polyps discovered at CTC has not been reached among all groups.[11,54–56] It is generally agreed that the presence of 3 or more small polyps increases the risk of developing CRC.[57] In the recent C-RADS consensus proposal, 6 mm was suggested as the minimum size for reporting polyp lesions for the purposes of screening.[11] This viewpoint was endorsed by the European Society of Gastrointestinal and Radiology in a recent consensus statement that recommends polyps 4 mm or smaller should be ignored, and a significant minority amongst the faculty would not report 5 mm polyps, even when multiple.[58] The practice guidelines of the ACR for the performance of CTC in adults state that the reporting of polyps 5 mm or smaller is not recommended due to the lower specificity associated with lesions of this size.[23] Current American College of Gastroenterology (ACG) recommendations state that patients with polyps 6 mm or larger and patients with 3 or more polyps of any size should be offered colonoscopy and polypectomy.[6] The ACG also recommends that polyps of any size detected with moderate to high confidence should be reported, as patients and referring physicians deserve to be aware of the test results.

The referral of patients to endoscopy for diminutive polyps ($\leq$5 mm) could lead to a large number patients being referred to endoscopy,[59] and compromise productivity at subsequent endoscopy. Moreover, current CTC acquisition parameters (principally slice thickness and radiation dose) are tailored to the detection of polyps 6 to 10 mm in diameter, but thinner slices or increased dose might improve performance.[19,20] Based on these considerations it is recommended that all polyps 6 mm or larger should be reported, but that smaller lesions need not be reported and should only be reported when reader confidence is very high. Extracolonic findings (many of which are incidental findings) are common. In a recent systematic review involving 3488 patients, 40% of the patients had one or more extracolonic abnormality. Extracolonic cancers were detected in 2.7%, and 0.9% had an aortic aneurysm.[60] Approximately 1% to 2% of patients will have highly important findings requiring medical or surgical intervention.[61,62] Whereas the incidence of extracolonic findings far surpasses the incidence of colorectal lesions 6 mm or larger,[60,63,64] the great majority of these findings are not clinically significant and require no additional medical workup (eg, hiatal hernia, cholelithiasis, renal calculi). The detection and interpretation of extracolonic findings at CTC have typically been performed by radiologists, who have completed formal training programs and passed written and oral subspecialty examinations, and who are trained in the use of CT in a variety of practice settings (eg, trauma, CT angiography, oncologic staging). In addition, the occasional use of intravenous contrast will allow the identification of lesions unseen without intravenous contrast, and the characterization of nonspecific abnormalities. These instances require extensive expertise in recognizing abnormalities of the lungs, solid organs, retroperitoneum, and the extracolonic gastrointestinal tract. Therefore, all extracolonic findings should be reported and a radiologist should be consulted to properly examine the extracolonic portion of the study.

Development of a standardized method of reporting CTC will be influenced by local practice, referral patterns, and methods of information dissemination (paper vs electronic). The report should encompass elements of preprocedure documentation, patient demographics, indications, technical descriptions, findings, clinical assessments, and recommendations for follow-up. In particular, the preprocedure element should include patient education and a discussion of possible complications (eg, perforation) as well as the risk of missing significant lesions. Review of available alternatives to CTC for colonic evaluation is appropriate. At the author's institution a consent form is administered similar to that used for endoscopic procedures, wherein information about alternative screening tests, complications, and limitations of CTC are included.

Technical Quality Control

Technical quality control should encompass both the CT scanner and the CTC workstation. In addition to routine quality control, facilities performing CTC must ensure that all rooms containing x-ray devices are appropriately shielded for radiation in accordance with all federal and state regulations. Annual testing should include uniformity testing of CT number as well as spatial resolution, with visibility to 5 lp/cm bar pattern clearly resolved. Daily testing should include manufacturer or water phantom testing of CT number and noise, depending on state regulatory requirements. The CTC workstation monitor should undergo weekly SMPTE (Society of Motion Picture and Television Engineers) or equivalent video test pattern testing, showing a lack of aliasing of bar patterns and other artifacts with 95% and 5% squares visible.[65] Retrospective, sporadic review of CTC parameters and reports can also ensure that appropriate technique and practice patterns are being followed. In particular, retrospective review of technical parameters in average-sized patients should measure compliance with standard acquisition protocols, ensuring low-dose, high-spatial-resolution technique.

Professional Quality Control

Professional quality assessment monitors outcomes relating to established metrics within a practice. It is anticipated that over time national benchmarks for CTC performance will be established, which can serve to improve quality and potentially guide reimbursement.[66,67] A National Radiology Data Registry (NRDR) is under development, which could serve as an "overarching" registry where modality-specific data (eg, positron emission tomography scans and CT colonography) could be entered.[68] For internal quality assessment purposes, practices should establish mechanisms to track endoscopic findings in patients referred to colonoscopy, so that true-positive rates, false-positive rates, and sensitivity in referred patients can be calculated. The number of "inadequate" exams, in which full assessment of the colorectum is precluded by excess stool or fluid, or luminal collapse, should also be recorded. The adequacy of the preparation, the appropriateness of the follow-up recommendations, and the prompt notification of the patient and the referring physician should also be tracked. Any complications at CTC should be recorded, along with any predisposing conditions (such as obstructing lesions, concomitant colonic disease, or type of insufflation).[69] Random CTC reports should be reviewed to ensure compliance with guidelines,

Jan 08	Colon Cancer	Jan	Feb	Mar	Apr	May	Jun	Jul
60.2%	2009 Screening	69.1%	69.6%	70.6%	71.6%	72.1	72.2%	72.8%
+12.8	90th 68.4 Denominator	9020	9020	9011	8963	8417	8561	8513

Fig. 2. Impact of offering CTC on CRC screening compliance.

that they include information summarizing technique, polyp location and size, and the presence of significant extracolonic pathology. Such measures may permit identification of trends or outcomes which will alert physicians that changes may need to be made in patient educational materials, patient preparation regimens, or interpretation techniques.

IMPACT OF CTC ON COLONOSCOPY PRACTICE

It is too early in the life of CTC to determine whether it will have a significant impact on CRC screening compliance or colonoscopy practice. Early indications from programs such as the CHI and the University of Wisconsin, however, indicate that CTC may have a beneficial effect on CRC screening adherence while having a neutral effect on colonoscopy volume.[70] Since its inception, more than 9000 screening CTC examinations have been performed in the CHI, with a current average of 10 to 15 per day. From 2005 to 2007 the annual number of colonoscopies performed for CRC screening in the NNMC Endoscopy Unit remained stable at 2432, 2843, and 2605, respectively.

A recent analysis of data from the CHI and University of Wisconsin programs determined that CRC is the most common cancer found with CTC, with a prevalence of 0.30% among asymptomatic, average-risk patients undergoing screening CTC.[71] The mean size of these lesions was 3.3 cm (±1.6 cm) and 55% were diagnosed at stage I. All but one patient (stage IV at diagnosis) remain alive over a mean follow-up period of 21 months. The prevalence of extracolonic cancers was 0.40%, with renal cell carcinoma and lung cancer being the most commonly encountered. All renal cell cancers and 50% of the lung cancers were stage I at the time of diagnosis and all of these patients remain alive, with a mean follow-up of 20 months. CRC screening adherence in the enrolled patient population has increased, recently surpassing 72% (Fig. 2). When CTC is included, more than 82% of enrolled beneficiaries could be considered compliant with current CRC screening recommendations.

A multicenter study assessing patient attitudes and the impact on colonoscopy screening volumes at programs involving CTC screening was recently reported.[70] Preliminary data from 3 United States centers that perform CTC screening were

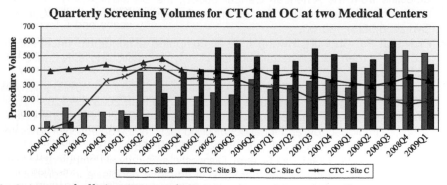

Fig. 3. Impact of offering CTC on colonoscopy volume. OC, optical colonoscopy.

analyzed. Survey data from adults undergoing CTC screening were gathered from 2 centers, and focused on the likelihood of undergoing CRC screening if CTC had not been available and the reasons for choosing CTC. Procedure volumes for integrated CTC and colonoscopy screening programs were also assessed to determine the impact of CTC implementation on colonoscopy screening. Between 36.4% and 37.2% of respondents indicated they would not have undergone colonoscopy screening if CTC had not been available. Convenience of CTC, its increased safety margin, and avoidance of colonoscopy were the leading reasons for choosing CTC at both sites where patients were surveyed. Colonoscopy screening volumes fluctuated somewhat by quarter, but in general were not negatively affected by the coexistence of CTC screening (**Fig. 3**). At one of the sites, a synergistic effect of adding the CTC option was suggested. These findings indicate that integration of CTC, along with commensurate efforts to educate the population and providers and ease the process of obtaining CRC screening, into a gastroenterology practice setting results in greater compliance with CRC screening guidelines without significantly affecting the volume of screening colonoscopy.

SUMMARY

CTC has been shown to be a viable option for CRC screening and is gaining acceptance from patients, clinicians, professional societies, and third-party payers as a test that is ready to be utilized more extensively. Setting up a CTC practice is a complex undertaking, as the optimal care and delivery of this modality of CRC screening necessarily involves several medical specialties with different skill sets and medical legal perspectives. These partnerships are possible, however, and have proven to be successful in several large programs throughout the United States. It may very well turn out that the practice of CTC remains confined to larger group practices, academic centers, and managed care organizations. As with any new technology, there are valid concerns regarding the misuse of CTC and many as yet unanswered questions about the impact of CTC on the practice of both gastroenterology and radiology, as well as its impact on society in terms of CRC screening compliance and possible decrements in CRC morbidity and mortality.

REFERENCES

1. Levin B, Lieberman DA, McFarland B, et al. Screening and surveillance for the early detection of colorectal cancer and adenomatous polyps, 2008: a joint guideline from the American Cancer Society, the US Multi-Society Task Force on Colorectal Cancer, and the American College of Radiology. CA Cancer J Clin 2008;58(3):130–60.
2. Pickhardt PJ, Choi JR, Hwang I, et al. Computed tomographic virtual colonoscopy to screen for colorectal neoplasia in asymptomatic adults. N Engl J Med 2003;349:2191–200.
3. Johnson CD, Chen MH, Toledano AY, et al. Accuracy of CT colonography for detection of large adenomas and polyps. N Engl J Med 2008;359:1207–17.
4. Graser A, Stieber P, Nagel D, et al. Comparison of CT colonography, colonoscopy, sigmoidoscopy, and fecal occult blood tests for the detection of advanced adenomas in an average risk population. Gut 2009;58:241–8.
5. Regge D, Laude C, Galatola G, et al. Diagnostic accuracy of computerized tomographic colonography for the detection of advance neoplasia in individuals at increased risk of colorectal cancer. JAMA 2009;301:2453–61.

6. Rex DK, Johnson DA, Anderson JC, et al. American College of Gastroenterology guidelines for colorectal cancer screening 2008. Am J Gastroenterol 2009; 104(3):739–50.
7. Centers for Medicare and Medicaid Services. Decision memo for screening computed tomography colonography (CTC) for colorectal cancer (CAG-00396N). Available at: http://www.cms.hhs.gov/mcd/viewdecisionmemo.asp?id=220. Accessed June 4, 2009.
8. Dhruva S, Phurrough SE, Salive ME, et al. CMS' landmark decision on CT colonography-examining the relevant data. N Engl J Med 2009;360:2699–701.
9. Marks DH. Blue cross blue shield technology evaluation center assessment of CTC TEC assessment program. Available at: http://www.bcbs.com/blueresources/tec/vols/24/ct-colonography-virtual.html. 2009;24:1–26. Accessed September 1, 2009.
10. Available at: http://www.bethesda.med.navy.mil/patient/health_care/medical_services/gastroenterology/gastroproser.aspx. Accessed September 1, 2009.
11. Zalis ME, Barish MA, Choi JR, et al. CT colonography reporting and data system: a consensus proposal. Radiology 2005;236:3–9.
12. Shinners TJ, Pickhardt PJ, Taylor AJ, et al. Patient-controlled room air insufflation versus automated carbon dioxide delivery for CT colonography. AJR Am J Roentgenol 2006;186:1491–6.
13. Burling D, Taylor SA, Halligan S, et al. Automated insufflation of carbon dioxide for MDCT colonography: distension and patient experience compared with manual insufflation. AJR Am J Roentgenol 2006;186:96–103.
14. Young BM, Fletcher JG, Earnest F, et al. Colonic perforation at CT colonography in a patient without known colonic disease. AJR Am J Roentgenol 2006;186:119–21.
15. Hara AK, Johnson CD, MacCarty RL, et al. CT colonography: single- versus multi-detector row imaging. Radiology 2001;219:461–5.
16. Kalra MK, Naz N, Rizzo SM, et al. Computed tomography radiation dose optimization: scanning protocols and clinical applications of automatic exposure control. Curr Probl Diagn Radiol 2005;34:171–81.
17. Kalra MK, Rizzo SM, Novelline RA. Reducing radiation dose in emergency computed tomography with automatic exposure control techniques. Emerg Radiol 2005;11:267–74.
18. Laghi A, Lannaccone R, Panebianco V, et al. Multislice CT colonography: technical developments. Semin Ultrasound CT MR 2001;22:425–31.
19. Taylor SA, Halligan S, Bartram CI, et al. Multi-detector row CT colonography: effect of collimation, pitch, and orientation on polyp detection in a human colectomy specimen. Radiology 2003;229:109–18.
20. Wessling J, Fischbach R, Meier N, et al. CT colonography: protocol optimization with multi-detector row CT—study in an anthropomorphic colon phantom. Radiology 2003;228:753–9.
21. Yee J, Akerkar GA, Hung RK, et al. Colorectal neoplasia: performance characteristics of CT colonography for detection in 300 patients. Radiology 2001;219:685–92.
22. Laghi A, Iannaccone R, Carbone I, et al. Detection of colorectal lesions with virtual computed tomographic colonography. Am J Surg 2002;183:124–31.
23. Radiology ACo. ACR practice guideline for the performance of computed tomography (CT) colonography in adults. 2002 (Res. 2) ACR Practice Guideline 2005; 29:295–9
24. Tolan DJ, Armstrong EM, Burling D, et al. Optimization of CT colonography technique: a practical guide. Clin Radiol 2007;62(9):819–27.

25. Dachman AH, Kelly KB, Zintsmaster MP, et al. Formative evaluation of standardized training for CT colonographic image interpretation by novice readers. Radiology 2008;249:167–77.

26. Young PE, Ray QP, Hwang I, et al. Gastroenterologists' interpretation of CTC: a pilot study demonstrating feasibility and similar accuracy compared with radiologists' interpretation. Am J Gastroenterol 2009;104(12):2926–31.

27. ACR practice guideline for the performance of computed tomography (CT) colonography in adults. Available at: http://www.acr.org/SecondaryMainMenuCategories/quality_safety/guidelines/dx/gastro/ct_colonography.aspx. Accessed September 15, 2009.

28. Rockey DC, Barish M, Brill JV, et al. Standards for gastroenterologists for performing and interpreting diagnostic computed tomographic colonography. Gastroenterology 2007;133:1005–24.

29. Available at: https://nrdr.acr.org/portal/CTC/Main/page.aspx. Accessed September 15, 2009.

30. 42 U.S.C. § 1320a-7b(b). Available at: http://www.aaasc.org/advocacy/documents/WDC99_937585_1.PDF. Accessed September 15, 2009.

31. 42 U.S.C. § 1320a-7b(b). United States Code: Title 42, 1320a-7b. Criminal penalties for acts involving Federal health care programs and 42 USC §1395nn, United States Code: Title 42, 1395nn, Limitation on certain physician referrals. Available at: http://www.ama-assn.org/ama/no-index/physician-resources/3882.shtml. Accessed September 15, 2009.

32. United States Code: Title 42, 411.351. Financial relationships between physicians and entities furnishing designated health services. Definitions. Available at: http://www.gpoaccess.gov/cfr/retrieve.html. Accessed March 10, 2010.

33. United States Code: Title 42, 411.351. Financial relationships between physicians and entities furnishing designated health services. Financial relationship, compensation, and ownership or investment interest. Available at: http://www.gpoaccess.gov/cfr/retrieve.html. Accessed March 10, 2010.

34. Dachman AH, Kuniyoshi JK, Boyle CM, et al. CT colonography with three-dimensional problem solving for detection of colonic polyps. AJR Am J Roentgenol 1998;171:989–95.

35. Macari M, Milano A, Lavelle M, et al. Comparison of time-efficient CT colonography with two- and three-dimensional colonic evaluation for detecting colorectal polyps. AJR Am J Roentgenol 2000;174:1543–9.

36. Barish MA, Soto JA, Ferrucci JT. Consensus on current clinical practice of virtual colonoscopy. AJR Am J Roentgenol 2005;184:786–92.

37. Pickhardt PJ. Three-dimensional endoluminal CT colonography (virtual colonoscopy): comparison of three commercially available systems. AJR Am J Roentgenol 2003;181:1599–606.

38. Cotton PB, Durkalski VL, Pineau BC, et al. Computed tomographic colonography (virtual colonoscopy): a multicenter comparison with standard colonoscopy for detection of colorectal neoplasia. JAMA 2004;291:1713–9.

39. McFarland EG, Brink JA, Pilgram TK, et al. Spiral CT colonography: reader agreement and diagnostic performance with two- and three-dimensional image-display techniques. Radiology 2001;218:375–83.

40. Macari M, Bini EJ, Xue X, et al. Colorectal neoplasms: prospective comparison of thin-section low-dose multi-detector row CT colonography and conventional colonoscopy for detection. Radiology 2002;224:383–92.

41. Fidler JL, Johnson CD, MacCarty RL, et al. Detection of flat lesions in the colon with CT colonography. Abdom Imaging 2002;27:292–300.

42. Pickhardt PJ, Lee AD, McFarland EG, et al. Linear polyp measurement at CT colonography: in vitro and in vivo comparison of two-dimensional and three-dimensional displays. Radiology 2005;236:872–8.
43. Young BM, Fletcher JG, Paulsen SR, et al. Polyp measurement with CT colonography: multiple-reader, multiple-workstation comparison. AJR Am J Roentgenol 2007;188:122–9.
44. United States Code: Title 42, 411.351. Financial relationships between physicians and entities furnishing designated health services. Exceptions to the referral prohibition related to compensation arrangements; subparts (d) Personal service arrangements and (l) Fair market value compensation. Available at: http://www.gpoaccess.gov/cfr/retrieve.html. Accessed March 10, 2010.
45. Fajardo LL, Hurley JP, Brown BP, et al. Business plan to establish a CT colonography service. J Am Coll Radiol 2006;3:175–86.
46. Pickhardt PJ, Taylor AJ, Kim DH, et al. Screening for colorectal neoplasia with CT colonography: initial experience from the 1st year of coverage by third-party payers. Radiology 2006;241(2):417–25.
47. Pickhardt PJ, Hassan C, Laghi A, et al. CT colonography to screen for colorectal cancer and aortic aneurysm in the Medicare population: cost-effectiveness analysis. AJR Am J Roentgenol 2009;192(5):1332–40.
48. Heresbach D, Chauvin P, Hess-Migliorretti A, et al. Cost-effectiveness of colorectal cancer screening with computed tomography colonography according to a polyp size threshold for polypectomy. Eur J Gastroenterol Hepatol 2009. [Epub ahead of print].
49. Vijan S, Hwang I, Inadomi J, et al. The cost-effectiveness of CT colonography in screening for colorectal neoplasia. Am J Gastroenterol 2007;102(2): 380–90.
50. Lansdorp-Vogelaar I, van Ballegooijen M, Zauber AG, et al. At what costs will screening with CT colonography be competitive? A cost-effectiveness approach. Int J Cancer 2009;124(5):1161–8.
51. Available at: http://www.ama-assn.org/ama/no-index/physician-resources/3882.shtml. Accessed September 15, 2009.
52. Federal Register, 2001;66:55269. Available at: http://www.gpoaccess.gov/cfr/retrieve.html. Accessed March 10, 2010.
53. Knechtges PM, McFarland BG, Keysor KJ, et al. National and local trends in CT colonography reimbursement: past, present, and future. J Am Coll Radiol 2007;4: 776–99.
54. Van Dam J, Cotton P, Johnson CD, et al. AGA future trends report: CT colonography. Gastroenterology 2004;127:970–84.
55. Rex DK. PRO: patients with polyps smaller than 1 cm on computed tomographic colonography should be offered colonoscopy and polypectomy. Am J Gastroenterol 2005;100:1903–5.
56. Ransohoff DF. CON: immediate colonoscopy is not necessary in patients who have polyps smaller than 1 cm on computed tomographic colonography. Am J Gastroenterol 2005;100:1905–7.
57. Winawer SJ, Zauber AG, Fletcher RH, et al. Guidelines for colonoscopy surveillance after polypectomy: a consensus update by the US Multi-Society Task Force on Colorectal Cancer and the American Cancer Society. Gastroenterology 2006; 130:1872–85.
58. Taylor SA, Laghi A, Lefere P, et al. European Society of Gastrointestinal and Abdominal Radiology (ESGAR): consensus statement on CT colonography. Eur Radiol 2007;17:575–9.

59. Rex DK, Lieberman D. ACG colorectal cancer prevention action plan: update on CT colonography. Am J Gastroenterol 2006;101:1410–3.
60. Xiong T, Richardson M, Woodroffe R, et al. Incidental lesions found on CT colonography: their nature and frequency. Br J Radiol 2005;78:22–9.
61. Hara AK, Johnson CD, MacCarty RL, et al. Incidental extracolonic findings at CT colonography. Radiology 2000;215:353–7.
62. Gluecker TM, Johnson CD, Wilson LA, et al. Extracolonic findings at CT colonography: evaluation of prevalence and cost in a screening population. Gastroenterology 2003;124:911–6.
63. Miao YM, Amin Z, Healy J, et al. A prospective single centre study comparing computed tomography pneumocolon against colonoscopy in the detection of colorectal neoplasms. Gut 2000;47:832–7.
64. Robinson P, Burnett H, Nicholson DA. The use of minimal preparation computed tomography for the primary investigation of colon cancer in frail or elderly patients. Clin Radiol 2002;57:389–92.
65. 147 NRN. Structural shielding design for medical x-ray imaging. Bethesda (MD): National Council for Radiation Protection & Measurements; 2004. p. 20814–30945.
66. Johnson C, Swensen S, Applegate K, et al. Quality improvement in radiology: White Paper report of the Sun Valley Group Meeting. J Am Coll Radiol 2006;3:544–9.
67. Swensen SJ, Johnson CD. Radiologic quality and safety: mapping value into radiology. J Am Coll Radiol 2005;2:992–1000.
68. Moser JW, Wilcox PA, Bjork SS, et al. Pay for performance in radiology: ACR White Paper. J Am Coll Radiol 2006;3:650–64.
69. Limburg PJ, Fletcher JG. Making sense of CT colonography-related complication rates. Gastroenterology 2006;131:2023–4.
70. Pickhardt PJ, Baumel MJ, Cash BD, et al. Implementation of CT colonography screening: multi-center evaluation of patient attitudes and effect on colonoscopy screening volumes. Presented at the 10th International VC Symposium. Washington, DC, October 26–28, 2009.
71. Pickhardt PJ, Meiners RJ, Wyatt K, et al. Colorectal and extracolonic cancers detected at CT colonography screening in over 10,286 asymptomatic adults. Radiology, in press.

Index

Note: Page numbers of article titles are in **boldface** type.

Gastrointest Endoscopy Clin N Am 20 (2010) 399–406
doi:10.1016/S1052-5157(10)00026-7
1052-5157/10/$ – see front matter © 2010 Elsevier Inc. All rights reserved.

giendo.theclinics.com

Moving?

Make sure your subscription moves with you!

To notify us of your new address, find your **Clinics Account Number** (located on your mailing label above your name), and contact customer service at:

Email: journalscustomerservice-usa@elsevier.com

800-654-2452 (subscribers in the U.S. & Canada)
314-447-8871 (subscribers outside of the U.S. & Canada)

Fax number: 314-447-8029

**Elsevier Health Sciences Division
Subscription Customer Service
3251 Riverport Lane
Maryland Heights, MO 63043**

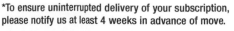

Printed and bound by CPI Group (UK) Ltd, Croydon, CR0 4YY

03/10/2024

01040458-0005